CONTESTING ILLNESS: PROCESSES AND PRACTICES

Edited by Pamela Moss and Katherine Teghtsoonian

The past decade has witnessed important changes in, and vigorous debates about, the ways in which people in the industrialized West understand and experience illness. These changes include a significant increase in the number of people diagnosed with chronic illness, the development of policies promoting fuller patient participation in the management of their own health, widespread support for treatment protocols that depart from accepted norms, and the emergence of new health activist movements. These developments pose a variety of challenges to conventional understandings of illness and its remedies, and have often met with considerable resistance.

Contesting Illness addresses the need to develop a critically informed analysis of emerging trends and of the multiple ways in which they are affecting, and being shaped by, conventional framings of illness and its treatment. The volume brings together a diverse group of scholars, working within a variety of theoretical frameworks and methodological approaches, who share a thematic focus on *contestation* as a conceptual tool with which to analyse the relation between power and illness. Some authors focus on a particular contested illness, that is, illness that is dismissed as illegitimate – framed as 'difficult,' psychosomatic, or even non-existent – by researchers, health practitioners, and policy-makers operating within conventional paradigms of knowledge (for example, chronic fatigue syndrome, fibromyalgia, environmental illness). Others analyse strategies for contesting how power shapes and is shaped by illness. That is, they identify processes and practices of critical engagement – by researchers, activist communities, those who have been diagnosed with illness or experience themselves as ill – with established understandings of the etiology, diagnosis, symptomatology, and treatment of illness. A fascinating and innovative contribution to current debates on health care and social and political relationships of power, *Contesting Illness* offers valuable insights into the assumptions, practices, and interactions that shape our definitions of and responses to illness in the twenty-first century.

PAMELA MOSS is a professor in the Studies in Policy and Practice Program at the University of Victoria. KATHERINE TEGHTSOONIAN is an associate professor in the Studies in Policy and Practice Program at the University of Victoria.

EDITED BY PAMELA MOSS AND
KATHERINE TEGHTSOONIAN

Contesting Illness

Processes and Practices

UNIVERSITY OF TORONTO PRESS
Toronto   Buffalo   London

ISBN 978-0-8020-9365-3 (cloth)
ISBN 978-0-8020-9512-1 (paper)

Library and Archives Canada Cataloguing in Publication

Contesting illness: processes and practices / edited by Pamela
Moss and Katherine Teghtsoonian.

Includes bibliographical references and index.
ISBN 978-0-8020-9365-3 (bound)
ISBN 978-0-8020-9512-1 (pbk.)

1. Chronic diseases – Social aspects. 2. Chronic diseases – Government policy.
3. Chronically ill. I. Teghtsoonian, Katherine Anne II. Moss, Pamela, 1960–

K634.C66 2007   362.196'044   C2007-904637-1

Cover illustration: *Chasm* by Heather Keenan

We wish to acknowledge the land on which the University of Toronto Press
operates. This land is the traditional territory of the Wendat, the Anishnaabeg,
the Haudenosaunee, the Métis, and the Mississaugas of the Credit First Nation.

This book has been published with the help of a grant from the Canadian
Federation for the Humanities and Social Sciences, through the Aid to Scholarly
Publications Programme, using funds provided by the Social Sciences and
Humanities Research Council of Canada.

University of Toronto Press acknowledges the financial support of the
Government of Canada, the Canada Council for the Arts, and the Ontario Arts
Council, an agency of the Government of Ontario, for its publishing activities.

 Canada Council
for the Arts
Conseil des Arts
du Canada

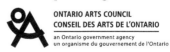 ONTARIO ARTS COUNCIL
CONSEIL DES ARTS DE L'ONTARIO
an Ontario government agency
un organisme du gouvernement de l'Ontario

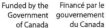 Funded by the
Government
of Canada
Financé par le
gouvernement
du Canada
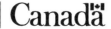  Canadä

For the women in my family who experience illness – PM

For my parents and grandparents – KT

Contents

Acknowledgments

The success of this project lies in the hands of the following people who contributed work to the book and participated in the Illness and the Contours of Contestation workshop, held November 2005, in Victoria, British Columbia, Canada: Stephanie Abel, Jan Angus, Kristin Barker, Pia Bülow, Peter Conrad, Joyce Davidson, Alexa Fankboner, Maya Gislason, Rachel Gold, Helen Gremillion, Tori Kelly, Sally Kimpson, Maren Klawiter, Steve Kroll-Smith, Katherine Lippel, Chris Martens, Michael Orsini, Janette Perz, Annie Potts, Michael Prince, Mary Ellen Purkis, Melody Quinn, Carolyn Schellenberg, Sharon Dale Stone, Jane Ussher, Catherine van Mossel, Zulis Yalte, and Steve Zavestoski. Thanks also to Phil Brown and Janet Price, both of whom had planned to participate but were not able to attend.

Our gratitude goes to several people involved in the project that has led to this book. Thanks to Heather Keenan and Barbara Egan for their assistance in putting together the applications for funding. Thanks to Maya Gislason for her superb organizing skills, her insight into the vision of the project, and her calm approach to problem-solving. Thanks to Stephanie Abel for capably arranging publicity and implementing the details for the workshop. Thanks to Rachel Gold and Catherine van Mossel for assisting in preparing the final manuscript. Thanks especially to our editor at University of Toronto Press, Virgil Duff, who was enthusiastic about the topic of power and illness and who understands the value of interdisciplinary knowledge. Thanks to staff at the University of Toronto Press responsible for editing, design, and pulling the entire book together, including Kate Baltais, Harold Otto, Anne Laughlin, Ani Deyirmenjian, and John Beadle.

For financial support, we thank the Social Sciences and Humanities Research Council of Canada (grant no. 646-2004-1531) and the Institute of Gender and Health (IGH) of the Canadian Institutes of Health Research for core funding for the workshop. We also thank the Office of the Vice-President, Research, the Office of the Dean of the Faculty of Graduate Studies, and the Office of the Dean of the Faculty of Human and Social Development, University of Victoria, for additional funding. We are grateful to the Office of the Dean in the Faculty of Human and Social Development and the Studies in Policy and Practice program, University of Victoria, for in-kind support.

Pamela thanks her colleagues for the intellectual space to pursue inter-disciplinary research. Thanks to Michael Prince, who is a co-investigator on the project on which my chapter is based. Thanks to my colleagues with whom I have shared bits and pieces of my work from time to time: Jody Berland, Karen Falconer Al-Hindi, Martha McMahon, Margo Matwychuk, Mary Ellen Purkis, and Katherine Teghtsoonian. Thanks to Karl for his support as I made my way through the entire project – from helping me hone my arguments about power and illness to making my breakfast (nearly) every morning.

Katherine would like to thank colleagues and students in the Studies in Policy and Practice program: you've provided me with rich opportunities to stretch beyond the disciplinary and theoretical traditions in which I was trained. Thanks especially to Pamela Moss and Mary Ellen Purkis for conversations and collaborations that have drawn me into new and productive avenues of inquiry. Many thanks to Bruce for his interest, engagement, and support throughout my work on this project and in my life beyond it.

Contributors

Jan Angus is Associate Professor in the Lawrence S. Bloomberg Faculty of Nursing at the University of Toronto, Canada. She uses qualitative methods to examine the barriers and supports that condition health-related decisions. She draws on social theories of gender, class, and the body to highlight the tactics employed by people as they confront structural patterns of advantage and disadvantage in experiences of chronic illness. Much of her work relates to issues arising from cardiovascular disease, including prevention, risk modification, and recovery from surgical treatment. She has published in several international journals such as *Sociology of Health and Illness*, *Social Science and Medicine*, and *Nursing Inquiry*.

Pia H. Bülow is Assistant Professor in the Department of Health and Society at the University of Linköping, Sweden. Her teaching and research interests focus on social interaction and narratives, especially institutional encounters and illness narratives. In her dissertation, entitled *Making Sense of Contested Illness: Talk and Narratives about Chronic Fatigue*, she examined sense-making processes about Chronic Fatigue Syndrome in interactions between experts and groups of sufferers, among sufferers, and in research interviews with individual sufferers. Her work has appeared in *Discourse and Society*, *Health*, and *Narrative Inquiry*.

Peter Conrad is the Harry Coplan Professor of Social Sciences in the Department of Sociology and Chair of the Health: Science, Society, and Policy program at Brandeis University. He has published ten books, including the award-winning *Deviance and Medicalization: From Badness to Sickness* (with Joseph W. Schneider) (1992) and the *Handbook of Medical Sociology*, 5th edition (co-edited with Chloe Bird and Allan Fremont)

(2000) and over a hundred journal articles and chapters. His newest book is *The Medicalization of Society* (2007). He received the Leo G. Reeder Award from the American Sociological Association (2004) for 'outstanding contributions to medical sociology.'

Joyce Davidson is Assistant Professor of Geography and cross-appointed in Women's Studies, at Queen's University, in Kingston, Ontario. Following the publication of *Phobic Geographies* (2003), she has developed a research and teaching program focused on health, embodiment, and emotion. Her current research examines virtual reality therapies for Autism Spectrum and Anxiety Disorders. Organizer (with Laura Cameron) of the First and Second Interdisciplinary Conferences on Emotional Geographies (Lancaster University 2002, Queen's University 2006), she has co-edited special issues on this subject for *Gender, Place, and Culture* (with Liz Bondi) and *Social and Cultural Geography* (with Christine Milligan). She has also co-edited *Emotional Geographies* (with Liz Bondi and Mick Smith, 2005). Davidson has published in sociology and philosophy as well as geography journals, and is co-author of *Subjectivities, Knowledges, and Feminist Geographies* (2002).

Helen Gremillion is Associate Professor and Peg Zeglin Brand Chair in the Department of Gender Studies at Indiana University. Her research and teaching interests include gender and science, constructionist theories of the body and of sexualities, medical anthropology, consumer culture, and feminist ethnographies. Her current research analyses therapeutic modalities that apply theories of gender and power elaborated in poststructuralist accounts of identity formation. She has published her work in a number of journals, including *Signs*, and in *Feeding Anorexia: Gender and Power at a Treatment Center* (2003).

Joshua Kelley is currently working on his doctoral degree at the University of Nevada at Las Vegas. He completed his BA and MA degrees at the University of North Carolina at Greensboro. His master's thesis, entitled 'Infant as Idea: The Birth of a New Composite Person,' examines the emergence of the infant as an idea in public discourse during the beginning of the twentieth century.

Maren Klawiter is Assistant Professor in the School of History, Technology, and Society at the Georgia Institute of Technology. She received her doctorate in Sociology from the University of California, Berkeley, in 1999. From 1999 until 2001 she was a fellow at the University of Michigan, in the Robert Wood Johnson Scholars in Health Policy Research Program. She teaches graduate and undergraduate courses in medical sociology; gender, science, and technology; culture; and social theory. Her research focuses on the medicalization of risk, lay participation in science, illness experiences, health- and disease-based social movements, the pharmaceutical industry, and the politics of cancer prevention. Her book, *The Biopolitics of Breast Cancer: Changing Cultures of Disease and Activism*, is forthcoming.

Steve Kroll-Smith is Professor of Sociology at the University of North Carolina in Greensboro. He has edited or authored five books on environmental hazards and disasters, health and the environment, and sociologists as expert witnesses. He is the current editor of *Sociological Inquiry* and the 2004 recipient of the American Sociological Association's Distinguished Contribution Award in the study of Environment and Technology. Kroll-Smith's latest book, *Volatile Places: Communities and Environmental Controversies* (2006), is co-authored with Val Gunter. He regularly contributes to the growing scholarship on the sociology of sleep.

Katherine Lippel is Professor of Law in the Civil Law Section of the Faculty of Law of the University of Ottawa and holds the Canada Research Chair on Occupational Health and Safety Law. She is a member of the Quebec Bar. Her research interests focus on work and mental health; interactions between law and medicine in the field of occupational health and safety; women's occupational health; and regulatory issues in occupational health and safety. In 2005 she received a prize for academic excellence from the Canadian Association of Law Teachers (CALT). Lippel's recent publications include two books on workers' compensation law and several articles on psychological harassment, therapeutic jurisprudence in the field of workers' compensation, precarious employment and occupational health and safety regulations, and gender-based analysis of compensation systems.

Pamela Moss is Professor in Studies in Policy and Practice at the University of Victoria, British Columbia. Her research coalesces around themes of power and body in different contexts – feminist methodology, constructs of contested illness, and activist practices. She draws on feminism and poststructural thinking to make sense of women's experiences of changing environments and uses autobiographical writing analytically in her empirical and theoretical work. She is active in feminist politics around issues about chronic illness and invisible or unapparent disabilities. Her recent books include *Autobiography in Geography* (2001), *Feminist Geography in Practice* (2002), *Women, Body, Illness* (with co-author Isabel Dyck, 2002), *Feminisms in Geography: Rethinking Space, Place, and Knowledges* (with co-author and co-editor Karen Falconer Al-Hindi, 2007).

Michael Orsini is Associate Professor in the School of Political Studies and Principal Scientist with the Institute of Population Health at the University of Ottawa. His research interests are in the area of health policy and politics, in particular the role of interest groups and social movements in policy processes. He recently co-edited a collection of papers entitled *Critical Policy Studies* (2007). He has published articles in *Social Policy and Administration*, the *Canadian Journal of Political Science*, and *Policy and Society*, among others.

Michael J. Prince is Lansdowne Professor of Social Policy at the University of Victoria, British Columbia. A political scientist by training and political animal from family upbringing, Prince is a frequent adviser and researcher to community agencies and government agencies on various public policy and governance issues. In 2006, on behalf of national disability organizations, Prince chaired the national task force on building the research and knowledge mobilization capacity of the disability community in Canada. His current research interests include Aboriginal peoples and Canadian state relations; intersections of health, gender, and culture in understanding contested illness; and the participation of marginalized groups in electoral systems and other forms of political action.

Annie Potts teaches courses on sexuality, human–animal studies, and the horror genre in the School of Culture, Literature, and Society at the University of Canterbury, Aotearoa/New Zealand. She was the lead researcher of a major study, funded by the Health Research Council of New Zealand, on the social impact of Viagra. Annie is the author of *The Science/Fiction of Sex: Feminist Deconstruction and the Vocabularies of*

Heterosex (2002), and co-editor of *Sex and the Body*, a volume showcasing research on sexuality, gender, and the body, with contributions by leading Australasian scholars (2004).

Mary Ellen Purkis is Associate Professor in the School of Nursing and Dean of the Faculty of Human and Social Development at the University of Victoria, British Columbia. She completed her doctoral work at the University of Edinburgh in 1993. Her research interests focus on organizational aspects of contemporary health care practice. She has drawn on ethnographic field studies to examine the practices of nurses in public health units, surgical units, cancer care, and home care.

Sharon Dale Stone is Associate Professor of Sociology at Lakehead University, Ontario, where she is also affiliated with the Women's Studies, Gerontology, and Masters of Public Health programs. Her research focuses on experiences of living with chronic impairments and issues that arise as a result. She has recently published *A Change of Plans: Women's Stories of Hemorrhagic Stroke* (2007). She is also working with team of academic researchers and community activists to investigate the experiences of injured workers with the workers' compensation system.

Cheryl Stults is a doctoral candidate in the Sociology Department at Brandeis University. She received her undergraduate degree in Sociology from Brigham Young University and an MA in Sociology from Boston College. Her academic interests are concentrated in medical sociology, methods (qualitative and quantitative), and science and technology. Her research interests include studying the impact of the Internet on illness, menopause and hormone replacement therapy, and examining the processes of 'risk scares' as they pertain to certain medical treatments.

Katherine Teghtsoonian is Associate Professor in Studies in Policy and Practice at the University of Victoria, British Columbia. Her scholarly agenda flows from an engagement with feminist and other critical literatures, and addresses the multiple ways in which neoliberal ideological framings and advanced liberal technologies of rule have shaped public and organizational policies in Canada and in other industrialized democracies. Alongside her ongoing work on women's policy agencies within government, she is pursuing research focused on government and organizational policies intended to address 'mental illness.'

Jane M. Ussher is Professor of Women's Health Psychology, and Director of the Gender Culture and Health Research Unit: PsyHealth, at the University of Western Sydney, Australia. She is the author of a number of books, including the following: *The Psychology of the Female Body* (1989); *Women's Madness: Misogyny or Mental Illness?* (1991); *Fantasies of Femininity: Reframing the Boundaries of Sex* (1997); and *Managing the Monstrous Feminine: Regulating the Reproductive Body* (2006). Her current research focuses on women's sexual and reproductive health, with particular emphasis on premenstrual experiences and gendered issues in caring.

Catherine van Mossel is a doctoral student in the Faculty of Human and Social Development at the University of Victoria, British Columbia. In her master's thesis, she explored resistance to privatization through an analysis of the framing and counter-framing of the debate in a public consultation process on the future of health care in British Columbia. She is building on this earlier work, and on her considerable practice and activist experience in the health care and social service sectors, in developing her current interests regarding the effects of 'evidence-based' policy-making and 'knowledge translation' on policy, practice, and those who live with illness.

CONTESTING ILLNESS:
PROCESSES AND PRACTICES

1 Power and Illness: Authority, Bodies, and Context

PAMELA MOSS AND
KATHERINE TEGHTSOONIAN

As the twenty-first century unfolds, we are witnessing important changes in, and vigorous debates about, the ways in which people in the industrialized West understand and experience illness. These changes include a significant increase in the number of people diagnosed with chronic illness (see World Health Organization, 2005), the development of policies promoting fuller patient participation in the management of their own health (Badcott, 2005; Wilson, 2001), widespread support for treatment protocols that depart from conventional norms (e.g., alternative and complementary medicine; see Chaffin, Thoennes, Boucher, & Pronk, 2003; Ng, Wong, Hong, Koh, & Goh, 2003; Snow, Hovanec, & Brandt, 2004), and the emergence of new health activist movements (Brown et al., 2004; Orsini, 2002). These developments pose a variety of challenges to conventional understandings of illness and its remedies – and they have met with significant resistance. Pharmaceutical companies, for example, continue to reinforce the idea that illness is something fixable, or even avoidable, through the consumption of prescription drugs (Moynihan & Cassels, 2005). Biomedically trained practitioners often refuse to assign diagnostic labels to the growing number of persons with symptoms that have no easily identifiable etiology (Edlow, 2003; Ware, 1992), and governments and employers do not readily accept claims for illness-related income support benefits in cases where etiology is complex or poorly understood (Brown et al., 2001; Dumit, 2000). Both types of refusal only add to the suffering of individuals who are ill (see Bendelow, 2006; Hydén & Sachs, 1998; Lippel, 1999). There is thus a pressing need to develop a critically informed analysis of emerging trends and of the multiple ways in which they are affecting, and are being shaped by, conventional framings of illness and its treatment.

The contributors to this book take up these tasks through an exploration of the intersections between power and illness. In so doing, they draw on a wide range of critical theoretical perspectives, including constructivism, feminism, political economy, and poststructuralism. Scholars working within and across these theoretical frameworks elaborate important insights into the ways in which power relations, organizational structures, and everyday practices constitute experiences and interpretations of illness, health, and access to services (e.g., Cohen, 2005; Fee, 2000; Hayes & Glouberman, 1999; Jung, 2002; Nguyen, 2005; Petersen & Bunton, 1997; Stoppard, 2000; Vickers, 2001; Ware & Kleinman, 1992). These theoretical perspectives also provide conceptual resources for analysing how particular combinations of bodily sensations and experiences come to be understood as an indication that individuals (or groups of individuals) ought to be considered unhealthy, diseased, or ill (e.g., Craddock, 2000; Moss & Dyck, 2002; Nettleton, 2006; Young, 2000).

In addition to building on the insights from a number of critical theoretical literatures, the contributors pull together conceptual and empirical insights from a range of disciplines including anthropology, geography, nursing, political science, psychology, and sociology. They draw on knowledge generated from their own home disciplines, from studies in related disciplines, and from literatures emerging from the growing number of interdisciplinary fields of inquiry (e.g., women's studies and cultural studies). The intersections among these disciplinary and interdisciplinary knowledges about illness hold the chapters together – and produce interesting, unexpected conversations between them – in ways that promote curiosity rather than propose definitive answers.

Individually and collectively, the chapters reveal that illness is positioned within multiple sets of power relations and that it both constitutes and is constituted by various social relations and processes. The analyses capture both the material aspects of being ill, by attending to the particulars of the experiences that this entails, as well as the discursive elements that contribute to shaping the constitution of illness itself. Each contribution addresses a specific combination of intellectual, political, cultural, and social concerns through a range of concepts relevant to power in order to interrogate critically the deceptively obvious meanings attached to illness and health. Together, these insights foster an understanding of the ways in which power and illness shape and reflect the relationships among individuals, their bodies, and their environments.

In this introductory chapter, we provide a framework for understanding contestation as a dimension of power that facilitates a critical
exploration of multiple facets of contemporary understandings and
experiences of illness. We follow this discussion with a brief overview
of the history of this book project. We then introduce individual chapters through three themes: authority, bodies, and context. In discussing
authority, we draw attention to multiple forms and sites of authority
that shape and define what illness is and what it means to be ill and
then note that there are material consequences to these authoritative
and regulatory policies and practices. Our discussion of bodies
sketches out a relationship between the materiality of the sensorial
bodily experiences that individuals feel and the discursive constructs
that articulate and give meaning to an ill body. By introducing context
as an organizing theme, we are able to incorporate discussions of structural and institutional mechanisms, as well as of particular spaces and
locations, and to explore the relationships between these and possibilities for collective action. We close with a discussion of alternate ways
of conceptualizing thematic linkages across the chapters and extend an
invitation to readers to contribute to an ongoing set of discussions
about power and illness by developing their own reading(s) of these
theoretical, conceptual, and empirical connections.

Power, Illness, and Contestation

Over the past three decades, scholars working with a range of theoretical perspectives have contributed to the development of a relational
notion of power (e.g., Mykhalovskiy, McCoy & Bresalier, 2004; Perrow,
1986; Rose, 1999; Young, 1990). Although individual analyses of power
vary in their emphasis and focus, key elements of a conceptualization
of power as located within various sets of social relations include an
understanding that power operates in and through multiple sites and
forms, that the constitution of power and its effects must be explained
rather than assumed, and that power is inevitably intertwined with
resistance. Michel Foucault (1990), for example, insists that power
must be understood as circulating through all aspects of one's location
and relationships in society, rather than as emanating from political
institutions, structures, or bureaucracies. Thus, 'power is everywhere;
not because it embraces everything, but because it comes from everywhere' (ibid.: 93). Similarly, Chantal Mouffe (1992) understands power
to be located in multiple sets of social relations and constitutive of the

social and the political. She argues that focusing on only one set of relations to the exclusion of others reflects a failure to understand how extensively power as a process shapes society, polity, and economy. Tracing power across numerous sets of social relations brings into view key sites and relationships that are crucial in shaping understandings and experiences of health and illness. Interactions between persons with illness and the health care system, between material ill bodies and discursive constructions of ill bodies, and between individuals and health care practitioners thereby become available for critical scrutiny and analysis (e.g., see Åsbring & Närvänen, 2004; Martin, 1994; Petersen, 2003; Werner & Malterud, 2003).

A relational notion of power also situates power as something that itself needs explanation, rather than positing it as a force or influence that is of interest because it helps to explain other things. Conceptualizing power in relational terms opens up space for researchers to explore the multiple processes and relationships through which power is constituted and expressed. For example, understanding how women come to embody health surveillance practices sheds light on the mechanisms through which notions of obligation and responsibility construct good citizenship in health care (Howson, 1998). Instead of using power as a conceptual tool to explain *why* health surveillance exists, the analysis focuses on *how* power is able to operate through health surveillance to create health-conscious citizens.

Finally, a relational notion of power entails critical interest in and empirical attention to various forms and sites of resistance to its operation. The complex workings of power spawn intricate networks of experiences and actions that disrupt, deflect, or redirect anticipated or intended developments. For example, people experience health-related practices and policies in paradoxical ways – what may seem effacing (like a diagnosis of cancer) can become empowering, and what may seem empowering (e.g., workplace-based or public health initiatives) may be contested in a variety of ways (Crossley, 2004; Hunt, 2000; McGillivray, 2005; Mitchell, 2000).

From the inception of this project, we identified contestation as a key dimension of power that could serve as a thematic link across a wide-ranging set of literatures and experiences and open up space for innovative and insightful analyses. Conceptualized as a process, contestation addresses not only the constitution of illness, for example, through diagnosis and policy, but also the mechanisms through which social practices, discourses, and institutional processes support, enhance, undermine, and break open conventional understandings of illness. Contestation is visible in what has come to be known as contested illness. By *contested illness* we mean illness that is dismissed as illegitimate – framed as 'difficult,' psychosomatic, or even non-existent – by researchers, health practitioners, and policy-makers operating within conventional paradigms of knowledge (see Abbey & Garfinkel, 1991; Bülow & Hydén, 2003; Dumit, 2006; Kroll-Smith, Brown, & Gunter, 2000; Moss & Dyck, 1999).[1] Contestation also manifests in *practices of critical engagement* – by researchers, by activist communities, by those who have been diagnosed with illness, or by those who experience themselves as ill – with both established and emerging understandings of the etiology, diagnosis, symptomatology, and treatment of illness. The reach of contestation, then, extends beyond contested illness to include illnesses that are conventionally understood to be straightforward and unproblematic. Although many of the authors consider a particular form of contested illness or examine contested illness more generally as a site of inquiry (see Conrad & Stults, Chapter 17), all of them are involved in exploring practices of critical engagement.

Contested illness does not conform to conventional framings of what being ill involves or how it ought to be understood. Rather, such illness generates heated debate regarding etiology (on the relationship between bodies and environments, see Kroll-Smith & Kelley, Chapter 16), the existence of a disease process as an entity to be diagnosed (on Chronic Fatigue Syndrome and Myalgic Encephalomyelitis, see Bülow, Chapter 7, and Moss, Chapter 9, respectively) and the identity one ought to assume after presenting with a set of symptoms (on Premenstrual Syndrome, see Ussher, Chapter 10). And, although other forms of illness may have long-standing or taken-for-granted premises regarding diagnosis and treatment, they are not exempt from contestation. For example, the emergence of risk categories as a type of diagnosis assigned to individuals who may not be experiencing any symptoms (on risk of heart disease, see Angus, Chapter 5) and the problematic relationships between standardized treatment protocols and the 'choices' offered to individuals receiving a diagnosis (on cancer, see Purkis & van Mossel, Chapter 8) demonstrate that there is significant potential for contestation between patients and physicians around established diagnoses. Similarly, there is considerable room for contestation regarding appropriate approaches to treatment for conventional illness where competing goals and priorities originating in different professional paradigms – for example, biomedicine, law, management – collide (on controversial illness, see Lippel, Chapter 3; on depression, see Teghtsoonian, Chapter 4).

All of the contributors address, or engage in, practices of critical engagement by contesting in a variety of ways conventional framings of how power and illness articulate. Using power conceptualized in relational terms, the authors draw attention to the mutually constitutive relationships between people's experiences of being ill and the discursive and policy contexts within which they engage with health care systems, practitioners, and each other (on Hepatitis C, see Orsini, Chapter 6; on disease regimes, see Klawiter, Chapter 15). Contributors are also well-situated to identify and re-read conventional assumptions about particular bodies: autism, for example, is less frequently diagnosed among girls than boys because of gendered assumptions about behaviour that inform clinical practice (Davidson, Chapter 13); stroke survivors are not chronically ill, but may have residual effects from an acute and threatening episode of illness and sometimes consider themselves (partially) disabled (Stone, Chapter 11); and young women with anorexia are not always white and middle class (Gremillion, Chapter 12). By employing a relational notion of power, the authors are able to highlight the political aspects of individual and collective action, for example, refusing pharmaceutical remedies (Potts, Chapter 14) and pursuing disability claims for illness in the face of institutional resistance (Prince, Chapter 2).

Drawing on theory in critical, non-conventional, and unexpected ways, the contributors unsettle traditional and tacit assumptions of what it means to be ill and bring into question a variety of established practices that are used to diagnose and treat illness. Through their analyses, they enrich a relational notion of power by focusing on one dimension – that of contestation. They fashion a complexly contoured understanding of this concept that can be applied in various settings, across multiple topics, and through diverse theoretical frameworks. As a whole, the collection contributes to a fuller understanding of the conceptual and empirical strategies used to contest (conventional) understandings of the intersections between power and illness.

History of This Book

The individual chapters began as invited papers presented at a workshop in November 2005, that was held in Victoria, British Columbia, Canada.[2] The two-day workshop consisted of 30 invited participants, of whom 20 were involved in 19 presentations. Participants included students and faculty from our home institution and English-speaking researchers from Australia, Canada, Aotearoa/New Zealand, Sweden, and the United States. We identified researchers outside the University of Victoria who were working on related topics through the literature with the intention of bringing together a diverse, multidisciplinary group of scholars interested in power, illness, and contestation. Participants were at various stages in their careers – ranging from second-year graduate students to scholars with over 40 years of academic experience. We circulated the papers to all participants in advance of the workshop.[3] Authors presented their papers in a series of thematically organized panels. For each panel, a discussant provided both general and specific comments: the former were intended to facilitate the group's exploration of contestation as a form of power and its relationship to illness; the latter, to assist the authors in preparing revised manuscripts for publication.

Through two plenary sessions, one held at the end of each day, participants collectively identified emerging empirical, conceptual, and theoretical themes from across the papers and panel discussions. Individual authors reflected on these themes in revising their papers. We as editors built on them in editing and organizing their contributions, with a view to bringing into focus key dimensions of the ways in which power and illness interact with and shape each other. The results of this process are presented as chapters in this book.[4] Individually and collectively, the chapters highlight the points of contact and the boundaries between power and illness. Through their analyses of concrete examples in various empirical settings, the contributors are able to find or create space – metaphorically and literally – to engage with these intersections.

Organizing Themes

We have arranged the chapters to coincide sequentially with the themes of authority, bodies, and context. This particular configuration of three themes emerged from our reading of the authors' revised workshop papers. The discussion in each chapter brings to the fore a specific feature of one of these themes. Each author also weaves threads drawn from one or more of the other themes into her or his analysis, so that these resonate across chapters and straddle the borders between clusters. As a collection, these contributions highlight the significance of contestation as a multifaceted dimension of power that can be used to address issues arising in a number of different disciplinary and interdisciplinary literatures concerning contemporary experiences of, and responses to, illness.

Authority

There are many forms of authority – and multiple challenges to them – that shape how illness and ill bodies are identified, experienced, and treated. For example, the state regulates key aspects of experiences of health and illness through a variety of different types of policies. Governments make decisions about which practitioners' services and forms of treatment, if any, are to be paid for using public funds (Armstrong et al., 2002; Commission on the Future of Health Care in Canada, 2002). They also establish (or forego) policies and programs through which people who require financial assistance as a result of illness or disability may be entitled to state-provided benefits, and define the eligibility requirements for such benefits (Office of the Auditor General, 2004). These multiple expressions of formal political authority in the area of health have, of course, been the focus of extensive contestation and debate (Esmail, 2006; Fuller, Fuller, & Cohen, 2003; Gilmour, 2002).

A second form of authority, biomedical knowledge, circulates within and interacts with a number of sites: policies and programs established by governments, legal proceedings, framings of ill bodies, and our intimate self-understandings. Although there are competing ways to capture what has gone awry in an ill body that lead to quite different sets of treatment choices (e.g., homeopathy, traditional Chinese medicine, shamanism, and Ayurvedic medicine), biomedicine retains a dominant positioning (see, e.g., Baer, 2001; Mizrachi, Shuval, & Gross, 2005; Shannon, 2002). Clinicians, health care practitioners, policy-makers, medical and health researchers, physicians, surgeons, insurance agents, lawyers, and government bureaucrats engage in practices that arise out of, are compliant with, and are regulated by biomedical interpretations of illness, health, and disability (Thomas-MacLean & Stoppard, 2004). A particularly authoritative element in the corpus of biomedicine is the *diagnosis*. In some cases, receiving a formal diagnosis provides welcome relief for individuals who experience illness (Karp, 1996; Lillrank, 2003). At the same time, diagnosis may complicate attempts to contest hegemonic constructions of illness because, as a practice, diagnosis itself reflects and expresses a range of exclusions and marginalizations (Caplan, 2004; Shaw & Proctor, 2005; Song, Jason, & Taylor, 1999).

Diagnoses offer explicit and authoritative models for engaging with any one particular person presenting as ill; diagnoses are often central to institutional interactions with ill bodies including, for example, those involving physicians, employers, family members, psychiatrists, insurance claims analysts, and staff responsible for administering government programs (Brown, 1987; Moss, 1999). Yet, as the discussion threaded through the initial cluster of chapters demonstrates, this form of knowledge has to contend with challenges from groups or individuals drawing on different types of expertise grounded in other forms of knowledge. For example, legal principles and precedents as well as quantitative calculations of economic performance in both the public and private sectors may generate truth claims that are at odds with those flowing from biomedically authorized knowledge. The bodily based expertise held by people who are ill has enjoyed a far less privileged status than any of these more conventionally accepted knowledges.[5] Nevertheless, chapters in this cluster show that this form of expertise constitutes an important resource on which people who are ill draw – individually and collectively – in contesting versions of and decisions about their lives that flow from more widely legitimated institutional sites and discourses.

Michael J. Prince (Chapter 2) focuses his empirical discussion on the Canada Pension Plan Disability (CPP-D) program, established by the Canadian federal government to provide financial support to adults who are unable to continue in paid employment because of illness or disability. Prince's analysis complicates conventional understandings of CPP-D income support benefits as unproblematically accessible to those who are 'entitled' to them by virtue of having contributed financially to the program while previously employed. Prince shows how, rather than receiving them as a formal entitlement of citizenship, many individuals are able to secure disability benefits only through a process rife with contestation. In Chapter 3, by analysing case law in the province of Quebec around claims for workers' compensation benefits, Katherine Lippel explores the relationship between contestation regarding particular diagnoses in the medical arena and contestation over medical issues in the legal arena. She draws attention to the importance of analysing the dynamics that come into play when biomedical and legal knowledge claims intersect and, sometimes, conflict. Lippel's analysis also highlights the processes through which individual workers' experience of illness, including their understanding of its relationship to their workplace, is often displaced by the interests and understandings expressed through the more privileged discourses of biomedicine and law. Katherine Teghtsoonian (Chapter 4) also takes up the intersection of different forms of knowledge claims in her discussion of emerging discourses circulating around efforts at managing depression in the workplace. Her analysis focuses on two documents that are intended to assist Canadian employers in developing policies and practices that will allow them to identify and respond to depression among their employees. Teghtsoonian identifies discursive strategies operating within the documents that frame individual workers as responsible for their own health and health practices while also subordinating their views, and the biomedical expertise of their family physicians, to the managerial and economic priorities of the employer. Jan Angus (Chapter 5) explores similar disjunctures between biomedical claims and the self-understandings of people who have been assigned a diagnosis: tensions emerge when individuals receive a diagnostic label based on their physician's assessment that their health status is 'at risk.' Angus notes that those deemed at risk for coronary heart disease (CHD) often have no symptoms, yet established medical practice urges them to alter their long-established patterns of tobacco use, physical activity, and/or dietary intake to reduce their long-term risk of CHD. Using data collected through interviews and focus group discussions with people who have been diagnosed as at risk for CHD, Angus explores their struggles with – and against – professionally and biomedically authorized accounts of their health status. Michael Orsini (Chapter 6) demonstrates that individuals' self-understandings and, by extension, collective political identities grounded in a specific illness, are not regulated only by professional and biomedical discourses. Orsini develops his analysis using the concept of *biological citizenship*, which involves the emergence of illness as an identity on the basis of which citizens might frame political demands, or be framed by state authorities as having particular duties and responsibilities with respect to their personal health. Drawing on extensive interviews with people diagnosed with Hepatitis C in Canada, Orsini argues that we need to rethink our understandings of both the concept of biological citizenship and of contestation.

Bodies

Embodied knowledge may well be the most popular, and perhaps effective, resource to draw on in contesting authoritative readings and practices of power and illness. Embodied knowledge emerges in situ, from sensations, emotions, thoughts, and subjectivities as well as cognition, physiology, and biology of both individual and collective bodies. It is true that in both conventional (medicalized) and embodied understandings of illness, bodies occupy a central place in understandings of how illness comes into being. However, understandings of illness arising from embodied knowledges are perhaps better able to highlight the mediation, negotiation, and articulation of the array of social relations constituting illness. As a result of insights emanating from embodied readings of illness, more nuanced and effective methods for dealing with the pain, discomfort, and distress experienced by persons who are ill can be developed, including integrated treatment regimes.

The bodies from which embodied knowledges emerge are simultaneously material and discursive (Grosz, 1994; Williams & Bendelow, 1998). Materially, bodies are concrete entities, multiple biological systems interacting with each other, producing and reproducing sensorial experiences and corporeal flows. Discursively, bodies comprise cultural, social, economic, and political meanings, embedded in power relations through which ideas and notions about bodies solidify and create ill, healthy, and disabled bodies. Exploring experiences of being ill and of being assigned a diagnostic category can bring into focus concrete examples of a synchronized material and discursive body.

Understandings of bodies as both material and discursive have generated studies that show how experiences of contested illness can have an enormous impact on the lives of individuals and their families (see, e.g., Barker, 2005; Moss & Dyck, 2002). In addition to their bodily experience of illness, people must often cope with scepticism on the part of employers, health care providers, and insurance administrators that can result in being denied access to paid sick leave or other income support benefits and/or being subject to surveillance and scrutiny (Dyck, 1995; Ellis, 2000; Harding, 1997; MacEachen, 2000). Such experiences often undermine the strategies that people use to cope with being ill and contribute to the further deterioration of their already challenging and already fluctuating health status (Bülow, 2004; Crossley, 1998; McCormick & Adelman, 2004; Wendell, 2001). Through the activities of work, reflection, dialogue, and interaction, among others, the ill body (as a site from which embodied knowledge arises) both constitutes and is constitutive of the experience of the categories assigned to an ill body – read diagnosis or lack of diagnosis – and the ill body itself. As this middle cluster of chapters demonstrates, through understanding ill bodies as constituted by and constitutive of the social relations through which elements of expertise and contestation are negotiated, one can trace the 'fixing' (in time and place) of bodies as 'ill' (materially and discursively) within the various contexts of identity work, biomedical authority, diagnostic categories, bodily sensations, and differentiating illness and disability.

Pia Bülow (Chapter 7) maps out key elements in the narratives of Swedish women who have sought a diagnosis of Chronic Fatigue Syndrome (CFS). She reveals the ways in which the contested status of CFS within medical and lay communities is reflected in women's efforts to preserve a moral sense of self. Bülow draws attention to the 'identity work' that women undertake while attempting to make sense of their bodily sensations and their relationships with others within a context where the diagnosis they receive (or seek) is poorly understood. Mary Ellen Purkis and Catherine van Mossel (Chapter 8) demonstrate that the challenges that people face in accessing appropriate care and managing identities persist even when people receive a diagnosis that is conventionally understood to be legitimate, obvious, and serious. Through analysis of interviews conducted with persons diagnosed with cancer, they detail the ways that the social practices of cancer care operate to ensure large-scale compliance by patients with established treatment protocols, which themselves produce significant illness, and do so under conditions where evidence of treatment effectiveness is limited. Their analysis draws attention to a tension between the material aspects of ill bodies and the discursive constructs through which they are regulated. In Chapter 9, Pamela Moss addresses this tension by proposing the possibility and promise of *rethinking* diagnosis as a set of practices. Moss argues that diagnostic categories need to rearticulate embodied knowledges that arise from illness experience with other dimensions of diagnostic practices in order to depict illness in embodied ways. Her discussion of the diagnosis experiences of women in Ireland and British Columbia, alongside her comparative analysis of competing sets of criteria for identifying Myalgic Encephalomyelitis, suggests new ways of thinking about diagnosis. Like Moss, Jane M. Ussher (Chapter 10) insists on the theoretical and practical importance of both the discursive and the material in considering women's bodily distress and strategies for addressing it. Ussher identifies a set of interconnected 'truths' that together define Premenstrual Dysphoric Disorder as a psychiatric illness, frame the female reproductive body as a cause of disorder, and serve to regulate women's subjectivities by leading them to interpret premenstrual change as evidence of individual pathology. Ussher proposes an alternative framing of women's experience of premenstrual change that situates it in the wider context of their lives, rather than viewing it as rooted in pathological characteristics of individual women. Sharon Dale Stone (Chapter 11) also insists on the importance of depathologizing women's experience, as she argues against a conflation of illness and disability that promotes the idea that disability is inimical to health and long life. Interpreting data from interviews conducted with women who have experienced significant effects from hemorrhagic stroke, Stone argues that women's experiences of life and sense of self post-stroke do not conform to conventional notions of disability as inevitably involving a diminished life marked principally by tragedy. Stone argues that established conceptualizations of health and illness would be more effective if they were grounded in embodied knowledges and the experiences of those who are ill.

Context

The context within which power and illness interact, articulate, and shape each other matters. Context itself denotes the contingent groupings of social relations as they manifest as spaces (e.g., public, private, corporeal, material, and discursive), places (e.g., home, workplace, a physician's office, and hospitals), and environments (e.g., natural, historical, social, political, and cultural). In addition to the forms of knowledge, economic interests, and cultural understandings that are prevalent in any one setting, the context within which power and illness articulate – and within which contestation may or may not emerge – is also crucially shaped by the marginalizations and exclusions organized around identity, class, gender, ability, age, and expressions of sexuality (e.g., Burman, Chantler, & Batsleer, 2002; Kimerling, Ouimette, & Wolfe, 2002; Richie, 1999; Thorson & Diwan, 2003). All of these aspects of context permeate and shape the ways in which bodies become ill, come to be understood as ill, and undergo treatment for being ill. And, of course, these aspects of context are linked, interacting with and shaping each other, generating new configurations over time in particular places.

An effective strategy to comprehend the contextual dimensions of the social constitution of illness involves addressing context at multiple scales. Even though scales themselves are socially constructed (Marston, 2000), it is nevertheless appropriate to think about multiple contexts in terms of size, impact, and magnitude. Researchers, mostly implicitly, work at a specific scale of analysis, for example, at the bodily, personal, or familial scale; at the local or regional community scale; at the scale of the organization, the state, or even global capital. All of these are pertinent when examining illness (e.g., Craddock, 2001; Philo & Wolch, 2001). Increasingly, scale as an analytical tool has come under critical scrutiny (e.g., Brenner, 1998; Marston & Smith, 2001; Peck, 2002). Here, however, we use scale only as a descriptor to make sense of how researchers come to understand the context within which power and illness interact.

Ill bodies take on specific characteristics, and are interpreted and regulated in different ways, depending on the discursive, institutional, and physical contours of a particular place at any one time. For example, because diagnostic categories are socially constructed, they can reflect and sustain marginalizing and exclusionary assumptions regarding illness, treatment, and appropriate social roles (Fassin, 2003; Gremillion, 2003; Horsfall, 2001; Metzl, 2003; Song, Jason, & Taylor, 1999; Stoppard, 2000). Such understandings of the experience of illness shape how persons who experience illness act and are regulated via diagnosis and treatment (e.g., Moreira, 2004; Ussher, 1997) and within consumer culture (Doel & Segrott, 2003; Metzl & Angel, 2004). The chapters in this third cluster provide nuanced readings of key aspects of context that shape the possibilities for change at a number of different scales: in clinical practice with, understandings of, and treatment for bodies that may or may not be ill; in the possibilities for connection and support among individuals who are ill; and in the likelihood that such connections will lead to collective action.

Helen Gremillion (Chapter 12) draws attention to the importance of racialized and classed constructions of personhood, health, and illness in shaping the ways in which experiences of disordered eating among young women come to be diagnosed, understood, and treated. In her analysis of the literature about anorexia, and drawing on her participant observation in an inpatient eating disorders treatment program, Gremillion demonstrates that the patients deemed most fit for treatment are generally white and middle class. Non-white, working-class patients are, by contrast, labelled 'difficult' and excluded from full participation in therapies even though their resistance to treatment protocols is not significantly greater. Joyce Davidson (Chapter 13) also explores systemic exclusions in the diagnosis and treatment of women, at both a personal and collective scale, through her analysis of the gendered dimensions of autism as a diagnosis and set of experiences. She discusses the ways in which gendered expectations regarding behaviour and interpersonal relationships limit the likelihood that young girls or women will receive a diagnosis of Autistic Spectrum Disorder (ASD). Through her reading of autobiographical accounts by women with ASD, she argues that women's stories about their experiences are a significant source of expertise that ought to be understood as credible and legitimate by the gatekeepers of diagnosis and treatment. Annie Potts (Chapter 14) draws attention to similar disjunctures across competing sources of knowledge in her discussion of the processes through which medical experts and their allies have developed a new set of diagnoses addressing 'female sexual dysfunction' that frame women's sexuality in primarily biomedical terms. Potts links this biomedicalization of women's sexuality to the global economic interests of pharmaceutical companies, a key constitutive force within the context where women's sexual lives have come to be framed as problematic. She also notes the discursive and political strategies through which a biomedical framing has been challenged by feminist scholars and activists, including their emphasis on the interpersonal, the cultural, and the sociopolitical as key contextual elements that shape women's experiences of their sexuality. Maren Klawiter (Chapter 15) introduces the concept of *disease regime* to explain how discourses and practices of public health and medicine have shifted over time in ways that have facilitated the development of the breast cancer movement in the United States. Klawiter identifies a series of changes in dominant approaches to the treatment of breast cancer during the twentieth century that have contributed to the transformation of the primary subjects of the disease regime from a relatively small number of temporarily sick and symptomatic women into a vast and permanent population of subjects at risk who occupy shifting positions on a breast cancer continuum. Steve Kroll-Smith and Joshua Kelley (Chapter 16) offer a conceptual framework through which to consider historical shifts in dominant cultural conceptions of the relationship between bodies and environments observable in the industrialized West over the past two centuries: from bodies *in* environments, through bodies *and* industrial environments, to industrial environments *in bodies*. Their analysis leads them to suggest the potential utility of reformulating our conception of impairment, extending it beyond its association with individual bodies to encompass the notion of impaired environments. They argue that this conceptual move offers an important opportunity to *imagine* ecological impairment as a conceptual development that would open up new spaces within which to address both damaged environments and ill bodies.

Multiple Readings and an Invitation

Although the themes of authority, bodies, and context have allowed us to explore intriguing and suggestive pathways through the debates, conversations, and arguments across the various chapters, this is not the only conceptual framework through which to read the authors' contributions. There are many alternative readings that could generate other, similarly productive thematic and conceptual connections. Chapter 17 offers one example. In it, Peter Conrad and Cheryl Stults present a reading of the themes and issues arising in the book's chapters through a different set of lenses from those that we have used in this chapter. They engage with the contributors' diverse conceptualizations of contestation in developing an insightful analysis of the relationship between contested illness and the medicalization of society. By identifying multiple contexts and relationships within which power circulates, they are able to show how pervasive medicalization is, as well as the diverse forms that resistance takes.

In yet another framing, all of the chapters in this volume can be read as expanding our empirical understandings of the multiple and reciprocal relationships among experience, diagnosis, and policy.[6] Several of the contributors illuminate how experiences of illness both shape and are shaped by the ways in which someone who is ill engages with discourses about particular illnesses (Bülow, Chapter 7; Orsini, Chapter 6; Ussher, Chapter 10). They also chart pathways that could integrate these experiences as embodied knowledges into the constitution and governance of ill bodies and their treatment (see Gremillion, Chapter 12; Klawiter, Chapter 15; Kroll-Smith & Kelley, Chapter 16). As well, the authors show that characteristic features of diagnosis, as a practice depicting a medically normalized body created through a standardized set of observations, are not to be taken at face value. The authors critically engage various aspects of diagnosis including debates over criteria in defining illness (Potts, Chapter 14), the links between diagnosis and the structuring of treatment options (Purkis & van Mossel, Chapter 8), the application (and non-application) of particular diagnoses to specific ill bodies (Davidson, Chapter 13), and the possibility of utilizing embodied knowledge as part of diagnosis (Moss, Chapter 9). The chapters dealing with the regulation and treatment of ill bodies can inform more effective and supportive health care practice and policy for persons who are ill. Critical analyses of the discourses shaping policy (Teghtsoonian, Chapter 4), as well as the implementation (Prince, Chapter 2) and adjudication (Lippel, Chapter 3) of policy, show the difficulties that arise when rules and processes reflecting hegemonic knowledges and interests collide with individual ill bodies.

This collection is distinctive in its focus on contestation as a conceptual tool with which to unpack the multifaceted relationships between power and illness. Positioning the authors' arguments in this way points to the need to scrutinize more extensively how power shapes the use of health as a normative and normalizing indicator of bodily status[7] alongside the use of illness to denote deviations from a standard, medicalized body. Twin premises underlie the conceptualization of the relationships between power and illness that runs through all the chapters: that illness is constituted through multiple mechanisms mediating social relations; and that illness and the experience of illness, in turn, profoundly shape social relations and practices of power. The authors, through their critical readings of the multiple manifestations of contestation as a dimension of power, demonstrate the potential of scholars working in diverse disciplinary locations coming together to talk about their own research in terms of distinct, yet complementary concepts. This collection indicates that there is a need for continued cross-, multi-, and interdisciplinary discussions in analyses of illness and health beyond those that focus on a shared empirical topic or theoretical orientation. More studies are also necessary to flesh out the ways in which discourse and materiality – as distinct processes and as a fused entity – constitute and are constituted by illness. Widening notions of what comprises discourse and materiality, while concentrating on a specific dimension of both, can lead to better understandings of *how* illness and power are constituted.

As editors, we invite the reader to think about the conceptual themes of authority, bodies, and context, as well as those of contested illness and medicalization, in the various empirical sites of experience, diagnosis, and policy examined in the chapters in this book. The contributors provide richly variegated and complex interpretations of the material conditions, circumstances, and bodily sensations of persons with illness or disability, as well as of the discursive constructs shaping engagements with health care systems, health care practitioners, medical diagnoses, and social health movements. In proffering these alternatives to biomedically authorized knowledge, the book ruptures and destabilizes conventional understandings of health by applying a relational notion of power to various readings of illness. These contributions themselves comprise a practice of critical engagement, contesting those established framings that so fascinate us and shape how we engage with health and illness. One of our principal goals for the collection as a whole is to stimulate you, the reader, to develop your *own* framing of the ways in which themes and concepts resonate across the chapters and, by extension, across disciplines and fields of study. We hope that you find this book as challenging and useful as we have in our efforts to rethink how we as social beings come to know, read, regulate, and treat ill bodies!

NOTES

1 For an alternative theorization of what psychosomatic means, see Wilson (2004).
2 We acknowledge the financial support for the workshop from the Social Sciences and Humanities Research Council of Canada (grant no. 646-2004-1531) and the Institute of Gender and Health at the Canadian Institutes of Health Research. We also thank the Offices of the Vice-President Research, the Dean of the Faculty of Graduate Studies, and the Dean of Human and Social Development at the University of Victoria.
3 Maren Klawiter was kind enough to accept a late invitation to the workshop when a participant at the last minute withdrew because of an unanticipated set of circumstances. She brought with her a completed manuscript to circulate at the workshop. A special thanks to Maren!
4 Some of the presenters were not able to contribute to the book because of other commitments. We appreciate the forbearance of all the presenters and contributors as we transformed the presentations at the workshop into print.
5 For an exception see the description and critique by Tyreman (2005a and 2005b).
6 Indeed these three concepts informed the structure of the original workshop.
7 Notwithstanding Stone's (Chapter 11) point that 'illness,' too, can be normalizing in the context of defining disability.

REFERENCES

Abbey, Susan E., & Garfinkel, Paul E. (1991). Neurasthenia and chronic fatigue syndrome: The role of culture in the making of a diagnosis. *American Journal of Psychiatry, 148*, 1638–1646.

Armstrong, Pat, Amaratunga, Carol, Bernier, Jocelyne, Grant, Karen, Pederson, Ann, & Willson, Kay. (2002). *Exposing privatization: Women and health care reform in Canada.* Aurora, ON: Garamond Press.

Åsbring, Pia, & Närvänen, Anna-Liisa. (2004). Patient power and control: A study of women with uncertain illness trajectories. *Qualitative Health Research, 14*(2), 226–240.

Badcott, David. (Ed.). (2005). Employing patient expertise: Introduction to the theme. *Medicine, Health Care and Philosophy, 8*(2), 147–148.

Baer, Hans. (2001). *Biomedicine and alternative healing systems in America: Issues of class, race, ethnicity, and gender.* Madison: University of Wisconsin Press.

Barker, Kristin. (2005). *The Fibromyalgia story: Medical authority and women's worlds of pain.* Philadelphia: Temple University Press.

Bendelow, Gillian. (2006). Pain, suffering and risk. *Health, Risk and Society, 8*(1), 59–70.

Brenner, Neil. (1998). Between fixity and motion: Accumulation, territorial organization and the historical geography of spatial scales. *Environment and Planning D: Society and Space, 16*(4), 459–481.

Brown, Phil. (1987). Diagnostic conflict and contradiction in psychiatry. *Journal of Health and Social Behavior, 28*(1), 37–50.

Brown, Phil, Zavestoski, Stephen, McCormick, Sabrina, Linder, Meadow, Mandelbaum, Joshua, & Luebke, Theo. (2001). A gulf of difference: Disputes over Gulf War-related illnesses. *Journal of Health and Social Behavior, 42*(3), 235–257.

Brown, Phil, Zavestoski, Stephen, McCormick, Sabrina, Mayer, Brian, Morello-Frosch, Rachel, & Gasior Altman, Rebecca. (2004). Embodied health movements: New approaches to social movements in health. *Sociology of Health and Illness, 26*(1), 50–80.

Bülow, Pia H. (2004). Sharing experiences of contested illness by storytelling. *Discourse and Society, 15*(1), 33–53.

Bülow, Pia, & Hydén, Lars-Christer. (2003). Patient school as a way of creating meaning in a contested illness: The case of CFS. *Health: An Interdisciplinary Journal for the Social Study of Health, Illness and Medicine, 7*(2), 227–249.

Burman, Erica, Chantler, Khatidja, & Batsleer, Janet. (2002). Service responses to South Asian women who attempt suicide or self-harm: Challenges for service commissioning and delivery. *Critical Social Policy, 22,* 641–668.

Caplan, Paula J. (2004). The debate about PMDD and Sarafem: Suggestions for therapists. *Women and Therapy, 27*(3/4), 55–67.

Chaffin, Jodi A., Thoennes, Jolene J., Boucher, Jackie L., & Pronk, Nicolaas P. (2003). Supporting herbal resource needs for health plan members: Complementary and alternative medicine by telephone. *Disease Management and Health Outcomes, 11*(8), 499–506.

Cohen, Lawrence. (2005). Operability, bioavailability, and exception. In Aihwa Ong & Stephen J. Collier (Eds.), *Global assemblages: Technology, politics, and ethics as anthropological problems* (pp. 79–90). Malden, MA, and Oxford: Blackwell.

Commission on the Future of Health Care in Canada. (2002). *Building on values: The future of health care in Canada*. Final Report. Saskatoon, Saskatchewan: Author.

Craddock, Susan. (2000). *City of plagues: disease, poverty, and deviance in San Francisco*. Minneapolis: University of Minnesota Press.

Craddock, Susan. (2001). Scales of justice: Women, equity, and HIV in East Africa. In Isabel Dyck, Nancy Davis Lewis, & Sara McLafferty (Eds.), *Geographies of women's health* (pp. 41–60). New York and London: Routledge.

Crossley, Michele L. (1998). 'Sick role' or 'empowerment'? The ambiguities of life with an HIV positive diagnosis. *Sociology of Health and Illness, 20*, 507–531.

Crossley, Michele. (2004). Making sense of 'barebacking': Gay men's narratives, unsafe sex and the 'resistance habitus.' *British Journal of Social Psychology, 43*(2), 224–244.

Doel, Marcus A., & Segrott, Jeremy. (2003). Self, health, and gender: Complementary and alternative medicine in the British mass media. *Gender, Place and Culture, 10*(2), 131–144.

Dumit, Joseph. (2000). When explanations rest: 'Good-enough' brain science and the new socio-medical disorders. In Margaret Lock, Allan Young, & Alberto Cambrosio (Eds.), *Living and working with the new medical technologies: Intersections of inquiry* (pp. 209–232). Cambridge: Cambridge University Press.

Dumit, Joseph. (2006). Illnesses you have to fight to get: Facts as forces in uncertain, emergent illnesses. *Social Science and Medicine, 62*, 577–590.

Dyck, Isabel. (1995). Hidden geographies: The changing lifeworlds of women with multiple sclerosis. *Social Science and Medicine, 40*, 307–320.

Edlow, Jonathan A. (2003). *Bull's eye: Unraveling the medical mystery of Lyme Disease*. New Haven, CT, and London: Yale University Press.

Ellis, Kathryn. (2000). Welfare and bodily order: Theorizing transitions in corporeal discourse. In Kathryn Ellis & Harley Dean (Eds.), *Social policy and the body: Transitions in corporeal discourse* (pp. 1–22). Basingstoke, England: Palgrave.

Esmail, Nadeen. (2006). Unhealthy move for Albertans: Third way transformed into old expensive way. Retrieved 15 June 2006, from http://www.fraserinstitute.ca/shared/readmore1.asp?sNav=ed&id=410.

Fassin, Didier. (2003). The embodiment of inequality: AIDS as a social condition and the historical experience in South Africa. *EMBO Reports, 4* (special issue), S4-S9.

Fee, Dwight. (Ed.). (2000). *Pathology and the postmodern: Mental illness as discourse and experience*. London: Sage.

Foucault, Michel. (1990). *The history of sexuality, volume 1: An introduction.* (Robert Hurley, Trans.). New York: Vintage Books. (Original work published in 1978.)

Fuller, Sylvia, Fuller, Colleen, & Cohen, Marcia. (2003). *Health care restructuring in BC.* Vancouver: Canadian Centre for Policy Alternatives, B.C. Office.

Gilmour, Joan M. (2002). Creeping privatization in health care: Implications for women as the state redraws its role. In Brenda Cossman & Judy Fudge (Eds.), *Privatization, law, and the challenge to feminism.* Toronto: University of Toronto Press.

Gremillion, Helen. (2003). *Feeding anorexia: Gender and power at a treatment center.* Durham, NC, and London: Duke University Press.

Grosz, Elizabeth. (1994). *Volatile bodies: Toward a corporeal feminism.* Bloomington and Indianapolis: Indiana University Press.

Harding, Jennifer. (1997). Bodies at risk: Sex, surveillance and hormone replacement therapy. In Alan Petersen & Robin Bunton (Eds.), *Foucault, health and medicine* (pp. 134–150). New York and London: Routledge.

Hayes, Michael J., & Glouberman, Sholom. (1999). *Population health, sustainable development and policy future.* Ottawa: Canadian Policy Research Networks.

Horsfall, Jan. (2001). Gender and mental illness: An Australian overview. *Issues in Mental Health Nursing, 22,* 421–438.

Howson, Alexandra. (1998). Embodied obligation: The female body and health surveillance. In Sarah Nettleton & Jonathan Watson (Eds.), *The body in everyday life* (pp. 218–240). London and New York: Routledge.

Hunt, Linda M. (2000). Strategic suffering: Illness narratives as social empowerment among Mexican cancer patients. In Cheryl Mattingly & Linda C. Garro (Eds.), *Narrative and the cultural construction of illness and healing* (pp. 88–107). Berkeley: University of California Press.

Hydén, Lars-Christer, & Sachs, Lisbeth. (1998). Suffering, hope and diagnosis: On the negotiation of Chronic Fatigue Syndrome. *Health, 2*(2), 175–193.

Jung, Karen Elizabeth. (2002). Chronic illness and educational equity: The politics of visibility. *NWSA Journal, 14*(3), 178–200.

Karp, David A. (1996). *Speaking of sadness: Depression, disconnection, and the meanings of illness.* New York: Oxford University Press.

Kimerling, Rachel, Ouimette, Paige, & Wolfe, Jessica. (2002). *Gender and PTSD.* New York and London: Guilford.

Kroll-Smith, Steve, Brown, Phil, & Gunter, Valerie J. (Eds.). (2000). *Illness and the environment: A reader in contested medicine.* New York and London: New York University Press.

Lillrank, Annika. (2003). Back pain and the resolution of diagnostic uncertainty in illness narratives. *Social Science and Medicine, 57,* 1045–1054.

Lippel, Katherine. (1999). Therapeutic and anti-therapeutic consequences of workers' compensation. *International Journal of Law and Psychiatry, 22,* 521–546.

MacEachen, Ellen. (2000). The mundane administration of worker bodies: From welfarism to neoliberalism. *Health, Risk and Society, 2*(3), 315–327.

Marston, Sallie A. (2000). The social construction of scale. *Progress in Human Geography, 24*(2), 219–242.

Marston, Sallie A., & Smith, Neil. (2001). States, scales and households: Limits to scale thinking? A response to Brenner. *Progress in Human Geography, 25*(4), 615–619.

Martin, Emily. (1994). *Flexible bodies: Tracking immunity in American culture from the days of polio to the age of AIDS.* Boston: Beacon Press.

McCormick, Coralie, & Adelman, Judith. (2004). *Navigating workplace disability insurance: Helping people with mental illness find the way.* Vancouver: Canadian Mental Health Association, B.C. Division.

McGillivray, David. (2005). Governing working bodies through leisure. *Leisure Sciences, 27,* 315–330.

Metzl, Jonathan Michel. (2003). *Prozac on the couch: Prescribing gender in the era of wonder drugs.* Durham, NC, and London: Duke University Press.

Metzl, Jonathan M., & Angel, Joni. (2004). Assessing the impact of SSRI antidepressants on popular notions of women's depressive illness. *Social Science and Medicine, 58,* 577–584.

Mitchell, Martin. (2000). Disciplinary interventions and resistances around 'safer sex.' In Kathryn Ellis & Harley Dean (Eds.), *Social policy and the body: Transitions in corporeal discourse* (pp. 139–159). Basingstoke, England: Palgrave.

Mizrachi, Nissim, Shuval, Judith T., & Gross, Sky. (2005). Boundary at work: Alternative medicine in biomedical settings. *Sociology of Health and Illness, 27*(1), 20–43.

Moreira, Tiago. (2004). Coordination and embodiment in the operating room. *Body and Society, 10*(1), 109–129.

Moss, Pamela. (1999). Autobiographical notes on chronic illness. In Ruth Butler & Hester Parr (Eds.), *Mind and body spaces: Geographies of illness, impairment and disability.* New York and London: Routledge.

Moss, Pamela, and Dyck, Isabel. (1999). Body, corporeal space, and legitimating chronic illness: Women diagnosed with M.E. *Antipode, 31,* 372–397.

Moss, Pamela, and Dyck, Isabel. (2002). *Women, body, illness: Space and identity in the everyday lives of women with chronic illness.* Lanham, MD: Rowman and Littlefield.

Mouffe, Chantal. (1992). Feminism, citizenship, and radical democratic politics. In Judith Butler & Joan W. Scott (Eds.), *Feminists theorize the political* (pp. 369–384). New York and London: Routledge.

Moynihan, Ray, & Cassels, Alan. (2005). *Selling sickness: How the world's biggest pharmaceutical companies are turning us all into patients.* New York: Nation Books.

Mykhalovskiy, Eric, McCoy, Liza, & Bresalier, Michael. (2004). Compliance/adherence, HIV, and the critique of medical power. *Social Theory and Health, 2*, 315–340.

Nettleton, Sarah. (2006). 'I just want permission to be ill': Towards a sociology of medically unexplained symptoms. *Social Science and Medicine, 62*, 1167–1178.

Ng, T.P., Wong, M.L., Hong, C.Y., Koh, K.T.C., & Goh, L.G. (2003). The use of complementary and alternative medicine by asthma patients. *QJM: An International Journal of Medicine, 96*, 747–754

Nguyen, Vinh-Kim. (2005). Antiretroviral globalism, biopolitics, and therapeutic citizenship. In Aihwa Ong & Stephen J. Collier (Eds.), *Global assemblages: Technology, politics, and ethics as anthropological problems* (pp. 124–144). Malden, MA, and Oxford: Blackwell.

Office of the Auditor General of British Columbia. (2004). *Audit of the government's review of eligibility for disability assistance.* Victoria, BC: Office of the Auditor General.

Orsini, Michael. (2002). The politics of naming, blaming and claiming: HIV, Hepatitis C and the emergence of blood activism in Canada. *Canadian Journal of Political Science, 35*(3), 475–498.

Peck, Jamie. (2002). Political economies of scale: Fast policy, interscalar relations, and neoliberal workfare. *Economic Geography, 78*(3), 331–360.

Perrow, Charles. (1986). *Complex organizations: A critical essay* (3rd ed.). New York: Random House.

Petersen, Alan. (2003). Governmentality, critical scholarship, and the medical humanities. *Journal of Medical Humanities, 23*(3/4), 187–201.

Petersen, Alan, & Bunton, Robin. (Eds.). (1997). *Foucault, health and medicine.* New York and London: Routledge.

Philo, Chris, & Wolch, Jennifer. (2001). The 'three waves' of research in mental health geography: A review and critical commentary. *Epidemiologia e Psichiatria Sociale, 10*(4), 230–244.

Richie, Beth E. (1999). The social construction of the 'immoral' Black mother: Social policy, community policing, and effects on youth violence. In Adele E. Clarke & Virginia L. Olesen (Eds.), *Revisioning women, health and healing: Feminist, cultural, and technoscience perspectives* (pp. 283–299). New York and London: Routledge.

Rose, Nikolas. (1999). *Powers of freedom: Reframing political thought.* Cambridge: Cambridge University Press.

Shannon, Scott. (Ed.). (2002). *Handbook of complementary and alternative therapies in mental health.* San Diego: Academic Press.

Shaw, Clare, & Proctor, Gillian. (2005). Women at the margins: A critique of the diagnosis of Borderline Personality Disorder. *Feminism and Psychology, 15,* 483–490.

Snow, Lynn A., Hovanec, Linda, & Brandt, Jason. (2004). A controlled trial of aromatherapy for agitation in nursing home patients with dementia. *The Journal of Alternative and Complementary Medicine, 10,* 431–437.

Song, Sharon, Jason, Leonard A., & Taylor, Renee R. (1999). The relationship between ethnicity and fatigue in a community-based sample. *Journal of Gender, Culture and Health, 4*(4), 255–268.

Stoppard, Janet M. (2000). *Understanding depression: Feminist social constructionist approaches.* New York and London: Routledge.

Thomas-MacLean, Roanne, & Stoppard, Janet M. (2004). Physicians' constructions of depression: Inside/outside the boundaries of medicalization. *Health: An Interdisciplinary Journal for the Social Study of Health, Illness and Medicine, 8*(3), 275–293.

Thorson, Anna, & Diwan, Vinod K. (2003). Gender and tuberculosis: A conceptual framework for identifying gender inequalities. In Matthew Gandy & Alimuddin Zumla (Eds.), *The return of the white plague: Global poverty and the 'new' tuberculosis* (pp. 55–69). New York and London: Verso.

Tyreman, Stephen. (2005a). An expert in what?: The need to clarify meaning and expectations in 'The Expert Patient.' *Medicine, Health Care and Philosophy, 8*(2), 153–157.

Tyreman, Stephen. (2005b). The expert patient: Outline of UK government paper. *Medicine, Health Care and Philosophy, 8*(2), 149–151.

Ussher, Jane M. (1997). *Body talk: The material and discursive regulation of sexuality, madness and reproduction.* New York and London: Routledge.

Vickers, Margaret H. (2001). *Work and unseen chronic illness.* New York and London: Routledge.

Ware, Norma C. (1992). Suffering and the social construction of illness: The delegitimation of illness experience in Chronic Fatigue Syndrome. *Medical Anthropology Quarterly, New Series, 6*(4), 347–361.

Ware, Norma C., & Kleinman, Arthur. (1992). Culture and somatic experience: The social course of illness in neurasthenia and chronic fatigue syndrome. *Psychosomatic Medicine, 54*(5), 546–560.

Wendell, Susan. (2001). Unhealthy disabled: Treating chronic illnesses as disabilities. *Hypatia, 16*(4), 17–33.

Werner, Anne, & Malterud, Kirsti. (2003). It is hard work behaving as a credible patient: Encounters between women with chronic pain and their doctors. *Social Science and Medicine, 57,* 1409–1419.

Williams, Simon J., & Bendelow, Gillian A. (1998). *The lived body: Sociological themes, embodied issues*. New York and London: Routledge.

Wilson, Elizabeth A. (2004). *Psychosomatic: Feminism and the neurological body*. Durham, NC, and London: Duke University Press.

Wilson, Patricia M. (2001). A policy analysis of the Expert Patient in the United Kingdom: Self-care as an expression of pastoral power? *Health and Social Care in the Community, 9*(3), 134–142.

World Health Organization. (2005). The impact of chronic disease in upper income countries. Retrieved 15 June 2006, from http://www.who.int/chp/chronic_disease_report/media/upper_income.pdf.

Young, Allan. (2000). History, hystery and psychiatric styles of reasoning. In Margaret Lock, Allan Young, & Alberto Cambrosio (Eds.), *Living and working with the new medical technologies: Intersections of inquiry* (pp. 135–162). Cambridge: Cambridge University Press.

Young, Iris Marion. (1990). *Justice and the politics of difference*. Princeton, NJ: Princeton University Press.

2 Claiming a Disability Benefit as Contesting Social Citizenship

MICHAEL J. PRINCE

In her book, *Illness as Metaphor*, Susan Sontag (1978: 3) calls illness 'the night-side of life, a more onerous citizenship.' Continuing the imagery, she adds: 'Everyone who is born holds dual citizenship in the kingdom of the well and in the kingdom of the sick. Although we all prefer to use only the good passport, sooner or later each of us is obliged, at least for a spell, to identify ourselves as citizens of that other place' (ibid.). This figure of speech resonates with prevailing beliefs regarding chronic illnesses and a great many experiences in accessing disability benefits (Prince, 2001 and 2002) and thus offers an obvious point of departure for understanding contestation and social citizenship. Besides portraying health and illness as a simple dichotomy (see Orsini, Chapter 6, this volume), Sontag's passage pathologizes illness while pointing out some biases that are no doubt dominant in contemporary cultures about wellness and disability. However, referring to citizenship in 'the kingdom of the well' and 'the good passport' conveys the formal status and actual practice of citizenship as unproblematic, as something that everyone holds and uses. Experience, both historically and still today, reveals that citizenship is a contested status for many individuals and social groups (Adamoski, Chunn, & Menzies, 2002; Prince, 2004; White & Donohue, 2003). Social citizenship, fully understood in practice, is not only a formal status of membership in a community or a firm solution to certain needs, but also a field of possible acts and relations of power that include action and resistance, participation and apathy, empowerment and exasperation (Cruikshank, 1999: 62; Foucault, 1980: 41). In what ways are social policies spaces for contestation, and how do individuals go about contesting aspects of policies and practices relating to personal experience, professional expertise, and program eligibility?

In this chapter, I examine how working-age adults who are participating in the formal labour market and experiencing significant impairments are governed by a public program established to provide disability income security as an earned right. For persons with mental or physical disabilities, claiming social insurance benefits can be understood as an experience of contested illness as well as contested citizenship. To investigate this theme, I cover four topics. I first briefly explore the meaning of *contestation* and how it relates to deliberative democracy, oppositional politics, and citizenship. I then examine disability as a contested field of identity politics and social policy. Next, I discuss social citizenship and diagnoses in action in relation to a public disability insurance program. Finally, I look at the interactions between individuals and officials as a multifaceted series of power relations. My empirical analysis is based on the particulars of, and experiences with, the Canada Pension Plan Disability (CCP-D) program.[1] The chapter concludes with a discussion of the implications of these practices in claiming disability income security for our understanding of citizenship, social policy, and power.

Thinking about Contestation

Contestation as a form of power easily relates theoretically to conflict approaches to research inquiry, and to the belief that struggle is endemic to social experiences, structures, and relations. As an analytical perspective, contestation holds the promise of considering structural contexts and the subjectivity of actors, at one and the same time.[2] Mark Warren (1999) offers a conception of politics quite useful for the purposes of this analysis that focuses on the intersection of power and conflict. The domain of politics includes 'contested relations of power' that deal with social identities, material resources, and state-centred activities (ibid.: 219). Along with these cultural, economic, and state forms of manifest conflict, Warren (ibid.) draws attention to 'suppressed politics,' in which 'routines and relations of power [are] uncontested owing to vulnerability or hegemony.' In such circumstances, although conflict is not perhaps widely apparent, power is involved nonetheless, and any resolution and decisions are 'displaced onto civil society organizations' (ibid.: 225). Warren's notion of suppressed politics, of uncontested relations of power, relates to what I would call *potential contestables*. These are social goals, practices, beliefs, and outcomes that are taken for granted and considered 'normal,' yet have the capacity in the future for being mobilized as a political issue and thus openly questioned and challenged. This is the stuff, of course, of agenda setting and the work of social movements.

Contestation also links to deliberative citizenship and democracy, concepts used recently in political science, social policy, and critical and philosophical studies. Like contestation, the notion of deliberation addresses political participation and shares an interest in enhancing the voices of groups traditionally marginalized from public and community spheres.[3] Contestation differs from deliberation, though, in terms of the understanding of power relationships that it reflects. Deliberation in public policy making is normatively seen as 'governed by norms of equality and symmetry; all have the same chances to initiate speech acts, to question, to interrogate, and to open debate' with consensus 'freely reached, not coerced' (Benhabib, 1996: 70). In contrast, contestation is commonly imagined in terms of power imbalances and struggles against domination and oppression.

As a relation of power, contestation implies controversy, resistance, dissent, and opposition to a dominant force, but other relationships and outcomes can occur. Contestation has an internal subjective side, in which resistance is contemplated and initiated, as well as an external dimension of power as imposition and restriction. More than this is involved though. Contestation is a relational phenomenon, a dynamic interaction between individuals or groups and their immediate settings and larger institutional contexts. Contestation is both 'outside in' and 'inside out' (Grosz, 1994), with the simultaneous experience and exercise of initiation and imposition. Contestation plays out through multiple processes and can result in several diverse power effects.

The concept of contestation is significant in challenging the construction of persons with disabilities or chronic illnesses as passive victims living in the kingdom of the sick or as deserving beneficiaries of readily available social rights. The notion also directs attention to particular features of the medical, bureaucratic, and financial discourses and structures, among others, that construct and condition identities along with access to welfare state social benefits and services (Prince, 2004). Contestation thus offers a more dynamic and problematic image of citizenship rights than is often presented in the social policy literature. The opportunity to claim benefits is important not only because of what it offers in financial support to individuals with disabilities and family members, but also because it involves members of a political community in pursuing and thus exercising the rights of citizenship. Contestation and citizenship, therefore, are intertwined, played out together in formal public policy structures, concrete programs, and myriad local sites of interactions between individuals and officials.

Disability as a Contested Field

Individuals, advocates, and groups in the disability field are struggling to change outmoded attitudes held by the public and the mass media (Enns, 1999) to remove barriers to participation and to gain access to much-needed supports and services for everyday living. There is also resistance, if not outright opposition, by numerous public authorities (Crown corporations, health and social service ministries, and school districts) to claims by individuals and families. Disability activists and groups *advocating* for integration and services seek a seat at the table of policy-makers in pursuit of equal participation and social justice (Boyce et al., 2001; Puttee, 2002).

Debates and disputes about disabilities – and thus people's identities – and about eligibilities for and exclusions from public services, have characterized income security programs from the modern beginnings of the provision of social services. Injured workers, wounded veterans, people with mental health conditions, and those with physical disabilities have advanced political claims to gain state recognition of their status and a meaningful response to their needs and interests. The contestation of illness and disability are intertwined with the politics of need interpretation. As Nancy Fraser (1987: 119) notes, since 'needs are irreducibly interpretive,' a politics of explaining and understanding needs arises. The interpretation of social needs in welfare systems are, in principle, contestable and thus subject to critique and struggle. Fraser (1987: 104) asserts that 'the interpretation of people's needs is itself a political stake, indeed sometimes the political stake.' A question to ask then is: whose interpretation of a person's illness is authoritative? Or, on whose terms does the welfare state deal with a person with a disability?

Quite often, contestations are linked to the incompleteness, incoherence, and thus inequities among programs, laws, and services of both a generic kind and those tailored for persons living with impairments, chronic illnesses, and disabilities. For instance, income programs and support measures in Canada offer different eligibility criteria and levels of assistance, as well as appeal and redress mechanisms. Consequently, whether a person qualifies, and if so, for what and for how long, is often related to how and where the injury or disability came about, and the nature and cause of the health condition (Puttee, 2002; Rioux & Crawford, 1994). Eligibility can also be related to which department, agency, or level of government is delivering the program. Predictably, there are frustrations, clashes, and tensions over navigating state systems and gaining access to existing income programs and support measures (Bennett, 2003; Doe & Kimpson, 1999).

Contestations occur and may reoccur again and again around key life transitions from, for example, pre-school to school, childhood to adolescence, school to work, changing jobs, exiting the labour market, returning to employment, marriage or common law unions, childbearing and rearing, caregiving, retirement, and end-of-life issues. Far too frequently, because supports and services are tied to specific programs, budgets, and agencies, they do not follow individuals through various stages and transitions over the course of their lives.

Public attitudes and practices certainly reflect and contribute to the contested nature of illnesses and disabilities in relation to social policy. A 2004 public opinion poll of Canadians revealed that many people 'retain devaluing or exclusive ideas about who people with disabilities are and how they participate in Canadian society' (Kloosterman, Rietschlin, Stienstra, Spector, & Westmorland, 2005: 14). This prompted the federal government department that has lead responsibility for disability issues to concede: 'There remain negative public attitudes about persons with disabilities regarding the costs of inclusion and their potential contributions' (ibid.: 14). People with disabilities struggle against 'paternalistic attitudes' and conceptions of disability that emphasize medical conditions and that see impairments as personal abnormalities and thus personal tragedies. The advocacy community also struggles for acceptance of the view that disability is in large part a function of whether society recognizes and accommodates impairments by adapting built environments, social beliefs, and laws.

As well, there are significant ontological and epistemological dimensions to contestation. Questions of what is the nature of disability as a lived reality and how we know that reality are not self-evident or simply answered. In her work on corporeal feminism, Elizabeth Grosz (1994: 19) theorizes how the body is 'the site of contestation, in a series of economic, political, sexual and intellectual struggles.' Andrew Webster (2002: 144) writes of 'the contested, socially constructed and variable "pathways" of medical technologies' with many meanings and diverse needs vying for resources. Understanding health as 'inherently complex, multiple and dynamic,' challenges assumptions of rationality in policy making that rely on 'certainty, predictability, [and] clear cause and effect relations' (Ontario Public Health Association, 2003: 2).

Matters of illness, disorders, and disability engage assorted knowledge clashes. For example, there are discursive conflicts between expert professions, across academic disciplines as well as among lay people and experts regarding definitions and the framing of experiences; screening technologies, diagnostic scales, and assessment tools; symptoms, prevalence, and incidence; causal relationships and the influence of other factors; and the efficacy and desirability of different treatments, interventions, and controls. The more forms of knowledge that are in play in a given policy field, the greater the possibility of divergent perspectives especially if information sources are aligned with different value systems and interests endowed with authority (e.g., medicine, the legal process, private life insurance companies, the state bureaucracy). In circumstances such as AIDS/HIV (Corbett, 2004), cancer care (Clow, 2001), innovative health technologies (Plummer, 2003; Webster, 2002), schizophrenia (Schneider, 2003) and workers' compensation (Duncan, 2003; Lippel, Chapter 3, this volume), we see conflicting perspectives that flourish, are quite noticeable, and persist over extended periods of time.

Reports produced by governments and disability policy advocates today routinely employ a discourse of citizenship, participation, and inclusion as the normative reference for pursuing social reforms (Council of Canadians with Disabilities, 1998; Enns, 1999; Puttee, 2002). A dilemma of this strategy is that *citizenship* is itself a contestable notion. There is lack of clarity and agreement in the academic literature and among practitioners as to the meaning of citizenship. Unresolved issues and ambiguities persist, as White and Donohue (2003: 393) observe: 'The dependence of "citizenship" on myriad forms of "participation" and "community" means that what it is must remain uncertain.' Historical research exposes deeply contested visions of the Canadian citizen marked by contradictory processes of exclusion, resistance, and stratification by age, gender, race, and ability among other differences (Adamoski, Chunn, & Menzies, 2002). And contemporary research shows that persons with disabilities are making incremental gains at best, attaining 'citizenship by instalments' (Prince, 2001) in a 'hit-and-miss affair' (Prince, 2004).

Social Citizenship and Diagnoses in Action:
The Canada Pension Plan Disability Program

Social insurance programs are regarded as pivotal to the development of modern welfare states. Catherine Jones (1985: 70) explains that social insurance was a crucial departure from traditional public last-resort poor relief, 'in that, for the first time, beneficiaries were being required to contribute towards their own security in relation to (predictable) times of need ... and that, when they did call for such assistance, they could do so as a matter of right not as a question of charity.' 'Compulsory social insurance,' elaborates T.H. Marshall (1975: 53), 'was a novelty in three respects. It involved a new kind of interference in the affairs of industry, a new type of relationship between the citizens and government, and new problems of finance and administration.'

Social insurance programs include several features that traditional welfare state thinking holds will alleviate various aspects of contestation. These programs treat human needs as social circumstances rather than personal conditions so that benefits are available to applicants as a matter of right based on their record of employment and financial contributions through payroll deduction. These elements provide social insurance programs with the legitimacy of market liberalism and, it is expected, the avoidance of stigma associated with more intrusive and punitive welfare relief. In administrative terms, with highly formalized means for calculating eligibility, social insurance is commonly thought of in the academic literature to have the advantage of automatic decisions on eligibility with uniform rules, thus minimizing contact between applicants and program officials and curtailing discretion by officials (Heidenheimer, Heclo, & Adams, 1975: 193). By providing coverage of significant risks to a wide population group, social insurance is believed to enjoy mainstream political support to maintain if not expand benefits and defend such programs against the threat of retrenchment.[4]

CPP Disability (CPP-D) is Canada's largest public disability insurance program.[5] Established in the mid-1960s, its primary policy goal is to provide a degree of income protection or financial security that complements private insurance, personal savings, and employment benefit programs, by replacing a portion of the earnings of contributors who cannot work because of a severe and prolonged mental or physical disability. This aim reflects the social insurance nature of the program's design. Other policy goals of this program are the following: (1)

promoting a return to work by supporting at least some CPP disability beneficiaries to undertake gainful employment; (2) ensuring program integrity and accountability so that benefits are paid correctly, appeals heard fairly and promptly, and fraud and errors are avoided; and (3) ensuring the financial sustainability and affordability of the Canada Pension Plan for present and future generations (Prince, 2002). In 2005–06, $3.3 billion was paid to just over 380,000 people. As part of this substantial expenditure, the CPP-D program includes a national vocational rehabilitation program and other related return-to-work support services and incentives. The program also provides for a decision-making process on applications and a three-stage appeal system for adjudicating benefit claims.

The Practice of Social Insurance: Discursive Rules and Diagnoses

A 'right' to CPP disability benefits is a claim for financial resources by individuals based on certain criteria and duties that is mediated through a number of discursive systems. Eric Gorham (1995: 29) reminds us that 'society and the state do not simply give them [rights] to citizens *gratis*; citizens must subject themselves to the procedures and institutions necessary to ensure that the state can continue to provide rights.' In the case of the CPP-D program, applicants are subjected to disciplinary procedures, knowledge systems, and rules from administrative, medical, vocational rehabilitation, actuarial, financial, income security, and judicial discourses. These discursive practices regulate access to and shape the experiences of individuals seeking to obtain benefits for which they believe they qualify and to which they believe they are entitled. Applicants and their claims must engage multiple diagnostic processes, including self-assessments, medical examinations, legal deliberations, rehabilitation evaluations, and even actuarial considerations regarding the 'financial health' of the program itself. This multiplicity of discourses and associated diagnoses are integral to the nature of contestation in claiming benefits. Even successful applicants for disability insurance who become beneficiaries experience tension and stress.

For many working Canadians with disabilities, the experience of seeking this social right of income support is one of rejection and denial of benefits. The 'earned right' of CPP disability, even though based on contributions and work force participation, does not guarantee the automatic provision of benefits. Although labour force attachment is a prerequisite for entitlement to the CPP-D, as a work-related insurance plan, it is not a sufficient condition for eligibility. Further conditions must be satisfied for a worker with a disability to actually qualify and obtain financial support from the program. In addition to having made sufficient valid contributions to the CPP, the individual must be assessed by program officials as having a severe mental or physical disability that is prolonged in nature.

This is a crucial point: the CPP-D program insures against a specific category of disability – severe in condition and prolonged in duration, preventing a person, it is assumed, from being able to hold or pursue any gainful employment. A related point is that the CPP-D program does not provide partial benefits; a person either qualifies for the full benefit or gets nothing at all from the program. To determine if the person has a severe and prolonged disability, information is compiled from the applicant, the attending physician, and the applicant's employer to produce a profile of the applicant, which is then used to determine medical eligibility for the income benefit. And while the issue of determining employability 'is often treated as a technical matter, it is impossible to separate the issue of employability from considerations of who is or is not deserving' (Boychuk, 1998: 18). Labour market considerations, too, enter into decisions, informed by the relative strength of the economy and the extent of employment opportunities in a local area that may match the skills or background of an applicant.

The interplay of these eligibility requirements as presented, interpreted, and at times, negotiated and challenged, affects a person's ability to receive benefits. Accessing benefits is certainly not free of numerous kinds of interventions into the personal lives of individuals. And both the literature and the record of the CPP-D show that medical judgments and administrative decisions on eligibility are shaped not just by professional knowledge and expertise but also by economic factors, political calculations, service traditions, and bureaucratic constraints (Biklen, 1988; Clow, 2001; Prince, 2002; Torjman, 2002). With detailed investigations, reviews, and various encounters with complex organizations, for many people this social insurance program can feel a lot like a social assistance program.

The CPP is part of what Pierre Bourdieu (1998: 2) calls 'the left hand of the state,' located in Human Resources and Social Development Canada, a spending department, with traces 'of the social struggles of the past,' in contrast to 'the right hand of the state, the technocrats of the Ministry of Finance' and private sector interests. Over the 40-year history of the CPP, both hands of the state have influenced and continue to shape the scope and direction of disability policy. This bureaucratic dialectic inside the state, reflecting larger ideological interests and differences, is an important part of the contested terrain. This ideological arm-wrestling, so to speak, adds weight to the argument advanced here that the operation of social insurance programs is not straightforward or free of tension.

Individual–Official Interactions

Turning to consider ways in which people engage in claiming social rights, I situate contestation within interactions between applicants for disability insurance and officials charged with diagnosing applicants and with determining their eligibility for income protection. How do people experience social policies in their daily lives? What interpretations, responses, and social identities are produced? These questions deal with prime experiential aspects of citizenship for people as individuals and as members of families, workplaces, and communities (Neysmith, Bezanson, & O'Connell, 2005), with what has been called 'intimate citizenship' and the intersection of public and private decisions (Plummer, 2003).

Following Max Weber, we can view the state as a mechanism of coercion and bureaucratic administration and, at the same time, following Foucault, see the state as a mechanism of compliance and self-regulation. This connects analytically to what Mitchell Dean (1995) calls practices of governmental self-formation and practices of ethical self-formation. While recognizing that these are not absolute distinctions, Dean (1995: 563) defines practices of governmental self-formation as 'the ways in which various authorities and agencies seek to shape the conduct and capacities of specified political and social categories, to enlist them in particular strategies and to seek definable goals.' Practices of ethical self-formation involve 'techniques and rationalities concerning the regulation of the self by the self, and by means of which individuals seek to question, form, know, decipher and act on themselves' (ibid.).

Dean (1995: 567) describes social security programs as 'governmental-ethical practices' suggesting that these income support programs have a hybrid nature combining practices of governmental and ethical self-formation. On the governmental side are goals of income protection, perhaps the alleviation of poverty, and labour market participation, and on the ethical side are practices shaping 'the attributes, capacities, orientations and moral conduct of individuals' and defining 'their rights, obligations and statuses' (ibid.). This perspective fits agreeably with the CPP-D program. The practices and relations of power in this disability insurance scheme are simultaneously coercive (social control) and chosen (self-compliance), as well as accepted (service provision) and resisted (contestation).

Along with medical constructions and organizational processing, contested illnesses are linked through and through with self-descriptions, presentations of personal experiences, and lived realities to various institutional agencies. To establish eligibility, individuals engage in self-presentations that construct and negotiate their identities in exchanges with professionals and administrators (Schneider, 2003) and the multiple discourses within human service organizations (Spencer, 2001).

Interactions between clients and experts are not all experienced as an overt struggle. Many interactions over seeking the provision of services or benefits are mostly helpful, encouraging, and productive, giving clients a sense of satisfaction and well-being. Other interactions generate a sense of quiet unease or forceful anxiety with 'the wish to suggest other issues for attention other than those given priority by the professional' (Leonard, 1997: 170). In still other situations, the 'interaction will be experienced more negatively as one of monitoring, surveillance and control' of individuals by experts (Bennett, 2003; Leonard, 1997: 170). Depending on how serious the controls and constraints, the client may feel a sense of mistrust, crisis, or panic. This might provoke strong resistance by clients, individually or collectively through informal or formal associations, to challenge the knowledge claims of experts and to seek a more equitable relationship by advancing the legitimacy of their own accounts. In the case of the CPP-D program, many applicants seek out the help and support of co-workers, their employer or union, legal advocates, or their Member of Parliament.

Significant numbers of people each year do not exercise their legal right to appeal an initial negative decision on their application for public disability insurance benefits (Bennett, 2003). Reasons are no doubt several and shed light on the constraints and context of contestation. People decline contesting a negative decision on eligibility for disability benefits because of any number of reasons, factors, or considerations including the following:

- Poor personal health
- Concern that they may lose some other supports that they are currently receiving if they do appeal
- Conversely, they lack important supports, such as accessible transportation, that would enable their attendance at appeal hearings
- Family members or friends discourage them from contesting
- The family physician tells them that they do not meet the eligibility criteria
- Information about rights of redress is not easily accessible, and so they are unaware of the review and appeal mechanisms
- Negative experiences with bureaucrats may convince them they have little or no chance of winning against the government.

This list contains explanations rooted in personal factors and organizational processes plus a cultural frame of beliefs and assumptions about medical science, state authority, and individual responsibility. We see in action here a mix of governmental and ethical practices of self-formation.

In carrying out the official policy goals of income protection, return to work, program integrity, and financial affordability, the CPP-D administration enlists the participation of clients in several ways (Bennett, 2003). These techniques place the responsibility on clients for compiling documentation and completing detailed applications forms, as well as for paying for copies of medical records required to be completed by a physician; if they appeal a denial of benefits, clients must pay for any legal assistance or representation they have along with other possible costs such as travel expenses to attend hearings. Further techniques include a specified labour force attachment requirement for eligibility purposes; a compulsory payment of contributions or premiums from regular paycheques to the program's fund; a requirement that recipients report to program officials any favourable change in their condition; an allowance for recipients to undertake some paid work, take courses, or do volunteer activities without jeopardizing their benefits; and an offering, on a voluntary basis, of vocational rehabilitation services for recipients of benefits. These latter techniques give clients opportunities and incentives to invest in their own conduct.

Other techniques include program officials making periodic reviews of files and issuing guidelines and interpretive directives to officials in field offices and to physicians and other medical practitioners across the country. Surveillance of specific cases and the overall caseload is justified by authorities through a quality assurance discourse of 'ensuring program integrity and accountability,' so that fraud and errors are avoided and benefits are paid to those properly eligible (Bennett, 2003). In turn, applicants marshal support from members in their households and extended families, their physicians, lawyers, advocates, and sympathetic others in compiling the necessary information for claiming disability insurance. And when faced with an initial negative decision of their claim, many applicants request a departmental reconsideration, and if after that they are still not satisfied, they can file a formal appeal to a review tribunal and possibly after that stage to a court for final resolution (Prince, 2002). Even with state constructions of disability and regulations governing eligibility, clients are capable of an array of decisions, actions on their own behalf, responses, and end results in this network of power relations. Through these practices and methods then, power circulates through this disability insurance program, and applying for benefits remains a contested and problematic experience for many individuals and groups.

Consider the story of Sandy, and her struggles through self-regulation and formal application to qualify for CPP disability benefits. In her own words:

> I have fibromyalgia, chronic fatigue syndrome, myofascial pain syndrome, and many other known illnesses that fall under the umbrella of the 'invisible illnesses' ... I applied for CPP disability only after I had tried everything imaginable to cope with and/or improve my life in living with these illnesses ... I gave up all social activities, changed my lifestyle dramatically by down-sizing the home I lived in, curtailed all hobbies that I enjoyed (gardening, reading, visiting), and had to quit a job that I loved dearly because I was just unable to do it any longer ... My application has been in the 'process' now for almost 2 years and there is no need for this to go on that long ... Their failure to acknowledge our illnesses (request repeat letters, request further tests, paper us to death with routine form letters), and not treat us individually, only intensifies our feelings that we are being treated like liars, thieves, and cheats. (Bennett, 2003: 34–5)

This brief account powerfully discloses the politics of contested illnesses, of individuals morally coping through practices of self-regulation, and the mechanisms of governmental control in a rights-based social program. In such circumstances, which are not rare, people endure public disability insurance programs as profound frustration and disappointment to be sure, but also as domination in which they are in a subordinate role with state officials holding considerable power over and within them.

Conclusions

This chapter has examined how working-age adults with significant illnesses and impairments are governed by public entitlement programs. The underlying conceptual theme has been the notion of contestation and how it interrelates with citizenship and with social policies in the modern welfare state that deal specifically with chronic illness: Susan Sontag's 'kingdom of the sick.' Sontag (1978) is just one of many writers who portray citizenship as a formal status in society with certain entitlements and guarantees. The analysis has shown that citizenship is not a thing or an 'it,' not a singular or static entity, and not a fixed bundle of rights and duties held by individuals. Social citizenship is a dynamic field of ideas and values, rules and resources, claims and responses, structures and processes. People, including program officials, practise social citizenship through everyday encounters in myriad situations, forms, and contexts. Processes of application, assessment, administration, and adjudication are relations of authority interwoven with other associations in families, support networks, and workplaces, in which power relationships are active.

With compulsory contributions and labour force attachment requirements, social insurance programs are said to be 'earned rights' to income benefits and important elements of social citizenship in modern welfare states. The analysis here shows that these rights are not so automatic and obtaining them is not so free from struggle. In comparison with classic means-tested welfare programs, social insurance policies like the CPP-D are understood to have a far less 'intrusive and individualised form of disciplinary relationship between the state and the applicant for benefit' (Squires, 1990: 138) because the state administers these programs by relying on actuarial principles of 'averages and the application of the laws of probability' (ibid.) for the working population as a whole. However, in social insurance programs that address risks of illness, injury, and disability (workers' compensation, sickness benefits, compassionate care benefits, and public disability insurance), the state intervenes in every case, examining and verifying the information submitted by each applicant, and accepting or rejecting that information for the purposes of eligibility. Social insurance is not the identical twin of means-tested programs, but they are relatives, with a lot of common history. The differences between these two social policy techniques are not as great as has been claimed in the literature.

Social programs, especially of the income security kind, are often viewed in one of two ways: as benevolent, welfare-enhancing provisions or as blunt tools of coercive control. This analysis shows there are four modes of power that circulate in social programs, particularly major expenditure programs that have elaborate administrative structures and regulatory procedures. In addition to overt contestation, the other forms of power are service provision, coercion/control, and self-compliance. To properly understand contestation, these other forms must also be considered. The politics of social policy is a multidimensional phenomenon with different, shifting, although interacting contours of power relations that includes the authority and inertia of state agencies, the prestige and expertise of medical professionals, and the agency of individuals in diverse local milieus. Following Warren's (1999) concept of suppressed politics, some relations of power in welfare states are often uncontested, such as in service provision and self-compliance. In these circumstances, program goals, administrative practices, and eventual outcomes are accepted, internalized, and taken for granted, for the most part. If these relations and activities were to be recognized as irreducibly political issues intertwined with competing interpretations of needs, then they could be more widely questioned, shifting more of the experience of social citizenship from compliance through potential to actual contestation.

In contemporary welfare states, there is no single answer to the question of whose interpretation of a person's need (Fraser, 1987) or illness is authoritative. Even for rights-based social insurance programs, the analysis in this chapter shows that social policies can carry – that is, incorporate and transmit – several discourses, at the same time and in assorted combinations. These discourses range from the medical, through actuarial and bureaucratic-legal, to the personal and rehabilitative. Each is a complex of ideas, practices, forms of knowledge, and relations of power. Striking a balance among multiple discourses is an interesting belief that liberal politics and administrative bureaucrats are fond of expressing. Although various discourses interact and interlock, they tend to not comprise a coherent pattern and stable arrangement. Each contains certain core principles and preoccupations and promotes particular aims and relationships over others.

In view of these struggles and contested experiences, obtaining a disability pension is as much a personal accomplishment as it is a formal entitlement. Clients are not totally autonomous agents but neither are they simple creatures of state bureaucracies or constructions of medical experts. Seeing the receipt of social benefits as a personal accomplishment underscores the role of individuals' own actions and their interactions with others (including their supporters) in both their immediate settings and larger contexts. Whatever its structure, social provision is a disciplinary and political occasion.

NOTES

1 In using the CPP Disability program as a case study, I am interested in how this public disability insurance program constitutes relations of power among state officials, medical professionals, and individual applicants, and how contestation figures in these networks of roles and relationships. The prime focus is not on the CPP-D program as a form of income security as such, although this is an important backdrop to the inquiry, but rather to view the CPP-D program as a place of power-laden interactions over different meanings of illnesses, diagnoses, and experiences. From this perspective, the politics of social policy goes beyond the conventional focus on debates about financing or adjusting programs to meet a range of shifting needs to encompass the politics of *interpreting* needs (Fraser, 1987) and resisting definitions constructed and imposed by others (Rice & Prince, 2000; Schneider, 2003).
2 Contestation suggests a way of thinking about the world that at its core is critical and social constructivist. Realities such as medical diagnoses, judicial rulings, or administrative decisions are socially constructed and subject to multiple interpretations expressed in numerous formats, sites, and narratives. Various power relations, interests, and ideas that interact in local, specific milieus and that are mediated by larger external settings shape such realities. Outcomes then are contingent and accompanied by unintended consequences.
3 Governance is another popular concept that, like deliberation, implies a new way of doing politics and policy with a new relationship between the state and civil society, one that is more participatory and open and less hierarchical and conflictual. This notion of governance is not to be confused with Foucault's (1980) concept of governmentality.
4 On the political resiliency of social insurance programs, see Brodie (1995) and Rice and Prince (2000) and on the CPP-D specifically, see Bennett (2003), and Prince (2001 and 2002).

5   The province of Quebec has a distinct program, the Régime de rentes du
Québec, with fairly comparable features in retirement pensions and disability and survivor benefits. For details, see Torjman (2002) and Lippel (Chapter 3, this volume).

REFERENCES

Adamoski, Robert, Chunn, Dorothy E., & Menzies, Robert. (Eds.). (2002). *Contesting Canadian citizenship: Historical readings*. Peterborough, ON: Broadview Press.
Benhabib, Seyla. (Ed.). (1996). *Democracy and difference: Contesting the boundaries
of the political*. Princeton, NJ: Princeton University Press.
Bennett, Carolyn, MP. (2003). *Listening to Canadians: A first view of the future of
the Canada Pension Plan Disability Program*. Report of the Standing Commit-
tee on Human Resources Development and the Status of Persons with
Disabilities. Ottawa: House of Commons. Available online, http://
www.parl.gc.ca (accessed 15 May 2007).
Biklen, Douglas. (1988). The myth of clinical judgment. *Journal of Social Issues,
44*(1), 127–140.
Bourdieu, Pierre. (1998). *Acts of resistance: Against the tyranny of the market*.
(Richard Nice, Trans.). New York: New Press.
Boyce, William, Tremblay, Mary, McColl, Mary Anne, Bickenbach, Jerome,
Crichton, Anne, Andrews, Steven, Gerein, Nancy, & D'Aubin, April. (2001).
A seat at the table: Persons with disabilities and policy making. Montreal and
Kingston: McGill-Queen's University Press.
Boychuk, Gerald William. (1998). *Patchwork of purpose: The development of pro-
vincial social assistance regimes in Canada*. Montreal and Kingston: McGill-
Queen's University Press.
Brodie, Janine. (1995). *Politics on the margins: Restructuring and the Canadian
women's movement*. Halifax: Fernwood.
Clow, Barbara. (2001). *Negotiating disease: Power and cancer care, 1900–1950*.
Montreal and Kingston: McGill-Queen's University Press.
Corbett, Kevin. (2004, September). *Contesting AIDS/HIV: The lay reception of bio-
medical knowledge*. Paper presented at British Sociological Association, Medi-
cal Sociology Conference, University of York, York, England.
Council of Canadians with Disabilities. (1998, June). *Disability income, supports
and services project: Consultation report*. Winnipeg.
Cruikshank, Barbara. (1999). *The will to empower: Democratic citizens and other
subjects*. Ithaca, NY: Cornell University Press.

Dean, Mitchell. (1995). Governing the unemployed self in an active society. *Economy and Society, 24*(4), 559–583.

Doe, Tanis, & Kimpson, Sally. (1999). *Enabling income: CPP disability benefits and women with disabilities.* Ottawa: Status of Women Canada. Available online, http://www.swc-cfc.gc.ca.

Duncan, Grant. (2003). Workers' compensation and the governance of pain. *Economy and Society, 32*(3), 449–477.

Enns, Ruth. (1999). *A voice unheard: The Latimer case and people with disabilities.* Halifax: Fernwood.

Foucault, Michel. (1980). Prison talk. In Colin Gordon (Ed.), *Power/knowledge: Selected interviews and other writings, 1972–1977* (pp. 37– 54). London: Pantheon Books.

Fraser, Nancy. (1987). Women, welfare and the politics of need interpretation. *Hypatia: A Journal of Feminist Philosophy, 2*(1), 103–121.

Gorham, Eric. (1995). Social citizenship and its fetters. *Polity, 28*(1), 25–47.

Grosz, Elizabeth. (1994). *Volatile bodies: Towards a corporeal feminism.* Bloomington and Indianapolis: Indiana University Press.

Heidenheimer, Arnold J., Heclo, Hugh, & Adams, Carolyn Teich. (1975). *Comparative public policy: The politics of social choice in Europe and America.* London: St Martin's Press.

Jones, Catherine M. (1985). *Patterns of social policy: An introduction to comparative analysis.* London: Tavistock.

Kloosterman, Ruth, Rietschlin, John, Stienstra, Deborah, Spector, Aaron, & Westmorland, Marilyn. (2005, June). *Disability: Definition, framework and key knowledge gaps.* Issues Paper Series. Gatineau: Social Development Canada.

Leonard, Peter. (1997). *Postmodern welfare: Reconstructing an emancipatory project.* London: Sage.

Marshall, T.H. (1975). *Social policy in the twentieth century* (4th ed.). London: Hutchinson University Library.

Neysmith, Sheila, Bezanson, Kate, & O'Connell, Anne. (2005). *Telling tales: Living the effects of public policy.* Halifax: Fernwood.

Ontario Public Health Association. (2003). *Health in cities: The role of public health.* A position paper adopted by the OPHA. Toronto. Available online, http://www.opha.on.ca/advocacy/ppres.html (accessed 15 May 2007).

Plummer, Ken. (2003). *Intimate citizenship: Private decisions and public dialogues.* Montreal and Kingston: McGill-Queen's University Press.

Prince, Michael J. (2001). Citizenship by instalment: Federal policies for Canadians with disabilities. In Leslie A. Pal (Ed.), *How Ottawa spends 2001–2002, Power in transition* (pp. 177–200). Toronto: Oxford University Press.

Prince, Michael J. (2002). *Wrestling with the poor cousin: Canada Pension Plan Disability policy and practice, 1964–2001.* Paper prepared for the Office of the Commissioner of Review Tribunals, Government of Canada. Available online, http://www.ocrt-bctr.gc.ca/pubs/prince/index_e.html (accessed 15 May 2007).

Prince, Michael J. (2004). Canadian disability policy: Still a hit-and-miss affair. *Canadian Journal of Sociology, 29*(1), 59–82.

Puttee, Alan. (2002). *Federalism, democracy and disability policy in Canada.* Montreal and Kingston: McGill-Queen's University Press.

Rice, James J., & Prince, Michael J. (2000). *Changing politics of Canadian social policy.* Toronto: University of Toronto Press.

Rioux, Marcia H., & Crawford, Cameron. (1994). *The Canadian Disability Resource Program: Offsetting costs of disability and assuring access to disability-related supports.* North York, ON: Roeher Institute.

Schneider, Barbara. (2003). Narratives of schizophrenia: Constructing a positive identity. *Canadian Journal of Communication, 28*(2), 185–198.

Sontag, Susan. (1978). *Illness as metaphor.* Toronto: McGraw-Hill Ryerson.

Spencer, J. William. (2001). Self-presentation and organizational processing in a human service agency. In Jaber F. Gubrium & James A. Holstein (Eds.), *Institutional selves: Troubled identities in a postmodern world* (pp. 158–175). Toronto: Oxford University Press.

Squires, Peter. (1990). *Anti-social policy: Welfare, ideology and the disciplinary state.* London: Harvester Wheatsheaf.

Torjman, Sherri. (2002). *The Canada Pension Plan Disability Benefit.* Ottawa: Caledon Institute of Social Policy. Available online, http://www.caledoninst.org (accessed 15 May 2007).

Warren, Mark E. (1999). What is political? *Journal of Theoretical Politics, 11*(2), 207–231.

Webster, Andrew. (2002). Innovative health technologies and the social: Redefining health, medicine and the body. *Current Sociology, 50*(3), 443–457.

White, Robert, & Donohue, Jed. (2003). Marshall, Mannheim and contested citizenship. *British Journal of Sociology, 54*(3), 391–406.

3 Workers' Compensation and Controversial Illnesses

KATHERINE LIPPEL

Workers in Quebec have the right to compensation if they become incapable of working because of illness attributable to a work 'accident' or considered to be an 'occupational disease.' When the etiology of disease is controversial, as in the case of many musculo-skeletal disorders (MSDs), or when the existence of a disease is questioned by the medical establishment, as in the case of Chronic Fatigue Syndrome (CFS), Fibromyalgia, Sick Building Syndrome (SBS), and Multiple Chemical Sensitivity Syndrome (MCSS), it becomes difficult to access economic support from workers' compensation systems in the event of disability. In this chapter, I examine the workers' compensation appeal cases in Quebec with regard to these illnesses, looking at the different facets of controversy. Where relevant, I have noted gender issues surrounding compensation claims for these illnesses.

I draw on traditional legal analysis of case law and also rely on case law as a source of information about the behaviour of the different actors in the compensation system (Lippel, 2002a). My analysis is also informed by interview data from a qualitative study of the effects of the compensation process on workers' health (Lippel, Lefebvre, Schmidt, & Caron, 2007). Eighty-five injured workers (41 women and 44 men) were interviewed individually with regard to this question, and the medico-legal controversies were at the heart of many of their stories. Among these workers were women who suffered from controversial illnesses (Fibromyalgia, MCSS) and several workers, mostly women and some men, who suffered from different types of MSDs.

In the first part of this chapter, I describe workers' compensation legislation and its impact on the behaviour of the different actors. In this highly polarized context, actors can actively promote controversy with regard to illnesses that are not in themselves controversial. In the second part, I concentrate on compensation claims for illnesses known to be controversial either with regard to their existence, their cause, or their consequences. I address the issue of contested illness in the most literal of its meanings: lawyers, compensation boards, and medical examiners denying either the existence of the illness itself, its presence in the particular case, or its causes. The worker's body becomes itself the nexus of the contestation.

Workers' Compensation as Context for Examining Controversial Illness

The Politico-Legal Environment in Which Claims Are Made

In contrast to European countries such as the Netherlands (Pennings, 2002), Canada has no universal disability insurance covering either temporary or permanent disability. In the case of temporary disability, Employment Insurance (EI) benefits are available to workers who have contributed to the EI scheme for a sufficient number of hours. If those eligible show that they are unable to work for medical reasons they receive 55 per cent of their gross salary for a maximum of 15 weeks. Those who have contributed to the Quebec or Canada pension plans (QPP or CPP) may be eligible for some economic support in the case of severe and prolonged disability – a maximum of $1,054 per month in 2007 (Service Canada, 2007).[1] Partial disability is not covered by the social insurance (non-means-tested) safety net unless it falls within workers' compensation coverage. For many, particularly those who develop long-term disability, workers' compensation becomes the only source of income support available, and for these people, the stakes are high when recognition of their illness is at issue.

Workers' compensation coverage varies from province to province.[2] The vast majority of workers are covered in Quebec and British Columbia, but less than 70 per cent of Ontario employees are eligible for workers' compensation benefits. Many jobs traditionally occupied by women, like teaching and positions in the financial sector, are not covered by workers' compensation in Ontario. Some form of sickness benefits through insurance is available to less than 50 per cent of the Canadian salaried workforce, but only 14 per cent of temporary employees, and 17 per cent of part-time employees have access to complementary insurance benefits, while 58 per cent of full-time workers have access to some benefits (Marshall, 2003: 9, Table 2).

In Quebec, as in other Canadian provinces, workers who become ill because of their work may seek compensation from the workers' compensation board (the Commission de la santé et de la sécurité du travail, or CSST). If the board concludes that disability is attributable to an 'employment injury,' claimants will receive 90 per cent of their net salary for the duration of their disability and other benefits if they remain permanently disabled, including access to vocational rehabilitation.

Legal Framework and Burden of Proof:
Scientific Certitude and Compensation Board Culture

In Quebec, workers must prove on a balance of probabilities that their work, or a work accident, was a contributing cause of their illness in order to be eligible for workers' compensation benefits. They must also prove that their illness is totally disabling in order to access full income benefits, or that it has left them partially disabled, in which case they will receive compensation for lost earning capacity. In the legislative language, as set out in Section 2 of the *Act Respecting Industrial Accidents and Occupational Diseases* (AIAOD: s. 2), '"employment injury" means an injury or a disease arising out of or in the course of an industrial accident, or an occupational disease, including a recurrence, relapse or aggravation.' Some illnesses may be triggered by an accident, as in cases of Fibromyalgia that develops after initial trauma. Other illnesses develop directly because of working conditions. The Act identifies occupational illnesses that are presumed to be work related (AIAOD: s. 29 and Annex 1), and permits workers to claim for illnesses that are not listed, if they can show they were caused by work and are either 'characteristic of that work' or related to 'risks peculiar to that work' (AIAOD: s. 30).

Quebec law provides that the CSST is bound by the opinion of the treating physician regarding most medical issues including diagnosis, degree of disability, and treatment. However, both the CSST and the employer can contest any of these opinions, and medico-legal controversies are prevalent not only in the case of controversial diseases but in many cases where injury is more obvious. Litigation surrounding all workers' compensation issues, but particularly medico-legal issues, has been on the rise since the 1990s because employer premiums that fund the system are now directly linked to costs of compensation for individual workers (Lippel, 2006). As a result, a new industry has developed around workers' compensation litigation, and many medical experts, consultants, and lawyers now make their living contesting workers' claims for compensation.

Legally, workers have to prove that it is more probable than not that (1) they are suffering from an 'illness,' (2) they contracted the illness because of a work accident or in the course of employment, (3) the illness can be ascribed to employment risks or is peculiar to their work, in the case of occupational disease, and (4) the illness is disabling. Legal culture and the courts are clear that the worker need only prove these elements on a balance of probabilities, yet in science and to some extent in medicine there is a strong tradition relying on principles of scientific certitude. Because doctors and the scientific literature play an important role in the adjudication process, it often happens that compensation boards and even appeal tribunals import exigencies that are inappropriate in a legal context, exacting of workers levels of certainty approaching 99 per cent certitude when 50 + 1 per cent is the traditional burden of proof (Cranor, 1993; Jasanoff, 1995). In cases of civil liability, the Supreme Court of Canada has clearly stated that plaintiffs in civil law need only prove that causation is more probable than not (Snell, 1990). This approach is often strongly resisted by compensation boards whose dominant culture is medical, and medical experts who testify in appeal cases still feel they can recommend claim denial if scientific uncertainty surrounds the issues raised in the case. This collision of cultures between the medical and legal communities often gets played out in a context in which the person who is ill, and who is the least able to afford litigation, has to invest money, time, and energy in order to access compensation, as it is often only in appeal that the appropriate standard of proof is applied.

To better understand contested illnesses in the context of workers' compensation litigation, the first step is to pinpoint where the controversy lies. Sometimes the only controversy is that regarding causation: there is no challenge to the claim that the worker is disabled by a recognized illness, the only question is whether work or a work accident caused the illness, as in the case of many MSDs. In other cases, not only does the compensation authority question causation, but it also may question disability and even the existence of the illness itself, as in the case of multiple chemical sensitivities and, until recently, Fibromyalgia.

Creating Controversy: Repetitive Strain Injury and Other Musculo-skeletal Disorders

One of the most important medico-legal controversies in the past twenty years is that surrounding musculo-skeletal disorders (MSDs) associated with repetitive work. Often referred to as repetitive strain injuries (RSI), an umbrella term including most MSDs, these health problems have been increasing all over the industrialized world. Quebec legislation actually presumes that certain MSDs (tendinitis, tenosynovitis, and bursitis) are caused by repetitive work. And yet employer medico-legal teams have succeeded in instilling the idea that these diseases are controversial, insinuating doubt not only with regard to issues surrounding causation but in some cases attacking the legitimacy of the illnesses themselves by alluding to the idea that the illness is the product of 'mass neurosis.' In the words of a medical expert working with Canada Post: 'We find here the same mass neurosis as in Australia characterized by a mutual interactive influence among workers as well as personal physicians, favouring the propagation of ideas, concepts and dogmas which are only hypothetical and not proven and which on the contrary glorify victimization and are thus detrimental to society and the worker' (Canakis, 1994, as cited in translation in Messing, 1998).

In three 1994 test cases, Canada Post contested claims brought by workers doing highly repetitive work and succeeded in convincing the Commission d'appel en matière de lésions professionnelles (CALP), the appeal tribunal in Quebec at that time, that in two of the three cases (those brought by two women) that the injury was not caused by work. One decision of over 400 pages relied on epidemiological literature, almost to the exclusion of legal principles, to conclude that repetitive work in itself was not a cause of the workers' disease, regardless of the legislative presumption to the contrary. The Canada Post medico-legal team then organized a conference where representatives and experts were presented with the successful medico-legal approach (Lippel, Messing, Stock, & Vézina, 1999). Afterwards, there was a large increase in employer contestations of such claims. There is still a great deal of litigation surrounding these claims, even those for illnesses presumed to be work-related.

Alluding to 'mass neurosis' or questioning work relatedness has been particularly successful in cases brought forward by women. For example, a study of 314 appeal cases in Quebec showed that women workers seeking workers' compensation benefits for various MSDs were less often successful than men both for illnesses presumed to be work-related, such as tendonitis, and illnesses that were not covered by the legislative presumption, such as carpal tunnel syndrome (Lippel, 2003). These types of difficulties are not specific to Quebec and have been documented in the rest of Canada (Kome, 1998: 71–99) and in Australia (Bohle & Quinlan, 2000). In Australia, medical consultants still actively promote the controversial nature of MSDs and offer their services to help contest claims (Lucire, 2003). The effect of these allegations, questioning the presence or severity of pain, is to undermine the credibility and honesty of the worker, and controversy surrounding these claims promotes further ill health (Reid, Ewan, & Lowy, 1991). Nor are these types of difficulties new. On the contrary, they are often based on bias in the medical textbooks, sometimes dating back to the mid-twentieth century, as in the case of carpal tunnel syndrome (Dembe, 1996: 69–77).

It is of course possible that in a given case an MSD such as tendonitis or carpal tunnel syndrome has not been caused by work. However, when we talk about 'controversial illnesses,' these types of illnesses do not readily come to mind as the existence of the illnesses is not debated in the traditional medical community, and many studies and meta-analyses have shown that the illnesses are often caused by work (Bernard, 1997; Kuorinka & Forcier, 1995). The CSST itself makes the prevention of MSDs a priority and underlines that, in the year 2000, MSDs were responsible for 40 per cent of the costs of compensation and 38 per cent of occupational injuries (CSST, 2005).

If such mainstream (legitimate) illness can become the object of so much contestation, it is not surprising that claims for controversial illnesses are rarely accepted. I now turn to case law to examine four such illnesses: Fibromyalgia, Chronic Fatigue Syndrome (CFS), Multiple Chemical Sensitivity Syndrome (MCSS), and Sick Building Syndrome (SBS).

Controversial Illness

What makes an illness controversial? When the medical establishment questions the existence of a given diagnosis, or the consequences of the illness, these positions will necessarily have an adverse impact on cases brought by workers with the illness who are claiming compensation. Sometimes it is not the illness itself that is questioned, but the cause of the illness – either in general terms or in the specific case brought before the CSST. Even in those cases where claims are accepted as being work-related, the degree of disability that would justify compensation may in itself be questioned. Acceptance of these claims is infrequent, and many claims are refused because of issues of scientific uncertainty.

The uncertainty itself has been recognized as a reason justifying a worker's failure to claim within the prescribed delay of six months (*Commission scolaire de Val d'Or v. Moreau*, 1999, a case of MCSS; Labbé, 1999, a case of CFS), and some claims have been accepted years after the initial manifestation of the health problem, particularly in cases of Fibromyalgia (Fabris, 2004) but also for MCSS (Moreau, 2002). The controversial nature of the diagnosis, and the additional complexity associated with the controversy, have also served to justify the employer who had filed a contestation after the legal deadline (De Miranda, 2001).

Chronic Fatigue Syndrome

Some controversial illnesses have been a challenge for social security administrators responsible for disability pensions, such as the Quebec or Canada pension plans, or welfare systems predicated on disability (Prince, Chapter 2, this volume), but are essentially invisible to the workers' compensation system, because there have been few claims attributing the illness to work or a work accident. This is the case for Chronic Fatigue Syndrome (CFS), an illness that is recognized as a potential source of disability but whose cause is still largely unknown, although there appears to be some evidence that it can be triggered by both viral infection and physical trauma (Carruthers et al., 2003: 9–10), two potentially work-related events. Few judgments have been rendered by the appeal tribunal (la Commission d'appel en matière de lésions professionnelles [CALP] between 1985 and 1998 and la Commission des lésions professionnelles [CLP] since 1998) concerning claims by workers suffering primarily from CFS, although some cases involved both Fibromyalgia and CFS (C.H. Chauveau, 2000; Laliberté, 2002).

Among the few accepted claims was the case of a woman who had initially suffered from back problems after a work accident. Her condition deteriorated, and several specialists confirmed a diagnosis of Fibromyalgia. A psychiatrist also concluded that the worker suffered from a major depression resulting from CFS, itself a consequence of the Fibromyalgia; the CLP, in light of the strong evidence in the specific case, accepted the claim for all these diagnoses (Laliberté, 2002). In this case, five specialists (rheumatologists and physiatrists) had confirmed the diagnosis of Fibromyalgia, two had confirmed the link between the initial fall and injury and the Fibromyalgia, and a psychiatrist had confirmed the presence of CFS and depression, linking them both to her deteriorated physical condition attributable to the Fibromyalgia. No evidence to the contrary was brought forward by the opposing parties, and given the absence of health problems prior to the accident, the tribunal concluded that on a balance of probabilities the Fibromyalgia and CFS conditions constituted an aggravation of the initial injury, and ordered compensation.

The only other case of CFS to be accepted by the appeal tribunal was also associated with diagnoses of a psychiatric nature. In this case, a worker developed CFS and 'typical depressive syndrome' while she was confronted with chronic stress at work associated with overwork clearly arising from cutbacks in the federal civil service where she was employed. Although the worker's personality was raised as a possible cause of her disorder (she was evaluated by a psychiatrist to be a perfectionist), the tribunal held that objectively stressful working conditions, combined with the worker's personality, led to the development of the disability. As the 'thin skull' rule[3] applies in workers' compensation cases, the fact that the worker's personality could have contributed to the development of the illness was not an obstacle to compensation. The tribunal concluded that the stressful working conditions justified compensation for an occupational disease related to risks peculiar to the worker's employment. The worker's claim was not aggressively contested in appeal, and some doubt remains as to the nature of her illness, as the medical evidence in the specific case seems to suggest that burnout and CFS are synonymous. Without the evidence concerning the worker's mental health, it seems clear this claim would not have been accepted (Laflamme, 2000).

Fibromyalgia

Fibromyalgia is a syndrome that has been the subject of medical controversy not only as to its etiology, treatment, and consequences, but as to its very existence as a diagnosis. Designating a cluster of debilitating symptoms, the existence of Fibromyalgia was acknowledged by the World Health Organization in 1992. However, it remains controversial since some medical specialties still question its diagnostic validity, and issues such as causation and the syndrome's role in engendering disability remain hotly contested in the medical literature (Fabris, 2004; Guité & Drouin-Béguin, 2000).

The controversy surrounding Fibromyalgia is perhaps the most visible of those examined here. It has become particularly so since the Quebec Court of Appeal has had to intervene several times against administrative tribunal decisions concerning both automobile accident victims (Viger, 2000) and injured workers (Chiasson, 2002), decisions that had refused claims for compensation on the basis of the scientific uncertainty surrounding the diagnosis. The case law of the Court of Appeal is clear: when medical evidence and factual circumstances permit the tribunal to draw the conclusion that a work accident or a car accident probably caused the condition in the particular case, the fact that controversy persists in the medical community is not in itself a reason to set aside the opinion of the medical experts who supported the claim for compensation (Lippel & Fabris, 2003). Fabris (2004) examined the case law that followed the Appeal Court decisions and found that one of the two tribunals involved, the Tribunal administratif du Québec, responsible for appeals from the Société de l'assurance automobile du Québec (SAAQ), the administrative body responsible for the compensation of victims of car accidents, had, until recently, largely ignored the dicta of the Appeal Court. By contrast, the CLP, the administrative tribunal responsible for work-related injury, has followed the lead of the Court of Appeal and has now accepted several cases of Fibromyalgia, where it was shown that the condition developed after either physical or psychological (Côté, 2001) trauma.

Until recently (Radio-Canada, 2005), the Quebec College of Physicians and Surgeons had taken a conservative position with regard to Fibromyalgia, concluding that it could not be considered to be a disabling disease unless other diagnoses also applied to the patient. Thus, if psychological problems were diagnosed as well, Fibromyalgia could be considered as disabling (Fabris, 2004). Although injured workers fare slightly better than individuals injured in car accidents, people suffering from Fibromyalgia can expect to be confronted with sophisticated legal teams and a battery of expert witnesses paid for by the employer and sometimes by the compensation board itself.

In other provinces, such as Nova Scotia, compensation boards have tried to get around their obligations to Fibromyalgia patients by limiting their access to benefits through policy or regulation. In 2003, the Supreme Court of Canada held this approach to be in violation of

Section 15 equality provisions of the Canadian *Charter of Rights and Freedoms* (Nova Scotia, 2003), and concluded that such policies constitute prohibited discrimination on the basis of handicap. No further 'special arrangements' seem to have been developed with regard to this diagnosis.

Sick Building Syndrome

A variety of health problems are known to be associated with poor air quality, and illness can be ascribed to work if it can be shown that exposure to mould, micro-toxins, or chemicals in the workplace have caused a recognized illness. Symptoms vary, including gastrointestinal problems, respiratory problems, sore throat, headaches, and fatigue. Sick Building Syndrome is one of the many illnesses associated with poor air quality; others include MCSS, rhinitis (Beaudet, 2004; Dallaire, 2003; Nguyen, Beaudry, Donnini, & Renzi, 1999: 245–58; Scott, 2003; Teixeira, 2003), and 'psycho-organic syndrome' (Nguyen et al., 1999: 245–58).[4]

SBS has been recognized as a compensable illness in Quebec (Laliberté, 1993), and occasionally workers have succeeded in accessing compensation. However, the burden of proof is difficult to meet, as decision-makers require that other causes of their illness be excluded, given that the diagnosis is considered to be a diagnosis by default, applicable only when no other illness can be identified. According to one case, cited with approval by Nguyen and colleagues (1999: 248), workers who prove that they have been diagnosed with SBS by a physician and that norms governing air quality have not been respected must also provide evidence that the poor air quality caused their illness. Current case law insists that proof that exposure limits for a given substance have been violated is not necessary for compensation to be granted (Della Cioppa, 2001; Lemoy, 2003; Lippel, 2002b: 318–20), although it is very difficult to convince the tribunal of a causal link when no excessive exposure can be identified. If other workers have also experienced debilitating symptoms this can strengthen the case, on the condition that there is actual evidence of this fact and not simply allegations without medical evidence (Grant-Fontaine, 2001; Nguyen et al., 1999: 254–6).

In Quebec, employers are responsible for eliminating at source working conditions that compromise health. It is not sufficient to meet specific standards: the employer must also comply with the general duty clause insuring that working conditions are safe. Seemingly, federal legislation in Canada is less exacting, as it is sufficient to comply with the specific regulations (Beaudry, 2006: 4–9). The argument that compliance with specific regulatory norms undermines the validity of a compensation claim is thus particularly inappropriate in Quebec cases.

The workers who succeeded in accessing compensation for illness associated with poor air quality were those whose medical portrait included rhinitis (Beaudet, 2004; Teixeira, 2003) and those whose work environment had been shown either to be in violation of regulated exposure levels (Beaudet, 2004) or undergoing a change (construction, painting, demolition, or fire) at the time of the onset of their symptoms (Dallaire, 2003; Scott, 2003; Teixeira, 2003).

The diagnosis of SBS makes accessing compensation more difficult because of the controversy surrounding the diagnosis itself. However, when new evidence allowed a worker to specifically point at exposure to mould, the worker was then able to prove that the health problems were attributable to an allergy to mould, and the claim, which had previously been refused, was then accepted (Université McGill, 2004). The British Columbia Workers' Compensation Appeal Tribunal has also granted the right to compensation for respiratory problems related to exposure to mould (British Columbia Workers' Compensation Appeal Tribunal, 2005).

Multiple Chemical Sensitivity Syndrome

Multiple Chemical Sensitivity Syndrome (MCSS) has been defined in medical textbooks as:

> a diagnosis that has increasingly been given to patients with a wide variety of symptoms that they attribute to exposure at very low levels to a number of commonly encountered chemicals. The syndrome usually begins after a well-defined environmental event, such as a reaction to a more clearly toxic dose of an organic solvent, pesticide, or respiratory irritant. Some cases of MCS[S] begin as SBS. Affected persons commonly report symptoms such as fatigue, malaise, headache, dizziness, lack of concentration, memory loss, and 'spaciness' – symptoms that overlap somewhat with those of other diagnoses of uncertain etiology, such as chronic fatigue syndrome. The pathogenesis of MCS[S] is obscure, and no proven methods exist for its diagnosis, evaluation, and treatment. Case series suggesting a high prevalence of affective disorders indicate that

psychological factors may play a role in causing MCS[S] and/or in determining its severity; however, evidence does not support MCS[S] as a
purely psychogenic illness. A few studies of MCS[S] patients suggest that
the biologic mechanism of MCS[S] may involve neurogenic inflammation
of the nasal mucosa (as indicated by abnormal rhinolaryngoscopic findings) linked to central nervous system dysfunction. (Braunwald et al.,
2001, as cited in Moreau, 2002: par. 78)

Compensation was granted in a few decisions where the workers
were diagnosed with MCSS, but in many of those claims MCSS itself
was not recognized as a legitimate diagnosis, and occasionally workers
were compensated for various forms of rhinitis (De Miranda, 2001). In
all cases where compensation was granted, exposure to a contaminant
was proven and without such proof, the worker's claim had little
chance of succeeding (Gauthier, 2001).

The CLP has recognized a few claims for MCSS. In the case of
Moreau, a technician in a chemistry laboratory of a high school, MCSS
was recognized as a compensable disease 7 years after his withdrawal
from work and 5 years after his initial compensation claim. The final
favourable decision was rendered 10 years from the moment when he
first alerted his union as to his suspicions regarding the possible occupational cause of his health problems. The worker showed that he had
been exposed to a variety of chemicals on a daily basis for over 20 years
and that the conditions of that exposure were not always secure; the
evidence of at least seven physicians (including that of a toxicologist; an
ear, nose, and throat specialist; and a psychiatrist) was before the tribunal (Moreau, 2002).

In Lemoy (2003), MCSS and specifically 'rhinitis caused by chemical
sensitivity' were the accepted diagnoses in a case where the chemical
substances (particularly toluene) did not exceed the regulatory exposure
limits but where it was made clear that the worker's exposure to a low
level of toluene had triggered her disease. The worker, a secretary in a
print shop, brought forward clear evidence of exposure to toluene, a
determining factor in the acceptance of her claim. Six doctors confirmed
a diagnosis of MCSS or rhinitis caused by chemical sensitivity (Lemoy,
2003). This decision constitutes a breakthrough in that the CLP acknowledges that a medical controversy regarding the diagnosis of MCSS can
no longer justify refusal of a claim given the clear instructions of the
Court of Appeal in Chiasson (2002). The tribunal explicitly sets aside
previous case law that refused MCSS claims because of the controversial

nature of the diagnosis. Case law prior to Lemoy (2003) denied compensation to MCSS claimants because of the controversy surrounding the diagnosis (Lippel, 2002b: 284; Rolko, 1994; Vasseur, 1998).

The CSST itself has accepted cases including MCSS diagnoses prior to the intervention of the CLP. Although there is no public access to information regarding these cases, appeals regarding specific aspects such as permanent disability (Serigraffiti Inc., 2002) or access to rehabilitation (Carter, 2003) show that when the link between exposure and medical evidence is solid, some claims are accepted without litigation. The acceptance rate of such cases is impossible to determine as statistics on refusals by the CSST are not available.

Controversial Consequences: What Constitutes Disability?

Even when compensation is awarded, claimants may still be considered able to work, and the challenges with which injured workers are confronted are not dissimilar to those encountered by claimants of disability pensions, although injured workers may have to face up to medico-legal teams of both the employer and the CSST, an often insurmountable burden. Case law rarely addresses this issue, but a study of Fibromyalgia decisions (Fabris, 2004) has shown that doctors and decision makers rarely conclude that Fibromyalgia can be permanently disabling unless other diagnosed diseases are contributing to the worker's disability.

Conclusion

This analysis of Quebec case law suggests that it is extremely difficult to access workers' compensation benefits in Quebec for illnesses contested by the medical community, as the appeal tribunal is very demanding with regard to evidence. The scientific community, by nature, is more comfortable with a Type 2 error, which leads to the erroneous conclusion that there is no relation between work and a disease, than with a Type 1 error, where such a relationship is erroneously held to exist. This leads to scientists, doctors, and sometimes specialized tribunals favouring refusal of a claim until there is close to a scientific consensus on the issue of causation, while exacting no such consensus to justify denial of the claim. Yet the law posits that each hypothesis should be given equal weight and that which is slightly more plausible than the other should prevail (Cranor, 1993; Snell, 1990).

In those cases where compensation is granted, it is often after a very long struggle, as in the case of Moreau (2002), who finally obtained compensation more than a decade after he had initially alerted his union to problems with his health that he believed to be associated with chemical exposure. Without a union or access to legal counsel and costly medical expertise, it seems close to impossible to win compensation, and even in those cases where medical evidence is strong, it is rare to see compensation granted if the employer or the compensation board aggressively contests the claim. In most cases a large number of medical experts intervene, as appears from several judgments discussed. Interviews confirmed this: one worker reported that she had consulted 20 specialists for a case of MCSS. Aside from exposing workers to a multiplicity of examinations and tests, an experience often associated with controversial illness regardless of legal issues, arguments over the worker's credibility, and the legitimacy of the claim are brought to the forefront in a legal context, and this can exacerbate the disability associated with the initial illness, including mental health problems associated with chronic pain and disablement (Reid, Ewan, & Lowy, 1991). The fact that these diseases are being discussed in a legal context can also make them even more controversial, leaving the worker spiralling in a vicious circle where her insistence on the legitimacy of her claim becomes in itself an argument to prove that it is psychogenic[5] (Brunner, 2003; Mendelson, 1995 and 2002).

Claimants interviewed report on the stress associated with making a claim and going into appeal. Although this is true of most appellants (Lippel, 2006), those suffering from controversial illnesses were particularly marked by the process. A worker who tried to obtain compensation for MCSS told of the imbalance of power in the courtroom: the worker, alone with her union representative, was confronted by the employer and its lawyers and experts as well as the CSST and its lawyers and experts. Accessing the workplace to obtain evidence as to the nature of exposure is difficult in itself, while obtaining support from a competent occupational hygienist is costly and beyond the means of most workers. Both claimants with MCSS eventually developed psychiatric problems that exacerbated their disability and made it even more difficult to obtain compensation for the initial physical problem.

A woman suffering from Fibromyalgia after an initial diagnosis of back pain was told by several of her treating physicians not to inform the compensation board of her condition as they feared her benefits for back pain would be cut off. In her case, this turned out to be a successful strategy as she surprised the employer and the compensation board with the Fibromyalgia diagnosis only during the appeal hearing concerning other issues surrounding the claim. This eventually led to an out-of-court settlement. Nonetheless, it is ironic that the only way this worker thought she could obtain adequate support from the compensation board was to leave them in the dark as to the true nature of her illness.

Although the workers we met who were suffering from controversial illnesses were mostly women, decisions regarding MCSS, CFS, and SBS were not sufficiently numerous to justify a gender-based analysis. Both men and women were claimants, and most claimants failed to access compensation. We do know that appeals concerning MSDs are less likely to be accepted when the worker is a woman (Lippel, 2003), and although female claimants for Fibromyalgia are more numerous than male claimants, the small number of male claimants made it difficult to measure gender differences in success rates (Fabris, 2004).

The difficulties discussed here are neither exclusive to Quebec, nor are they exclusive to the workers' compensation arena. Insurance companies can set up obstacles to compensation, and they have been known to target claimants suffering from Fibromyalgia by having recourse to private detectives to observe their behaviour and perhaps question their disability (Lippel, 2005: 163, nn 8 and 10). Stress surrounding medico-legal issues and the process designed to determine the cause of the disease and its legitimacy as a 'proper' diagnosis have been found to further exacerbate the consequences of some of these illnesses, and new approaches have been put forward to better respond to the needs of the people who suffer from them (Bülow, 2003; Lax, 2002).

In the context of civil law litigation, controversy in the scientific arena has been the subject of enormous debate, particularly in the United States where, in the early 1990s, the Supreme Court forced judges into the role of scientific gatekeepers charged with keeping so-called junk science out of the court room. The result has been a systemic exclusion of evidence that could otherwise help plaintiffs, as the plaintiffs are those whose cases suffer when something is not proven, and as Jasanoff (2005: S52) points out, 'Scientists are […] at greater liberty to accept a verdict of "not proven" with regard to a given hypothesis or question.' In the United States, examples exist where scientists are themselves vulnerable to legal strategists who seek to discredit them, by undermining their credibility and their integrity as researchers, by attempting to force them to violate their confidentiality commitments (Picou, 1996), and by questioning the very legitimacy and relevance of their science, as in the case of epidemiologists who address risk but not causation (Givelber & Strickler, 2006).

Analogies with the U.S. context must be used sparingly because there 'the courts have an obligation to make whole the uncared-for victims of a robust culture of risk-taking' (Jasanoff, 2005: S57). Canadians, by contrast, tend to rely more on the regulatory framework to protect them from dangerous substances and practices. Nevertheless, scientific uncertainty in Canada, as in the United States, does not exist in a vacuum: 'The scientific knowledge that the law needs for its purposes is frequently unavailable until the legal process itself creates the incentives for generating it; nor are methods that technical communities regard as valid necessarily at hand until interested litigants seek out the expertise to help them win their case' (ibid.: S54).

Workers' compensation in Canada has often served as a forum where new risks in the workplace have been identified, and new obligations for prevention have been developed. Controversy in the scientific community serves to keep contested illnesses out of the compensation arena. It is often forgotten that this does not make the illness go away; it simply transfers the cost of the illness to the workers and their families and to taxpayers, who assume the cost of Medicare and social assistance.

Acknowledgments

The author wishes to acknowledge the financial support of the Fonds québécois de la recherche sur la société et la culture and that of the Social Sciences and Humanities Research Council of Canada. Research assistance for the preparation of this article was provided by Sophie Fabris, Marie-Claire Lefebvre, Geneviève St Georges, and Audrey Pederian. Particular thanks go out to Pamela Moss, Kathy Teghtsoonian, Steve Kroll-Smith, Clara Valverde, and Zulis Yalte, who provided helpful comments on previous versions of this chapter.

NOTES

1 See Michael J. Prince (Chapter 2, this volume) for an extended discussion of disability benefits.
2 This chapter focuses on the Quebec system; it is important to note that rules may differ in other jurisdictions in Canada.

3 The 'thin skull' rule, elaborated in the context of tort law, dictates that the defendant must take the victim as he or she is, even if he or she is more vulnerable than the average person. It has been extended to the field of workers' compensation law, notably in the case of Chaput (1992) (Lippel, 2002b: 339).

4 Occupational asthma is a disease explicitly recognized by Quebec workers' compensation legislation, but this disease falls outside the purview of this chapter as it is not deemed to be controversial, although claims are nonetheless often contested.

5 In an interview with a compensation system manager from outside Quebec we were told that the quest for confirmation of the existence of the physical origin of an illness (Chronic Fatigue Syndrome) in the context of a compensation claim was in itself a symptom of the psychogenic nature of the illness.

REFERENCES

Beaudry, Christian. (2006). Qualité de l'air en milieu de travail: Principaux aspects juridiques. In *Développements récents en droit de la santé et de la sécurité du travail, 239,* (pp. 3–19). Cowansville: Editions Yvon Blais.

Bernard, Bruce. (Ed.). (1997). *Musculoskeletal disorders and workplace factors.* Cincinnati: NIOSH.

Bohle, Philip, & Quinlan, Michael. (2000). Repetition strain injury: A case study of occupational injury. In Philip Bohle & Michael Quinlan (Eds.), *Managing occupational health and safety* (pp. 144–172), Melbourne, Australia: Macmillan.

Braunwald, Eugene, Fauci, Anthony S., Kasper, Dennis L., Hauser, Stephen L., Longo, Dan L., & Jameson, J. Larry. (2001). *Principles of internal medicine* (15th ed.). New York: Harrison's Press.

Brunner, Jose. (2003). Trauma in court: Medico-legal dialectics in the late nineteenth-century German discourse on nervous injuries [Electronic Version]. *Theoretical Inquiries in Law, 4*(2), article 8. Available online, http://www.bepress.com/til/default/vol4/iss2/art8 (accessed 15 Mai 2007).

Bülow, Pia. (2003). *Making sense of contested illness.* Linköping, Sweden: Tema Communications Studies, Linköping University.

Canakis, André. (1994, Dec.). *Mouvements répétitifs: La problématique. Littérature scientifique.* Document distributed during a colloquium on Les mouvements répétitifs: À quelles conditions représentent-ils un risque de lésions professionnelles?: L'expérience vécue des quatre causes-types de la Société canadienne des postes, organized by Robert Gilbert, Olivier Laurendeau, and François Lebire, in collaboration with Canada Post Corporation and held in Montreal.

Carruthers, Bruce M., Jain, Anil K., De Meirleir, Kenny L., Peterson, Daniel L., Klimas, Nancy G., Lerner, A. Martin, Bested, Alison C., Flor-Henry, Pierre, Joshi, Pradip, Powles, A.C. Peter, Sherkey, Jeffrey A., & van de Sande, Marjorie I. (2003). Myalgic Encephalomyelitis/chronic fatigue syndrome: Clinical working case definition, diagnostic and treatment protocols. *Journal of Chronic Fatigue Syndrome, 11*(1), 7–115.

Cranor, Carl F. (1993). *Regulating toxic substances: A philosophy of science and the law.* New York: Oxford University Press.

CSST. (2005). *Troubles Musculo-squelettiques.* Retrieved 25 Sept. 2005, from http://www.csst.qc.ca/NR/rdonlyres/7A11861B-9D81-40AF-89F8-6F10DDC1C4C8/296/dc_500_236.pdf

Dembe, Allard E. (1996). *Occupation and disease: How social factors affect the conception of work-related disorders.* New Haven, CT, and London: Yale University Press.

Fabris, Sophie. (2004). Fibromyalgie: l'accès aux indemnités prévues dans la *Loi sur les accidents du travail et les maladies professionnelles* dans un contexte d'incertitude scientifique et médicale. In *Développements récents en droit de la santé et de la sécurité du travail, 201* (pp. 275–306). Cowansville: Editions Yvon Blais.

Givelber, Daniel, & Strickler, Lori. (2006). Junking good science: Undoing *Daubert v Merrill Dow* through cross-examination and argument. *American Journal of Public Health, 96*(1), 33–37.

Guité, Marcel, & Drouin-Bégin, Agathe. (2000). *La fibromyalgie.* Sainte-Foy, PQ: Multimonde.

Jasanoff, Sheila. (1995). *Science at the bar: Law, science and technology in America.* Cambridge, MA: Harvard University Press.

Jasanoff, Sheila. (2005). Law's knowledge: Science for justice in legal settings. *American Journal of Public Health, 95* (Suppl. 1), S49-S58.

Kome, Penny. (1998). *Wounded workers: The politics of musculoskeletal injuries.* Toronto: University of Toronto Press.

Kuorinka, Ilkka, & Forcier, Lina. (Eds.). (1995). *Work related musculoskeletal disorders (WMSDs): A reference book for prevention.* London: Taylor and Francis.

Lax, Michael. (2002). Occupational medicine: Toward a worker/patient empowerment approach to occupational illness. *International Journal of Health Services, 32*(3), 515–549.

Lippel, Katherine. (2002a). Droit et statistiques: réflexions méthodologiques sur la discrimination systémique dans le domaine de l'indemnisation pour les lésions professionnelles. *Canadian Journal of Women and the Law, 14*(2), 362–388.

Lippel, Katherine. (2002b). *La notion de lésion professionnelle*. Cowansville: Editions Yvon Blais.

Lippel, Katherine. (2003). Compensation for musculo-skeletal disorders in Quebec: Systemic discrimination against women workers? *International Journal of Health Services, 33*(2), 253–281.

Lippel, Katherine. (2005). Les enjeux juridiques et sociaux du recours aux enquêteurs privés pour surveiller les victimes de lésions professionnelles. *Canadian Journal of Criminology and Criminal Justice, 47*, 127–173.

Lippel, Katherine. (2006). L'expérience du processus d'appel en matière de lésions professionnelles telle que vécue par les travailleuses et les travailleurs. In *Développements récents en droit de la santé et de la sécurité du travail, 239,* (pp. 119–180). Cowansville: Editions Yvon Blais.

Lippel, Katherine, & Fabris, Sophie. (2003). La fibromyalgie: peut-elle donner lieu à une indemnisation? *Le Médecin du Québec, 38*(7), 81–83.

Lippel, K., Lefebvre, M.-C., Schmidt, C., & Caron, J. (2007). *Managing Claims or Caring for Claimants: The Effects of the Compensation Process on the Health of Injured Workers*. Montreal: Services aux collectivités, UQAM.

Lippel, Katherine, Messing, Karen, Stock, Susan, & Vézina, Nicole. (1999). La preuve de la causalité et l'indemnisation des lésions attribuables au travail répétitif: rencontre des sciences de la santé et du droit. *Windsor Yearbook of Access to Justice, 17*, 35–85.

Lucire, Yolanda. (2003). *Constructing RSI: Belief and desire*. Sydney, Australia: UNSW Press.

Marshall, Katherine. (2003). Benefits of the job. *Perspectives on Labour and Income,* Statistics Canada, *4*(5), 7–14.

Mendelson, Danuta. (1995). The expert deposes but the court disposes: The concept of malingering and the function of medical expertise. *International Journal of Law and Psychiatry, 18*(4), 425–436.

Mendelson, Danuta. (2002). English medical experts and the claims for shock occasioned by railway collisions in the 1860s: Issues of law, ethics and medicine. *International Journal of Law and Psychiatry, 25*, 303–329.

Messing, Karen. (1998). *One-eyed science: Occupational health and women workers*. Philadelphia: Temple University Press.

Nguyen, Van Hiep, Beaudry, Christian, Donnini, Giovanna, & Renzi, Paolo. (1999). *La qualité de l'air intérieur: Aspects techniques, médicaux et juridiques* (2nd ed.). Cowansville: Editions Yvon Blais.

Pennings, Frans. (2002). *Dutch social security law in an international context*. The Hague: Kluwer Law International.

Picou, J. Steven. (1996, Summer). Compelled disclosure of scholarly research: Some comments on 'High Stakes Litigation.' *Law and Contemporary Problems*, *59*, 149–157.

Radio-Canada. (2005). Les personnes atteintes de fibromyalgie remportent une importante victoire. Retrieved 5 May 2005, from http://radio-canada.ca/regions/abitibi/nouvelles/200504/13/001-fibromyalgie.shtml.

Reid, Janice, Ewan, Christine, & Lowy, Eva. (1991). Pilgrimage of pain. The illness experiences of women with repetition strain injury and the search for credibility. *Social Science and Medicine*, 32(5), 601–612.

Service Canada. (2007). Canada Pension Plan CPP Payment Rates. Retrieved 20 Aug. 2007, from http://www1.servicecanada.gc.ca/en/isp/pub/factsheets/rates.shtml.

Legislation

AIAOD [Act Respecting Industrial Accidents and Occupational Diseases], R.S.Q. c. A-3.001 (*AIAOD*).

Case Law

BURDEN OF PROOF AND THIN SKULL RULE

Chaput v. Montréal (Société de transport de la Communauté urbaine de Montréal), [1992] C.A.L.P. 1253 (C.A.Q.).

Chiasson v. Reitmans Inc., J.Q. no 43 (C.A.Q., 2002).

Snell v. Farrell, [1990] 2 S.C.R. 311.

SAAQ [Société de l'assurance automobile] v. Viger, [2000] R.J.Q. 2209 (C.A.Q.).

CHRONIC FATIGUE SYNDROME

C.H. Chauveau v. Hamel, C.L.P.E, 2000LP-108, (Guylaine Tardif, 27 Nov. 2000, [refused]).

Daoust v. Extermination Denis Brisson Inc., CLP 88497-71-9705, (Mireille Zigby, 31 May 1999, [refused]).

Labbé v. Corporation Northern Village Kuujjuak and CSST, CLP 111146-01B-9903, (René Ouellet, 15 Nov. 1999, [deadline extended]).

Labbé v. Corporation Northern Village Kuujjuak and CSST, CLP 111146-01B-9903-2, (Jean-Maurice Laliberté, 9 April 2001, [refused]).

Laflamme v. D.R.H.C. Direction Travail, CLP 141372–07-0006, (Denis Rivard, 15 Nov. 2000, [accepted]).

Laliberté v. Top Billard de Laval Inc. (fermée), CLP 144600-61-0008, (Fernard Poupart, 9 August 2002, [accepted]).

Roger v. Équifax Canada and CSST, C.L.P.E. 2003LP-214, (Lucie Landriault, 20 Oct. 2003, [refused]).

FIBROMYALGIA

Chiasson v. Reitmans Inc., J.Q. no 43 (C.A.Q., 2002).
Côté v. P. Bélanger and C. Ranger Pharmaciens and C.S.S.T., [2001] C.L.P. 95.
Nova Scotia (Workers' Compensation Board) v. Martin, [2003] 2 S.C.R. 504.
SAAQ [Société de l'assurance automobile] v. [2000] Viger, R.J.Q. 2209 (C.A.Q.).

SICK BUILDING SYNDROME / MOULD / POOR AIR QUALITY

British Columbia Workers' Compensation Appeal Tribunal: WCAT-2005-01431, (Lynn M. Wilfert, 22 March 2005, [accepted]).
Beaudet v. EDM Laser, CLP 192373-31-0210, (Pierre Simard, 26 July 2004, [accepted]).
Dallaire v. Services ménagers Roy ltée and CSST, CLP 174333-02-0112, (Claude Bérubé, 21 Jan. 2003, [accepted]).
Della Cioppa v. Docteurs de l'Espace Inc., CLP 155730-72-0102, (Doris Lévesque, 18 Sept. 2001, [refused]).
Grant-Fontaine v. Cuirs Bentley Inc., CLP 146652-71-0009, (Danièle Gruffy, 19 Sept. 2001, [refused]).
Kaiser v. Travail Canada, CALP 22720-62-9011, (Simon Lemire, 27 July 1993, [accepted]).
Laliberté v. Hôpital Royal-Victoria [1993] CALP 699, (Gabrielle Lavoie, [accepted]).
Scott v. Centre d'Accueil St-Margaret, CLP 200717-72-0302 & 200719-72-0302, (Yolande Lemire, 16 Dec. 2003, [accepted]).
Teixeira v. Ameri-Source Publications Inc., C.L.P.E. 2003LP-181, (Thérèse Giroux, 30 Sept. 2003, [accepted]).
Université McGill v. Côté, CLP 221829-32-0312 et 224355-32-0401, (Rock Joli-coeur, 18 Nov. 2004, [accepted]).

MULTIPLE CHEMICAL SENSITIVITY SYNDROME

Carter v. Primeteck Électroniques Inc. and CSST, CLP 140851-62-0006-R, (Mireille Zigby, 6 March 2003, [benefit granted during rehabilitation process]).
Commission scolaire de Val D'Or v. Moreau, [1999] CLP 552, (Pierre Prégent, [deadline extended]).
De Miranda v. Concordia Auto Ltée and CSST, CLP 110241-73-9902, 140504-73-0006, 140618-73-006, (Francine Juteau, 31 July 2001, [accepted as a rhino-pharayngo-conjonctivitis but MCSS refused]).
Gauthier v. Hôpital Marie-Enfant and CSST, CLP 100786-73-9805-3, (Simon Lemire, 1 Oct. 2001, [refused]).
Lemoy v. Litho Associates Ltée and CSST, [2003] C.L.P. 634, (Lina Crochetière, [accepted]).

Moreau v. Commission scolaire de Val-D'Or, C.L.P.E. 2002 LP-44, (Pierre Prégent, [accepted]).

Rolko v. Dept. of National Defense, [1994] CALP 1341, (Margaret Cuddihy, [refused]).

Serigraffiti Inc. v. Cayouette, CLP 148264-71-0010 and 148805-71-0010, (Mirelle Zigby, 13 Feb. 2002 [accepted]).

Vasseur v. Ville de Montréal and CSST, CLP 92134-72-9710, (Lina Crochetière, 22 Dec. 1998, [refused]).

4 Managing Workplace Depression: Contesting the Contours of Emerging Policy in the Workplace

KATHERINE TEGHTSOONIAN

It is difficult not to notice the heightened profile that has been achieved in the Canadian context by the issue of 'mental illness in the workplace,' reflected as it has been in government discourse, reviews of relevant research literatures, and discussions within the business community (B.C. Business and Economic Roundtable on Mental Health, 2006; Bilsker, Gilbert, Myette, & Stewart-Patterson, 2004; Global Business and Economic Roundtable on Addiction and Mental Health [hereafter Global Roundtable], 2006; *HealthCarePapers*, 2004; Ministry of Health Services, 2002 and 2003; Senate Standing Committee, 2004a and 2004b). Almost invariably across these contexts, mental distress among employees has been presented as a widespread – and growing – phenomenon that generates considerable financial costs for employers, trends that are understood to signal a pressing need for research, analysis, and action (for typical examples see Dew, Keefe, & Small, 2005; Global Roundtable, 2005; Lesage, Dewa, Savoie, Quirion, & Frank, 2004: 4–5; see also Canadian Institutes of Health Research, 2005). While more recently addressing themselves to 'depression, anxiety, and addiction' in the workplace, many of these discussions originally focused on depression, which continues to be a crucial element in the configuration of employee troubles of interest.

Leaders in the business community have suggested that undiagnosed depressive illness among employees is of particular concern. If an individual's struggle with depression remains unidentified, they suggest, her diminished performance and productivity may be inappropriately framed as the result of insufficient work commitment or limited competence, rather than as symptomatic of mental illness. A number of organizations have therefore proposed various practical strategies to avoid this outcome, including training managers to address an employee's problematic work performance in ways that facilitate and encourage the employee's collaboration in seeking and accepting a diagnosis and treatment (B.C. Business and Economic Roundtable on Mental Health, 2006; Global Roundtable, 2006; Mental Health Works, 2006).

At first glance, such initiatives appear oddly juxtaposed to established narratives of contestation around depression (and other illness that is not readily apparent) that involve struggles between individuals who insist that they are ill in the face of the sceptical scrutiny of employers and insurance companies, who deny that such claims are valid (Dumit, 2000; Lippel, Chapter 3, this volume; MacEachen, 2000; McCormick & Adelman, 2004). However, as the discussion below will establish, this seeming paradox is resolved when we observe the central place reserved in these emerging initiatives for recommendations that employers implement a disability case management approach in dealing with employees requiring sick leave or disability benefits as a result of being diagnosed with depression. Rather than contesting the legitimacy of individuals' claims that they are ill, current initiatives encourage employers to relocate their scrutiny of employees' health status into decision-making processes regarding treatment and the timing of their return to work.

Employers' interest in managing aspects of employees' private lives is not new (Conrad & Walsh, 1992; Hansen, 2004; Miller & Rose, 1995), nor has it been restricted to issues of emotional well-being.[1] For example, Ellen MacEachen (2000: 322) notes an 'expanding sense of corporate jurisdiction over worker bodies' evident in managers' attempts to reduce employers' financial liabilities in workers' compensation claims for repetitive strain injuries developed on the job. These efforts have involved 'extensive regulation of worker bodies both on and off work time' (ibid.: 320) such that 'the worker body appeared to represent the property of the company, even when the worker was on "personal time" or off duty. The corporate expectation appeared to be that an employee's non-work time must be geared to regeneration and care of a worker body' (ibid.: 323).

In contesting these practices MacEachen (2000: 325) articulates a number of important questions: 'Whose body is it? Do managers have the right to ask workers not to use their bodies in certain ways in order to keep their bodies in a state of constant readiness for work? Who has authority over the body when the worker is not on paid work time? Is this body the corporation's in keeping? Or is it a personal body? ... [The evidence from this study] ... points to a blurring of boundaries between work and leisure, public and private, as the disciplined worker is expected to maintain optimal fitness and work readiness at all times.' MacEachen argues that the managerial practices and discourses that she observed while conducting her research reflect the insertion of neoliberal orientations into the ways in which employees' claims for workers' compensation are taken up in the workplace.

In this chapter, I suggest that questions and concerns similar to those raised by MacEachen regarding the location and permeability of the border between the public world of work and employees' private lives arise from a critical engagement with current proposals to address depression among employees. The strategies outlined in these proposals involve breaching that border in a variety of ways, while simultaneously constructing new borders intended to contain the biomedically grounded expertise of family physicians as well as the emerging expertise of the informed, 'empowered' patient/employee. In so doing, these strategies also reflect and operate as linkages to key elements of the neoliberal ethos that currently dominates political life in Canada, and in the industrialized West more generally.

Theoretical Framework, Conceptual Tools, and Empirical Terrain[2]

Scholars working within a Foucauldian framework have argued that a series of technologies of rule or governing practices described as 'advanced liberal' have come to be aligned with neoliberalism (Dean, 1999; Lemke, 2001; Rose & Miller, 1992). These practices do not operate through directly coercive strategies; rather they secure compliance through mechanisms that generate an alignment of the self-interested choices of individuals with the goals of those who govern (Dean, 1999; Foucault, 1983). As Nikolas Rose (1998: 155), following Foucault, has argued, 'governing in a liberal-democratic way means governing *through* the freedom and aspirations of subjects rather than in spite of them' (emphasis in original).

For some time now in the political arena in Canada the goals of those who govern have reflected the tenets of neoliberalism, including a reduced role for the state in the provision and funding of services; an emphasis on the individual as the normative unit of economic, social, and political life; and a privileging of market-oriented and corporate values and practices, including those of economic efficiency and productivity (Brodie, 1995 and 2002; Teghtsoonian, 2003). Key features of current framings of the problem of mental illness in the workplace are consistent with these orientations. For example, the intense interest in the workplace as an avenue through which the emotional well-being of employees ought to be addressed, by virtue of its focus, directs attention away from the role of the state in the funding and provision of relevant services (Bakan, 2005). Moreover, as the analysis in this chapter will suggest, the individualizing and corporate discourses that circulate in discussions of the problem and strategies for addressing it resonate with neoliberal norms and objectives.

Contemporary technologies of rule have included discourses of responsibilization that direct individuals to become 'enterprising selves' who are incited to work on themselves in various ways (Rose, 1998). As Thomas Lemke has argued, 'The strategy of rendering individual subjects "responsible" (and also collectives, such as families, associations, etc.) entails shifting the responsibility for social risks such as illness, unemployment, poverty, etc., and for life in society into the domain for which the individual is responsible and transforming it into a problem of "self-care"' (2001: 201). Rather than directing their energies to organizational or political change, 'responsibilized' employees diagnosed mentally ill are exhorted instead to undertake the work of self-care and self-management. Through their efforts to improve their psychological, spiritual, and physical selves, individual employees are understood to be enhancing their capacity to adapt successfully to their work environment. In so doing, they enact themselves as good neoliberal citizen-workers who take responsibility for making choices that ensure that they will be able to contribute as healthy, productive members of their workplaces and communities.

By focusing on the individual worker as the appropriate site and engine of action to address emotional distress, and in framing employment as a key obligation of citizenship, discourses of responsibilization resonate powerfully with central elements of neoliberalism. And yet, governing programs operate imperfectly. They are beset with a variety of complications borne of resistances from those they target, imperfect knowledge and analysis on the part of those who design and implement them, and contradictory relationships with other initiatives emanating from various sources that may disrupt or undermine their intended outcomes (Larner, 2000; Lemke, 2001; O'Malley, Weir, & Shearing, 1997). Technologies of rule thus accomplish their aims with varying degrees of success and coherence, and hold the potential to generate their own difficulties.

For example, there is a tension lodged at the heart of responsibiliza-tion projects: freely choosing individuals, including ill employees, may make choices that disrupt or disregard the goals of those who govern (Fullagar, 2002). Rose (1998: 155) argues that 'a potential, if always risky and failing, solution' to this dilemma can be located in 'the proliferation of experts' such as psychiatrists, physicians, and social workers who are able to 'direct the personal capacities and selves of individuals under the aegis of a claim to objectivity, neutrality, and technical efficacy rather than one of political partiality.' The liberal state was thus able to govern indirectly, *through* professionals' deployment of expert knowledge, thereby avoiding the need to intervene in more direct ways. However, experts 'have the capacity to generate ... *enclosures*: relatively bounded locales or types of judgment within which their power and authority is concentrated, intensified and defended' (Rose & Miller, 1992: 188, emphasis in original). As a result, experts have been articulated to gov-erning authority unevenly, through 'loose and flexible linkages' (ibid.: 184) that have entailed a significant degree of autonomy for practising professionals. The resulting scope for discretion thus replicates, in the relationship between experts' decisions and the goals of ruling authori-ties, the tension embedded in the responsibilization of individuals that the privileging of expertise seemingly addresses.

Other technologies of advanced liberal rule, including discourses of accountability, budget discipline, and the construction of 'calculating selves' and 'calculative spaces' (Miller, 1994), entail a series of responses to the dilemmas that this autonomy of experts poses for governments:

> Monetarisation has played a key role in breaching the enclosures of expertise within the machinery of welfare. For example, when contempo-rary British hospitals are required to translate their therapeutic activities ... into cash equivalents, a new form of visibility is conferred upon them ... Managers rather than [medical] consultants become the powerful actors in this new network, and power flows from the cabinet office to the operating theatre via a multitude of calculative and manage-rial locales, rather than in the other direction. This is not an attempt to impose a power where previously none existed, but to transform the terms of calculation from medical to financial ... Far from autonomizing the health apparatus, these new modes of action at a distance increase the possibilities of governing it. (Rose & Miller, 1992: 200)

Similarly, discussions about the importance of addressing mental ill-ness invariably involve the mobilization of a broad range of statistical evidence regarding the economic losses accruing to employers as a result of untreated, or inappropriately treated, depression. Depression among employees as a medical issue is thus rendered into a calculable problem that can be expressed through a corporate idiom and addressed via managerial practices within the workplace setting. And disability case management emerges as an organizational technology that works to circumscribe both the choices of responsibilized ill employees and the expertise of family physicians who treat them.

To begin an analysis of these developments, I explore two documents. The first, entitled *Depression and Work Function: Bridging the Gap between Mental Health Care and the Workplace* (Bilsker et al., 2004), was published by the Mental Health Evaluation and Community Consultation Unit (MHECCU), which was located within the Department of Psychiatry in the Faculty of Medicine at the University of British Columbia (UBC).[3] The second, entitled *Roadmap to Mental Health and Excellence at Work in Canada* (2005), was produced by the Global Business and Economic Roundtable on Addiction and Mental Health, a Toronto-based organization composed of and addressing itself to leaders in the Canadian business community.

The two documents differ significantly in the features of the workplace to which they direct their primary attention. As a result, they make visible the operation of different technologies of rule. *Depression and Work Function* focuses on the psychology and behaviours of individual employees as key targets of intervention, and in so doing deploys discourses of responsibilization. The *Roadmap to Mental Health and Excellence*, by contrast, draws attention to the ways in which organizational and managerial practices and policies may contribute to employees' mental distress; it mobilizes discourses of accounting and accountability in constructing a case for addressing these and in proposing particular strategies. Alongside these differences, the two documents share a strong enthusiasm for a disability case management approach to employees diagnosed with depression, viewing it as the cornerstone of a successful organizational response to the issue. My analysis shows how the different intervention strategies and technologies of rule articulated in each of these two documents constitute, through their links to disability case management, elements of a wider project that involves shaping the subjectivities and choices of ill employees – and of their managers and physicians – in ways that are congruent with the goals of corporate leaders and, more generally, neoliberalism as a governing program.

Responsibilization, Disability Case Management, and the Subordination of Biomedical Expertise

In *Depression and Work Function*, the principal focus of attention is the individual, that is, the employee diagnosed with – or at risk of developing – depression. Although there are passing references to structural conditions that are associated with higher rates of depression, such as 'being female' and 'living in poverty,' these are dismissed without further analysis on the grounds that 'only some are directly relevant to the work setting and within our control' (Bilsker et al., 2004: 27). Thus the authors indicate that they '[will not] recommend gender change as a way of reducing depression risk' (as if this constituted a significant avenue through which one might address the relationship between gender and depression), and reject the need to consider linkages between poverty and depression among workers with the questionable claim that 'few employed individuals in Canada (depressed or not) are living in poverty' (Bilsker et al., 2004: 27). With these brief rhetorical flourishes, the multiple gendered impacts of public policy and organizational structure, the circumstances of the working poor, and the need to develop responses to these realities are all erased.

The authors consider at greater length research findings that indicate a link between aspects of the structure of work and the workplace, workplace stress, and depression. However, they suggest that the relationships revealed by this research are 'complicated' both by the difficulty in separating out the relative contributions to depression of workplace-related stress and stress originating with an employee's home life, and by the fact that 'personal traits of workers affect their vulnerability to workplace stressors' (Bilsker et al., 2004: 29). Although one might imagine a variety of responses to this multiplicity of variables, the 'complication' is resolved by downplaying the potential utility of addressing organizational practices and emphasizing instead interventions designed '[to teach] employees skills to manage existing stresses more effectively' (ibid.: 34).

The rhetorical structure of this analysis is repeated elsewhere in the document, so that the potential relevance of organizational factors in generating workplace stress is acknowledged but then quickly followed up with a renewed emphasis on intervening at the level of the psyche of the individual worker. For example, a brief consideration of the contribution that management style and human resource policies can make to employees' emotional well-being soon gives way to the following passage: 'In addition to favourable environmental conditions, it is important that employees take an active role in maintaining their own health. Routine exercise, good nutrition and weight control, adequate sleep, sufficient leisure time, stress management, and avoidance of illicit drugs and excessive alcohol are all beneficial to both mental and physical health' (ibid.: 52).

Alongside prescribing particular modes of living for employees in their lives outside the work context, the document also recommends strategies through which they are to be responsibilized within the workplace. One such strategy involves the provision of 'resilience training,' which is 'designed to teach skills for dealing with work stressors so that employees have greater resilience when faced with changing patterns of workplace stress' (Bilsker et al., 2004: 51). The authors suggest that by working on their abilities in areas such as problem-solving, time-management, goal-setting, and mood management, employees will become better equipped to cope with problematic features of their work environment, presumably reducing thereby the need to address the latter as a source of emotional difficulties, stress, and illness.

Although the strategies described above are presented as preventive measures relevant for *all* employees, some responsibilizing interventions are targeted specifically at those who have been diagnosed with depression. For example, the document suggests the distribution of 'self-care' materials to employees recovering from depression, as well as to those experiencing 'depressive symptoms or mild disorder,' ideally accompanied by interventions from staff who have been trained 'in how to support employees in the application of self-care strategies' (Bilsker et al., 2004: 55). And for those who are on disability leave, there is a strong and consistent message that they – and their treating physicians – ought to make the resumption of their employment responsibilities the top priority in their recovery.

Although targeting the psychological profile of employees as a key site of interventions to prevent and respond to mental illness, and framing them as individually responsible for undertaking various health-supporting practices in all aspects of their lives, *Depression and Work Function* adopts a sceptical stance towards the empowerment of ill employees as critically informed consumers of health care information and services. The main purpose of 'empowerment' is framed instead as ensuring compliance with prescribed treatment protocols, with 'timely information and suitable counselling' deployed towards this end: '"Informed consumers" can then participate more actively in their own recovery and can help construct a more meaningful therapeutic plan. Compliance can also be facilitated in the workplace by an integrated performance management and case management process that continually monitors progress and securely links the employee, employer, and practitioner' (Bilsker et al., 2004: 60). This passage reveals a certain cynicism concerning the degree of choice and empowerment that ought to be afforded to ill employees. It seems to suggest that allowing employees to understand themselves as 'informed consumers' is fine, but that the range of practical alternatives available to them is to be tightly constrained by managerial practices – including disability case management – that 'securely link' the employee diagnosed with depression to those who know better.

In *Depression and Work Function*, the ill employee does not emerge as the only target of this sort of constraint. Indeed, the disability management approach that the authors advocate involves various measures designed to shape treatment decisions – including the assessment of readiness to return to work – made by the employee's family physician. As the authors note, the project that resulted in the publication of this document originated in 'a common concern that a gap existed between the usual treatment goals established by health practitioners and their patients, and the expectations regarding work function that are critical to the relationship between employer and employee' (2004: 5).[4] The image of a bridge between these two solitudes appears in the subtitle of the document – *Bridging the Gap between Mental Health Care and the Workplace*. The technology with which the bridge is to be constructed is the insertion of one or more additional practitioners (e.g., disability case managers, medical consultants) into the decision-making matrix, practitioners who are paid by the employer and equipped to import managerial rationalities and priorities into treatment and return-to-work decisions.

There are several passages in the document that can be read as attempts to breach the 'enclosed expertise' of biomedical authority by insisting that it be subordinated to a managerial expertise more in tune with the imperatives and priorities of the workplace. For example, the authors argue that 'management of depression in the workplace must begin with the workplace rather than the healthcare system' and offer, as an example of inappropriate treatment, 'recommendations of "stress leave" without concurrent provision of strategies to maintain or build resilience and coping skills' (2004: 45). Here, and throughout the document, the authors frame family physicians as not really understanding the particular requirements of the workplace, and as therefore poorly positioned to provide an accurate and informed assessment of whether and when the ill employee is ready to take on what configuration of tasks.

Ensuring that treatment is designed to prioritize an early return to work is one of the principal tasks of case managers. Thus the authors suggest that 'the ability to communicate effectively with the attending physician or mental health practitioner permits the case manager to monitor clinical progress and ensure that early return to work is an element of the therapeutic plan' (2004: 57), a strategy described elsewhere as 'establishing a successful therapeutic alliance with health care professionals' (ibid.: 62). Employers are also advised that 'some organizations create preferred provider arrangements to ensure access to mental health professionals who are informed and cooperative with early return to work initiatives' (ibid.). Such arrangements are intended to reduce from the outset the odds that practitioners will make treatment choices that are inconsistent with the interests and priorities of employers and insurance companies.

It might be argued that the strategies advocated in this document simply reflect the best science available, rather than the (political) displacement of biomedical expertise by managerial imperatives. Certainly the authors emphasize the importance of ensuring that interventions directed at employees diagnosed with depression be 'evidence-based' and well-supported by existing research. For example, after reviewing two studies that showed that changes intended to reduce organizational sources of stress resulted in less absenteeism and depression among employees, they conclude that 'more research is needed to clearly demonstrate that workplace modification can significantly reduce depression in employees' (Bilsker et al., 2004: 34). Here, and elsewhere in the document, the implication is that it would be imprudent to act on the basis of findings that can only be understood as preliminary, tentative, or ambiguous.

And yet, the implementation of disability case management strategies with respect to employees diagnosed with depression that is so strongly endorsed in the document appears to be based on practically no evidence at all. The authors note that while disability management programs have been successful with employees with physical illnesses or injuries, 'the relevance of disability management to disability caused by mental health disorders has been recognized only recently.

We *believe* that the staged and comprehensive model [of disability management] *could be* readily adapted for the work rehabilitation of depressed workers' (Bilsker et al., 2004: 44–5; emphasis added) but currently 'there is little evidence related to disability management for mental disorders' (ibid.: 60).[5] The authors' vigorous advocacy of this strategy, despite the absence of research substantiating the *belief* on which it rests, suggests that politics and interests – as much as neutral, scientific evidence and expertise – are at play in their assessment of different approaches to addressing employees' emotional distress.

Organizational Policies, Accountability, and Calculative Space

Roadmap to Mental Health and Excellence at Work in Canada, which was released as a draft document by the Global Business and Economic Roundtable during the summer of 2005, presents the group's collective thinking developed over several years. Whereas *Depression and Work Function* (Bilsker et al., 2004) dismisses or downplays research that suggests the potential utility of altering the organization of work or managerial practices in order to reduce employees' emotional distress, the Global Roundtable document takes these latter variables to be of crucial importance.

In outlining a strategy for supporting mental health in the workplace, the *Roadmap* urges business executives and managers to 'identify workplace practices which pose material risks to the health of both the employees and the organization and make needed changes' (Global Roundtable, 2005: 47), and to address a list of ten 'common management stress traps that snare employees' including 'unreasonable deadlines' and 'trivializing employee workload concerns' (ibid.: 48). The authors argue that employee distress must *always* be understood as a potential indicator of underlying problems in the workplace that need to be explored and addressed by managers (ibid.: 57–9). Thus, although the *Roadmap* shares with *Depression and Work Function* an interest in ensuring that employees take responsibility for ordering their lives in ways that support their ability to function as productive members of the workplace, the *Roadmap*'s authors insist that there is a complementary corporate responsibility to consider the context within which employees are asked to perform.

Although reflecting a greater willingness to acknowledge a role for organizational policy and managerial practices in undermining the mental health of employees, the Global Roundtable's *Roadmap* loudly echoes the analysis presented in the MHECCU document in its advocacy of disability case management for employees diagnosed with depression. One of the techniques it proposes as a component of such management is the Medical Affirmation Process (MAP). Framed as presenting a 'Fresh Take on Managing the Front End of Mental Disability' (Global Roundtable, 2005: 68), MAP involves the insertion of a physician or psychiatrist who is paid by the employer into the processes of diagnosis and treatment at the earliest stages of an employee's mental health challenges. The *Roadmap* argues that the approach envisioned in MAP constitutes a vast improvement over the established practice of costly independent medical assessments (also paid for by the employer) precisely because the latter occur 'downstream, after-the-fact' and can leave employers and insurance companies with the difficult task of 'sorting out the deadlock' that can occur between the employee's physician and the medical adviser hired by the company (ibid.: 69). MAP, instead, is designed to ensure that 'the parties – employers, insurers and employees – are unified by good information at the front-end of the disability leave' (ibid.).

In thinking about this proposal using the conceptual tools offered by the literature on governmentality, one could argue that MAP provides a technology through which the understandings of ill employees and their treating physicians can be aligned with the interests of employers and insurance companies in ensuring an early return to work and in particular approaches to treatment. The *Roadmap*, then, like *Depression and Work Function*, envisions the subordination of biomedical expertise to managerial discourses and imperatives. This outcome is also in alignment with the wider goals of governments informed by a neoliberal political rationality, which are to enhance productivity and competitiveness, and to maximize private responsibility for health and well-being.

Discourses of accounting and accountability occupy an important place in the *Roadmap*. For example, the document is replete with quantitative evidence of the prevalence and cost of mental illness, in terms of absenteeism, sick leave and disability benefits, and presenteeism ('employees on the job but not fully-functioning'), which is of particular concern since 'it costs employers 2x–3x more than absenteeism' (Global Roundtable, 2005: 44). In the section of the document directed specifically to CEOs, we learn that 'disability costs in your company, overall, are driven by the duration of the claims not their frequency or volume' (ibid.: 43), a circumstance that helps to explain the importance attached to an early return to work in both this document and in *Depression and Work Function*. Investors in the firm are encouraged to 'determine whether corporate directors and management have quantified and therefore grasp the impacts of employee absence, disability and downtime' (ibid.: 41). Along with investors, all those in positions of responsibility within the firm are encouraged to become 'calculating selves' (Miller, 1994), that is, to track and analyse quantitative indicators of the costs associated with employee mental illness, and to incorporate improvement on these measures into the firm's performance management systems. The problem of the ill employee thus comes to be represented by the costs she or he incurs, and addressing those costs in turn comes to be framed as a key focal point of organizational and managerial efforts.

To ensure that the proposed measures receive more than lip service, the *Roadmap* recommends that managers should be held accountable for the success of an ill employee's return to work, and argues further that 'the line manager and human resources personnel should receive financial incentives to bring about a successful RTW [return to work] wherein the employee comes back full-time gradually and remains successfully on the job for six months and counting' (Global Roundtable, 2005: 76). These provisions are undoubtedly designed to pre-empt discriminatory treatment directed towards a returning employee that might flow from stereotypical assumptions about mental illness, or from a failure to apprehend correctly the scope of the employer's duty to accommodate.[6] Unfortunately, the document does not explore the implications of the dynamic that these arrangements set up, as the career path and personal economic circumstances of others in the workplace come to depend – in part – on the performance of the recovering employee. In the workplace context, accountability mechanisms of this sort may well place additional pressure on the recovering employee by attaching financial consequences for others to her ability to remain on the job. Perversely, such a strategy may contribute to an *increase* in the phenomenon of 'presenteeism,' if recovering employees feel compelled to continue working while experiencing a relapse in order to avert financial consequences for their immediate superior.

The surveillance of employees, both on and off the job, that is involved in the proposed initiatives is presented as being in the interests of employee and employer alike. For example, the *Roadmap*'s authors argue that early detection of mental illness facilitates early treatment, which, in turn, is understood to support more rapid recovery and an earlier return to work if the employee has had to go on sick leave. To support early detection, the *Roadmap* encourages managers and supervisors to monitor employees' behaviour and performance for evidence of emerging mental illness, and describes in some detail the verbal and body language that could be used in raising with an employee the possibility that she or he may be experiencing 'health issues' (Global Roundtable, 2005: 55–7). There are some troubling aspects of these strategies. Although perhaps motivated by genuine concern for employee well-being, the proposed practices open the door to unlimited scrutiny of an employee's performance in the workplace. Because 'undetected mental illness' is something that is manifest empirically through an absence, the hypothesis that it is present can never be disconfirmed: if we have not discovered it, this may simply be because we have not looked hard enough.

It is also important to consider the possibility that some of the recommended strategies may result in significant and unwanted intrusions of the employer into the employee's private life. For example, the document emphasizes the need for managers and supervisors to remain in close contact with employees who are off work on sick leave or longer-term disability leave, arguing that 'guided work-to-home and home-to-work communication between the employee and his or her supervisor and co-workers … is absolutely vital' (Global Roundtable, 2005: 70). There is little sense that such communication may impede, rather than contribute to, the recovery of an ill employee or that it may be experienced by the employee as harassment rather than support. Although there may be nothing but the best of intentions behind a proposal to 'survey employees now off work on sick or disability leave to determine their experience, what worries them about returning to work' (ibid.: 58), it is arguably as likely that this sort of intervention will undermine someone's recovery as support it. As Coralie McCormick and Judith Adelson (2004: 30) have noted, 'even the idea of embarking on a return-to-work strategy can introduce significant stress to the lives of people who are already struggling to manage mental health symptoms.'

The *Roadmap* also suggests that, in addition to the workplace-based accommodation that an employer can provide to an employee recovering from diagnosed mental illness, 'an employee can make her own accommodations in other facets of her life which enhance the return to work experience for both employer and employee' (Global Roundtable,

2005: 74). This point is illustrated with a sample return-to-work plan developed by an employee, a 'young mother and wife,' recovering from bipolar disorder. Presented in the form of a list, it includes items such as 'I will do majority of housework on Saturday. I will delegate some to my daughters,' 'keep meals and clean-up during the week simple' and 'take my medication as directed' (ibid.: 73). The presentation of this plan as one that the Global Roundtable considers to be exemplary suggests the importance of further analysis, following MacEachen (2000), of its naturalization of both employers' proprietary interest in workers' dispositions of their physical bodies and energies while not in the workplace and of a particular gendered division of domestic labour.

Concluding Comments

The authors of these two documents suggest that the strategies they propose for responding to mental distress among employees will serve the interests of both the ill employee and the employer. And yet, this confluence of interest does not materialize naturally. Rather, as the discussion in the documents illustrates, extensive work is necessary to bring the employee's psychological profile and lifestyle choices into alignment with the employer's interest in reducing disability-related costs and, more generally, enhancing the productivity and competitiveness of the organization. Discourses of responsibilization urge employees to *work on themselves* in ways that enhance their ability to contribute in the workplace; they also construct as legitimate employers' interest in various aspects of employees' private lives, not only within the workplace but also outside the employment context. Discourses of accounting and accountability transform the problem of 'depression in the workplace' into one that is both calculable and amenable to corporate management. Both sets of discourses sustain the argument for disability case management as an organizational technology designed to constrain – under the guise of politically neutral, disinterested expertise – the decisions of family physicians and those of the ill employees for whom they care.

I have suggested that several features of the initiatives proposed in these documents can be understood as congruent with a neoliberal governing program. This is not to suggest that there is a unified driving force behind these initiatives, nor that they constitute the coherent implementation of an overarching plan. Nevertheless, we can trace within documents like those analysed in this chapter loose connections between the strategies they outline and a wider set of goals. Elsewhere, more explicit linkages are being developed. For example, 'the BC Minister of Mental Health, the BC Roundtable [a provincial group similar to the Global Business and Economic Roundtable on Addiction and Mental Health] and the UBC Mental Health Evaluation and Community Consultation Unit have agreed to form the BC Scientific Consortium on Mental Health in the Workplace,' chaired by the head of the MHECCU (B.C. Business and Economic Roundtable on Mental Health, 2005: 8).[7] Emerging sites such as these bear close watching, as locations that may serve as relays through which the goals of neoliberal governments come to be pursued 'at a distance' (Rose & Miller, 1992: 185–187), through relationships and decisions that are legitimized as flowing from ostensibly neutral – because scientifically informed – expertise.

Finally, it is worth underlining the absence of any significant discussion of structural inequities flowing from gender, racialized identity, or other dimensions of marginalization in these documents. This erasure of the role played by such structural inequities in shaping people's lives, including their experiences of emotional wellness or distress, is consistent with neoliberalism's privileging of the individual, and its concomitant antipathy to analysis or politics that attends to group-based identity. Neither is there any effort within the documents to explore systematically the relationship between distress within the workplace and the wider policy agendas currently being pursed by governments in Canada and elsewhere in the industrialized West.[8] Although such analysis was arguably beyond the authors' understanding of their task, this framing of the problem nevertheless removes from view linkages that require critical analysis if we are to fully understand, and respond appropriately to, the distress experienced by workers in the contemporary workplace.

Acknowledgments

I would like to thank everyone who participated in the November 2005 workshop, *Illness and the Contours of Contestation*, for a stimulating set of discussions. I am also grateful to Hester Lessard, Katherine Lippel, Melanie Hope, Pamela Moss, Steve Kroll-Smith, and Suzanne Maurice for their helpful feedback on earlier versions of this chapter.

NOTES

1 In recent times workplace-based initiatives have addressed many aspects of employees' lives conventionally understood as private, including spirituality, sexual behaviour, daytime napping, and exercise and other leisure activities (Adkins, 2002; Baxter & Kroll-Smith, 2005; Bell & Taylor, 2003; MacEachen, 2000; McGillivray, 2005).

2 In this chapter, I am trying to work in a space between the literature on governmentality and an approach that takes seriously the importance of critique as a form of engagement and standpoint. Scholars using conceptual tools flowing from Foucault's analysis of government, as the conduct of conduct, have argued that others – such as feminists – who have been engaged in the project of uncovering the interests served by seemingly objective and neutral processes and policies are missing an important part of the picture that would be revealed if the analysis were to be focused instead on *what is actually happening* and *how it actually happens* (Dean, 1999; Rose, 1987). Feminist and related critical analyses have something to offer, they suggest, but improperly ignore key features of the landscape. My approach in this chapter rests on a similar concern about the governmentality literature itself: it too has something to offer, but in marginalizing the insights that flow from critique, it fails to theorize important dimensions of *what is actually happening*. Rather than accept a binary construction of theoretical alternatives, I want to develop an analysis that draws on both approaches in exploring what is taking place as employers are instructed to be concerned about, and to act in response to their perception of, mental illness – particularly depression – among their employees. In other words, I want to develop an argument about whose interests are being served, and whose are not, alongside my use of some of the conceptual tools that have been developed within the literature on governmentality.

3 MHECCU has since closed. Several of the researchers that were associated with it are now affiliated with the Centre for Applied Research in Mental Health and Addiction (CARMHA), which was established in the Faculty of Health Sciences at Simon Fraser University in the wake of MHECCU's closure.

4 In considering the arguments presented in *Depression and Work Function*, it is useful to keep in mind the institutional locations of those involved in its production: two of the three sponsors of the project are involved in the business of health insurance (Great West Life and the Healthcare Benefit Trust), and three of the report's four authors have some affiliation with corporate health interests, as follows: (1) Principal, Gilbert Action Le Page, Occupational

Health Consultants; (2) Director and Occupational Medicine Consultant, Healthcare Benefit Trust; and (3) Occupational Physician, Khatsahlano Corporate Medical Services. Healthcare Benefit Trust is an organization that administers health benefits for those employed in the health care sector in the province of British Columbia.

5 *Belief* also appears to constitute the basis for the insistence on an early return to work following sick or disability leave for depression: we are told that employers 'typically believe that early and safe return to work is therapeutic' (Bilsker et al., 2004: 31).

6 My thanks to Katherine Lippel for this point.

7 The position of minister of state for mental health in the government of British Columbia has been eliminated. The B.C. Mental Health and Addiction Scientific Committee was established in October 2005 with two co-chairs, one of whom previously served as head of MHECCU. For further information about the committee see www.carmha.ca/research/index.html.

8 Interestingly, the founder and chair of the Global Roundtable, Bill Wilkerson, has argued elsewhere that significant levels of emotional distress and illness among Ontario public school teachers can be traced to policy decisions taken by the Ontario provincial government that have created unhealthy working conditions (see Harvey, 2004).

REFERENCES

Adkins, Lisa. (2002). Risk, sexuality and economy. *British Journal of Sociology, 53*(1), 19–40.

Bakan, Joel. (2005, Feb.). *The corporation*. Remarks presented to *Depression, Anxiety Disorders and Addictions in the Workplace*, Bottom Line Conference, Vancouver, B.C.

Baxter, Vern, & Kroll-Smith, Steve. (2005). Normalizing the workplace nap: Blurring the boundaries between public and private space and time. *Current Sociology, 53*(1), 33-55.

B.C. Business and Economic Roundtable on Mental Health. (2005). *Recognizing, treating and re-integrating employees with psychiatric disabilities: A proposed guide to national action for employers, insurers, unions, healthcare providers and employees – Discussion draft*. Retrieved 17 Aug. 2005, from http://www.bcmentalhealthworks.ca/files/WorkshopDiscussionPaper.pdf.

B.C. Business and Economic Roundtable on Mental Health. (2007). *Website*. Available online, http://www.bcmentalhealthworks.ca.

Bell, Emma, & Taylor, Scott. (2003). The elevation of work: Pastoral power and the new age work ethic. *Organization, 10*(2), 329–349.

Bilsker, Dan, Gilbert, Merv, Myette, T. Larry, & Stewart-Patterson, Chris. (2004). *Depression and work function: Bridging the gap between mental health care and the workplace*. Vancouver: Mental Health Evaluation and Community Consultation Unit. Retrieved 15 Feb. 2005, from http:// www.mheccu.ubc.ca/documents/publications/Work_Depression.pdf.

Brodie, Janine. (1995). *Politics on the margins: Restructuring and the Canadian women's movement*. Halifax: Fernwood.

Brodie, Janine. (2002). The great undoing: State formation, gender politics, and social policy in Canada. In Catherine Kingfisher (Ed.), *Western welfare in decline: Globalization and women's poverty* (pp. 90–110). Philadelphia: University of Pennsylvania Press.

Canadian Institutes of Health Research. (2005). *Mental health in the workplace: Delivering evidence for action – request for applications*. Retrieved 18 June 2005, from http://www.cihr-irsc.gc.ca/cgi-bin/print-imprimer.pl. [Archived; now available at www.irsc.gc.ca/e/28318.htm.]

Conrad, Peter, & Walsh, Diana Chapman. (1992). The new corporate health ethic: Lifestyle and the social control of work. *International Journal of Health Services*, 22(1), 89–111.

Dean, Mitchell. (1999). *Governmentality: Power and rule in modern society*. London and Thousand Oaks: Sage.

Dew, Kevin, Keefe, Vera, & Small, Keitha. (2005). 'Choosing' to work when sick: Workplace presenteeism. *Social Science and Medicine*, 60, 2273–2282.

Dumit, Joseph. (2000). When explanations rest: 'Good-enough' brain science and the new socio-medical disorders. In Margaret Lock, Allan Young, & Alberto Cambrosio (Eds.), *Living and working with the new medical technologies: Intersections of inquiry* (pp. 209–232). Cambridge: Cambridge University Press.

Foucault, Michel. (1983). The subject and power. In Hubert L. Dreyfus and Paul Rabinow (Eds.), *Michel Foucault: Beyond structuralism and hermaneutics* (2nd ed.) (pp. 208–226). Chicago: University of Chicago Press.

Fullagar, Simone. (2002). Governing the healthy body: Discourses of leisure and lifestyle within Australian health policy. *Health: An Interdisciplinary Journal for the Social Study of Health, Illness and Medicine*, 6(1), 69–84.

Global Business and Economic Roundtable on Addiction and Mental Health (Global Roundtable). (2005). *Roadmap to mental health and excellence at work in Canada – Summer draft*. Retrieved 17 Aug. 2005, from http://www.mentalhealthroundtable.ca/june_2005/RoadmapJune82005.pdf.

Global Business and Economic Roundtable on Addiction and Mental Health (Global Roundtable). (2007). *Website*. Available online, http://www.mentalhealthroundtable.ca.

Hansen, Susan. (2004). From 'common observation' to behavioural risk management: Workplace surveillance and employee assistance 1914–2003. *International Sociology, 19*(2), 151–171.

Harvey, Robin. (2004, 30 April). Depression haunts teachers. *Toronto Star online*. Retrieved 15 Sept. 2005, from http://www.thestar.com.

HealthCarePapers. (2004). *Special issue on mental health, 5*(2).

Larner, Wendy. (2000). Neoliberalism: Policy, ideology, governmentality. *Studies in Political Economy, 63*, 5–25.

Lemke, Thomas. (2001). 'The birth of bio-politics': Michel Foucault's lecture at the Collège de France on neo-liberal governmentality. *Economy and Society, 30*(2), 190–207.

Lesage, Alain, Dewa, Carolyn S., Savoie, Jean-Yves, Quirion, Rémi, & Frank, John. (2004). Mental health and the workplace: Towards a research agenda in Canada. *HealthCarePapers, 5*(2), 4–11.

MacEachen, Ellen. (2000). The mundane administration of worker bodies: From welfarism to neoliberalism. *Health, Risk and Society, 2*(3), 315–327.

McCormick, Coralie, & Adelman, Judith. (2004). *Navigating workplace disability insurance: Helping people with mental illness find the way.* Vancouver: Canadian Mental Health Association, B.C. Division.

McGillivray, David. (2005). Governing working bodies through leisure. *Leisure Sciences, 27*, 315–330.

Mental Health Works. (2007). *Website*. Available online, http://www.mentalhealthworks.ca.

Miller, Peter. (1994). Accounting and objectivity: The invention of calculating selves and calculable spaces. In Allan Megill (Ed.), *Rethinking objectivity* (pp. 239–264). Durham, NC, and London: Duke University Press.

Miller, Peter, & Rose, Nikolas. (1995). Production, identity, and democracy. *Theory and Society, 24*, 427–467.

Ministry of Health Services. (2002). Government of British Columbia. Ministry of Health Services. *British Columbia's provincial depression strategy: Phase 1 report*. Victoria: Author.

Ministry of Health Services. (2003). Government of British Columbia, Ministry of Health Services/Health Planning – Mental Health and Addictions. *Development of a mental health and addictions information plan for mental health literacy 2003–2005*. Victoria: Author.

O'Malley, Pat, Weir, Lorna, & Shearing, Clifford. (1997). Governmentality, criticism, politics. *Economy and Society, 26*(4), 501–517.

Rose, Nikolas. (1987). Beyond the public/private division: Law, power and the family. *Journal of Law and Society, 14*(1), 61–76.

Rose, Nikolas. (1998). *Inventing our selves: Psychology, power, and personhood.* Cambridge: Cambridge University Press.

Rose, Nikolas, & Miller, Peter. (1992). Political power beyond the state: Problematics of government. *British Journal of Sociology, 43*(2), 173-205.

Senate Standing Committee. (2004a). Senate of Canada, Standing Senate Committee on Social Affairs, Science and Technology, *Interim report – Report 1: Mental health, mental illness and addiction: Overview of policies and programs in Canada.* Ottawa: Author.

Senate Standing Committee. (2004b). Senate of Canada, Standing Senate Committee on Social Affairs, Science and Technology, *Interim report – Report 3: Mental health, mental illness and addiction: Issues and options for Canada.* Ottawa: Author.

Teghtsoonian, Katherine. (2003). W(h)ither women's equality? Neoliberalism, institutional change and public policy in British Columbia. *Policy, Organisation and Society, 22*(1), 26–47.

5 Contesting Coronary Candidacy: Reframing Risk Modification in Coronary Heart Disease

JAN ANGUS

Risk discourse, as a central component of health promotion, emphasizes the alignment of factors that may contribute to a range of potential negative outcomes for individuals or populations (Lupton, 1999; Petersen & Lupton, 1996). The emphasis on risk obviates the requirement for demonstrable signs or symptoms of disease and creates the possibility of a newly medicalized subjectivity: that of the person who is 'at risk' for disease or its recurrence (Petersen & Lupton, 1996). The 'at risk' body is the locus of personal and professional surveillance and is the site where people practise elaborate repertoires of risk-modification activities. Neoliberal rationalities of risk call for enterprising subjects who regulate their practices to manage health risk; the associated discourses present those who hesitate or fail to heed this call as irrational or irresponsible (Petersen & Lupton, 1996). One example is the accumulation of discourse and corresponding practices that cluster around the notion of cardiovascular risk, specifically as it relates to coronary heart disease (CHD).

The knowledges and practices associated with cardiovascular risk assessment and modification are characteristic of technologies of rule that encourage prudent self-management. Ideally, the 'at risk' individual recognizes her or his coronary candidacy and chooses to adopt specific lifestyle practices (Rose, 1998). The appeal is not simply to self-interest in a longer, healthier life. Embedded within the discourse is a moral vision of responsible citizenship. As Petersen argues: 'Given that the care of the self is bound up with the project of moderating individual burden on society, it is not surprising that since the mid-1970s, there has been a clear ideological shift away from the notion that the state should protect the health of individuals to the idea that individuals should take responsibility to protect themselves from risk' (1996: 48).

The dual objective of reducing danger to the self and modifying the potential burden to society is presented as achievable through practices of self-care and risk modification. However, risk 'is not a static, objective phenomenon, but is constantly constructed and negotiated as part of the network of social interaction and the formation of meaning' (Petersen & Lupton, 1996: 29). Personal candidacy for cardiovascular disease is interpreted (or misinterpreted) under complex social circumstances where 'the strain towards the single is counterbalanced by the heterogeneity of multiplicity' (Law, 2000: 18). Coronary candidacy is but one of many subject positions, one possible embodiment of the multiple forms of social conduct with which individuals must contend. I argue that the road to responsible cardiovascular health management is paved with points where individuals are woven (and weave themselves) into institutional relations (Law, 2000).

This chapter considers the everyday struggles inherent within entrepreneurial processes of interpreting, embodying, and balancing the discourse of cardiovascular health with other schemes of social conduct. I take up the point raised by Katherine Teghtsoonian (Chapter 4, this volume), that is, that 'technologies of rule … accomplish their aims with varying degrees of success and coherence, and hold the potential to generate their own difficulties' (this volume: 72). The biomedical literature on cardiovascular risk is replete with discussions of the barriers to successful risk assessment and modification. In the next section I provide an outline of the major issues related to risk within the literature on cardiovascular disease. I then turn to empirical illustrations from two qualitative studies that shed light on the forms and sites of contestation described by coronary candidates. I conclude that the 'strain towards the single' embedded within technologies of rule inspires tensions and contestations at the scale of the body and the everyday. Indeed, it is these conflicting demands that mobilize the enterprising self to interpret and reinterpret the meanings of coronary candidacy and develop risk modification projects.

The Components of Cardiovascular Risk Discourse

Several authors have noted the contribution of modifiable risk factors to the development of CHD, including hypertension, diabetes, smoking, body mass index greater than 27, a diet with more than 30 per cent of calories from fat, and a sedentary lifestyle (Bartley, Fitzpatrick, Firth, & Marmot, 2000; Choiniere, Lafontaine, & Edwards, 2000; Davey-Smith, 1997; Gonzalez, Artalejo, & Calero, 1998; Krieger, Chen, & Selby,

2001; Rutlege et al., 2003). Education and counselling interventions have been recommended for over a decade to encourage people with CHD to modify these risks (British Cardiac Society, British Hyperlipidemia Association, British Hypertension Society, & British Diabetic Association, 2000; Califf, Armstrong, Carver, D'Agostino, & Strauss, 1996; Grover, Paquet, Levinton, Coupal, & Zowall, 1998; Grundy et al., 1998; Heart and Stroke Foundation of Canada, 1999; Sebregts, Falger, & Bar, 2000; Wood, 1998). Although adherence to cardiovascular risk reduction practices such as exercise, dietary management, or smoking cessation may be high over the short term, long-term adherence is often low (Bellg, 2003; Orleans, 2000; Wing, 2000). For some people, the risk of CHD may seem less significant over time, or loss of contact with educators after program completion may reduce available support and encouragement (Wiles, 2001). Numerous cognitive, educational, and behavioural interventions have been developed and tested for their efficacy in improving adherence (Burke, Dunbar-Jacob, & Hill, 1998; Ebrahim & Davey Smith, 2000; Prochaska, DiClemente, Velicer, & Rossi, 1993). Indeed, the issues and experiences associated with maintaining health-related lifestyle changes are at least as complex and worthy of consideration as those that contribute to the development of CHD (White, 2000).

One problem noted in the literature is that people may resist the notion that they are at risk. At the core of informational campaigns or messages from health professionals is the warning that heart disease is associated with high morbidity and mortality rates, which generate economic burden and human suffering. These cautionary messages are tempered with an optimistic note: most risk factors can be modified in order to avoid dire consequences. The expectation is that once people realize that they might be at risk, they will take steps to avert the threat. Thus, in conventional thought, knowledge plays a pivotal role in reducing cardiovascular morbidity and mortality. The research literature also suggests this relationship in demonstrating a recurrent negative correlation between education and incidence of CHD (Choiniere, Lafontaine, & Edwards, 2000; Jaglal, Bondy, & Slaughter, 1999; Potvin, Richard, & Edwards, 2000; Wiles, 2001). However, it is important to recognize that the implementation of prescriptive health information is embedded within social relations of gender, class, ethnoracial group membership, and ability, and that these relations are embodied in a multiplicity of ways.

CHD is unquestionably a pathophysiological process that develops *within* the body. Risk of CHD occurs across a continuum from low (no presence of risk factors or signs of disease) to high absolute risk (presence of several risk factors or signs of disease, including history of myocardial infarction). Coronary heart disease develops over time. Atherosclerotic deposits gradually accumulate to the point where coronary arteries that perfuse the myocardium are increasingly obstructed and symptoms are experienced, including shortness of breath on exertion, fatigue, and chest pain. Hence, there may be considerable fluidity in individual subjectivities of coronary candidacy; people who are 'at risk' according to biomedical assessment schemas may renegotiate or reinterpret their susceptibility over time and in light of their personal experience.

The subject position of the coronary candidate entails adoption or cessation of specific, often habitual, practices. The practices and bodily states that confer coronary risk are highly prevalent in Western society: obesity, diets high in fat, smoking, and sedentary patterns occur widely. Although the prevalence of CHD increases the likelihood of contact with at least one person who has been visibly affected, the prevalence of modifiable risk factors also increases the likelihood of contact with instances of healthy longevity in those who violate preventive prescriptions. Sceptics may point to this fallibility of risk epidemiology as they deny their own candidacy (Davison, Davey Smith, & Frankel, 1991; Hunt, Emslie, & Watt, 2001; Preston, 1997). They may cite the example of a healthy elderly relative who has smoked a pack of cigarettes a day for his or her entire adult life, or a friend who exercised regularly but died prematurely of a coronary event.

Lay contestation of cardiovascular risk is therefore situated within three overlapping clusters of issues. First, although the diagnostic category 'coronary heart disease' is undeniably recognized in biomedical terms, lay acceptance of coronary candidacy or 'cardiovascular risk' must often occur in the absence of any physical experience of illness. Unlike contested diagnostic categories (e.g., Chronic Fatigue Syndrome, Multiple Chemical Sensitivity Syndrome), coronary risk is so well accepted by medicine and other interest groups (such as the pharmaceutical industry, public health practitioners, and the media) that the associated discourse is deeply embedded within multiple fields and sites of health-related activity. However, those at risk for CHD may not experience noticeable symptoms or functional impairment that would confirm the diagnostic label. The acknowledgment of candidacy requires acceptance of a frightening future wherein debilitating heart disease and death of a heart attack are possible outcomes, yet these outcomes may be difficult to map onto current bodily experiences. Second, acceptance of candidacy is accompanied by an obligation to modify risk, so that CHD will not develop or progress. In other words, acknowledging coronary candidacy is the first step towards risk consciousness or subjectivity. It requires health literacy skills, to be sure, but it also involves a process of responsibilization which may prompt various responses, including resistance (see Teghtsoonian, Chapter 4, this volume). Third, risk modification entails prescribed practices that often require the cooperation of others who share households and other everyday spaces. Information about new regimens must be accessed, interpreted, and implemented – *embodied* – often with some difficulty or inconvenience as 'habits' are broken and replaced.

Contesting Coronary Candidacy

To explore further these three dimensions of contested candidacy, I draw on data from two qualitative studies. One study consisted of interviews with 18 women who had undergone coronary artery bypass grafts (CABG), a surgical procedure to restore coronary circulation in cases where CHD has become a threat to survival (Angus, 2001). The focus of the study was on the challenges posed by recovery from open heart surgery within domestic spaces that called forth practices of homemaking and family care. Each woman participated in two interviews; one 4 weeks after returning home from the hospital, and one in the fourth month after the surgery. During the interviews the women spoke of conflicts and challenges as they balanced their obligations to modify further risk to themselves and their perceived responsibilities to create and maintain 'home' as the site of shared practices with others. Their risk modification projects were often subject to contestation by others, to the extent that some yielded to pressure and amended their approaches.

The second study consisted of a series of focus group discussions with people in urban, northern, and rural sites in Ontario at risk for CHD that were intended to illuminate the barriers to and supports for risk modification (Angus et al., 2005). Participants discussed the difficulties they experienced in their attempts to understand the meaning and implications of cardiovascular risk. Some contested their coronary candidacy based on a lack of physical symptoms or perceived success in eradicating one or more sources of risk. Others abandoned or struggled to continue risk modification projects after encountering contextual constraints.

I read these dimensions of coronary candidacy – absence of symptoms, obligation to modify risky behaviour, cooperation of household members – through the lens of *technologies of rule*. Even though there is extensive contestation by persons identified as candidates for CHD, there is also movement towards being more responsible for one's own health. Risk reduction is not situated as a means through which the state can protect health; rather, risk reduction becomes part of an individual's social conduct as a responsible citizen taking care of her or his health by occupying the subject position offered by coronary candidacy.

Reading the Absence of Symptoms

Some participants in the study of women's recovery from CABG initially rejected the meaning of their symptoms. The vulnerabilities associated with an illness as life-threatening as CHD did not fit with their previously defined, gendered images of themselves. Many understood themselves as active and reliable participants in an informal web or network of helping relations. They were the caregivers; others became ill. Long-established patterns of concealing their own feelings and reassuring others were described. Hence, some women not only rejected the prospect of illness because they themselves found it unpalatable; they sought to protect others from that alarming possibility as well. For example, one woman continued her customary grandparenting activities while she waited to have surgery; these practices assisted her to hide her worries from herself as well as others: 'Of course, you are so, you stay so strong, you know. I was so strong. I was doing things, I was babysitting for my daughter, and so maybe I forgot about myself sometimes.' About half of the women were concerned to protect others from worry and to 'get well' so that they could resume everyday life as it was before. Their assumption was that the disease could be hidden, the damage repaired, and most activities could go on as usual throughout the process. The women's narratives identified the conflicts between gendered identity and illness behaviour: they talked about obligations that were embedded within relations of gendered responsibility and that were not easily relinquished.

Another reason the women gave for their initial rejection of the possibility of CHD was a mistaken belief that the disease manifests itself less frequently in women than it does in men. For these women, heart disease was a 'man's problem.' They ignored physical cues of developing disease and were taken by surprise when more serious problems became manifest. One woman had shortness of breath and occasional chest pain for several months prior to her myocardial infarction:

> I was aware this was 99 per cent a man's problem. You hear, on TV or the paper, you'd maybe scan through the paper and say: 'Oh, gee, yeah, heart disease is becoming number one.' But to actually say I was totally aware of it, well, I may have heard it, but it went in one ear and out the other. And when I had my heart attack, my only reaction was: 'I've had a heart attack? Oh, *come on!*'

One woman believed that she was protected by her good dietary practices as well as her gender, explaining that her husband more closely fit the profile of the coronary candidate. Her history as a smoker with Type I diabetes did not appear to enter into the comparison; instead she understood that her role was to be concerned about her husband's health patterns rather than about her own.

Some of the men who participated in focus group discussions also admitted that they had not entertained thoughts of their own coronary candidacy: they gave the matter no thought and disregarded any information about cardiovascular risk that they may have received. Other male focus group participants sometimes recognized physical symptoms of disease as a clear (but late) indicator of candidacy, but a few ignored these warning signs until CHD was well advanced. These men described the gradual realization that their shortness of breath indicated the possibility of illness:

INTERVIEWER: So you said before that you walked. What made you start to walk?
PARTICIPANT 4: I kind of did to pass the time (laughter).
INTERVIEWER: So it was something you had done for a long time?
PARTICIPANT 4: Oh, yes, I really like to walk. But then I started to notice that the streets seemed longer. And later it kind of seemed that the blocks in between each light, they seemed to be longer, and I was kind of missing air before I got there.
PARTICIPANT 3: For me it happened when I was walking around ... And then I really noticed that I was short of breath.
INTERVIEWER: Oh, yes?

PARTICIPANT 3: I couldn't find it. I always knew that I wasn't getting any younger (group laughs). But I also knew at some point that I had no reason to be short of breath. And I went to the doctor, and I told him of all this. And he told me that they were going to send me for tests right away.

Coronary candidacy was gradually and reluctantly accepted in these cases. The wry humour the men used in recounting their stories indicates retrospective awareness of a strategy of procrastination, a strategy used until physical symptoms could no longer be attributed to other alternatives such as 'normal' ageing processes. With some men and women, myocardial infarction forced the issue.

Focus group participants who were at risk but pre-symptomatic also engaged in comparisons between themselves and acquaintances who actually had CHD. Some were disturbed by paradoxical cases of acquaintances or relatives who led healthy lives and yet still suffered heart disease. These instances highlighted the indeterminacy of risk calculations: perceived high risk did not immediately result in actual disease, nor did the apparent absence of risk factors guarantee immunity, as this woman's anecdote illustrates:

> My aunt wasn't very big, she didn't smoke, she was a nurse, ah, very busy. And ah, bang, that's it, the end of her career. I think from my own perspective, I look back and say, 'Good, I've got all the precursors to have a cardiac event, she had none, so what was in there?'

One woman remarked on the lack of clear indicators of risk in her own case, although she could 'case out' or calculate the level of risk in another participant. The speaker's mother died of heart disease but had no discernible risk factors, hence the problem was to discover in retrospect whether the disease was lifestyle-related or genetically determined:

> I guess what I'm asking for, give me scientific evidence, explain to me what it is. I mean, you, I could case out. You have … you're doing everything within your power to prevent further heart disease for yourself … Now, how do I know if my mother's was genetic or lifestyle?

Thus, while knowledge of modifiable risk factors conferred the option of reducing risk by changing certain health behaviours, familial tendencies could not be altered. This woman's musings point to the difference between understanding disease as preventable or as inevitable. Since heredity could not be altered, this woman seemed to be asking whether she should bother to engage in the rigors of lifestyle modification.

Acceptance of coronary candidacy was merely the first locus of contestation in study participants. After struggling to accept their level of risk, coronary candidates engaged in projects of risk modification to reduce the likelihood of further atherosclerotic disease. Risk modification involved changes in embodied practices, and these were enacted in the spaces of everyday life. Some initially accepted coronary candidacy but later contested the need for risk modification and renegotiated their understandings of risk.

Obligation to Modify Risky Behaviour

After the trauma of open heart surgery, most of the women interviewed for the study of recovery from CABG were anxious to avoid further threats to their cardiovascular health. The following woman's comments typify the enterprising subjectivity of the responsible coronary candidate. This woman reasoned that it made no sense to court further damage to her newly reconstructed heart. She explained that she should be the one that cared most about herself. Therefore if she truly did care, she would have no difficulty eating healthier food:

> I – the whole attitude changed, because I know now I've got only one heart, and I've got to look after it, even my eating habits have changed where I used to be – well, I wouldn't care about what I ate. If you don't care, who cares enough to do it for you? Because now I really watch, cut all the fat off because I'm eating a piece of meat, you know. Because now I don't want to have another [surgery].

Another woman brought out a pile of new 'heart healthy' recipe books and leafed through pages of colourful illustrations to show and explain her new diet:

> I add the tofu in the end and lots of onion and I have beans and – yes, the dry beans or the green beans – even potato, I cook potatoes in the beans and that, it makes your meal. And no meat, you see here, no meat. That's lots of onions, and everything. And zucchini, and sweet potatoes, you know, and maybe some tomato. That's all. And the fat would be just like you see, one tablespoon of oil. You cook it all together slow. That's my food.

Her words underscore the sensual, embodied nature of diet, taste, and culinary skill, and she appeared genuinely pleased with her accomplishment – one reward of creative self-care that some women cited.

In contrast, a small number of women rejected the discourses of risk modification that accompanied treatment for CHD. One woman brought out the same 'heart healthy' cookbooks and adamantly condemned the contents. Her comments also suggested that diet is a sensual enterprise and that motivation to change is not necessarily a simple cognitive matter of learning a new diet:

> I went to [doctor] and said, 'I have this book. If I start to eat all that stuff that's in that book, I'd be throwing up every day, I'm sure. It sounds terrible.' And he said, 'Well, you know, you do have to live. You don't have to go by that.' … So, I really haven't changed too much. Our diet wasn't that bad. I'm sure it's not the only cause. I think it's hereditary myself. Because I know all my – most of my aunts and uncles died because they had angina.

Her doctor's support for her stance on diet illustrates a paradoxical approach. In stating that she has to live, the doctor was not advocating that she prolong her life by restricting her diet; instead, he acknowledged that living requires sensory enjoyment of life itself. In this case, self-care was interpreted within the limitations of tolerance for dietary change. Even after bypass surgery, this woman contested the discursive emphasis on dietary or other changes, attributing her disease to heredity rather than modifiable risk factors. She renegotiated her risk profile, apparently with her physician's support.

Similarly, some focus group members questioned the need for long-term adherence to risk modification practices. They offered various arguments to justify reversals, often taking cues from their feelings of physical well-being. One man from a rural community explained:

> See it was easier at the beginning when you first had the heart attack. I mean, you had this big fear. And yeah, I lost a lot of weight right off the bat … and I started following practically the same habits again, it gets kinda, you know, 'What's the chance you're going to get a second heart attack?'

His story indicates that the fear associated with heart disease is a strong but sometimes short-term motivating force. In this instance, the odds of a second heart attack are portrayed as slim. The speaker is willing to gamble in order to return to previous eating habits, despite the danger of recurrence that persistently lurks in the background of his narrative.

Cooperation of Household Members

The difficulty of maintaining the discursive standard for 'heart healthy' behaviour was a recurrent theme in both studies. This is not surprising, since risk modification involves revision of everyday practices such as smoking, diets high in fat, or lack of exercise – all of which can have an impact on all members of a household. Cognitive knowledge, and discourses for that matter, may poorly equip people to solve problems such as cravings for foods or cigarettes, resistance of significant others to new practices, or challenges presented by the spatio-temporal organization of social life.

The first hurdle occurs at the level of the sensuous body, the source of cravings for the reinstatement of specific 'high risk' habits or preferences. Some of the most intensely enjoyable foods are also associated with heightened cardiovascular risk; most of the women interviewed following CABG spoke of their tastes for certain high cholesterol items and described in detail their strategies for managing cravings. However, even as they became more informed about the effects of certain foods on their health, they were forced to confront the difficulties associated with changing embodied preferences and tastes. Some described the strategies that they developed to deal with this problem, which included occasionally enjoying very small portions of forbidden treats. One woman said:

> If you cheat once in a while, just taking small amounts, it's better than, you know, having a craving and going completely off the diet altogether. And like you see, I make sometimes pirogi and even my grandchildren want. I'm making pirogi, and I put in it vegetables and everything, but I would eat just two, that's it. And I will never touch another one.

As this comment illustrates, there is a fine line between indulgence and losing control over dietary management. The line was maintained by this woman through strict self-management. Only a certain size of portion was deemed acceptable, and additional amounts were not permitted. Some women would simply not allow certain items to enter their homes, thus keeping temptations to a minimum.

In both studies, those who acknowledged coronary candidacy and worked to incorporate regimens of risk modification into their daily practices were faced with varying levels of resistance from others who shared local spaces and places. Change was problematic – and problematized. Following CABG, some women who changed their patterns of eating and exercise found that loved ones were reluctant to follow the same patterns; efforts to encourage risk subjectivity in these close others were rebuffed:

> Because I'll maybe worry about something happening to him too, and 'don't eat too much of that, don't take too much of it.' But butter, he loves butter on his potatoes and stuff. And he's like, 'Leave me alone!'

As a result, in some families, two different modes of food preparation and dietary patterns coexisted. For example, one man who participated in a rural focus group stated:

> And one of the problems I have is because of my diet, what I try to eat, I don't really impose that on anybody else. But living in a household – and there's a certain meal that's cooked at supper time and dinner and breakfast, you know. It's different than what I eat; it's almost like a special preparation just on my kind of food. I don't want to impose it on them ... Yeah, there's a big change – it's not only yourself that's gotta accept it, but your family's got to accept it ... I don't want to see my children get the same thing I did, or my wife.

He worried about the health of his loved ones, but his concerns and choices were not shared. Instead, two different meals were prepared to accommodate different tastes.

But in the same rural focus group, the comments of other men remind us that domestic spaces are inhabited by people's bodies in sensuous as well as active ways. Odours and objects in the home persistently call forth particular dispositions:

> And in the morning you get up and you got eggs frying. You got that egg – it smells good in the morning and it's, you know, it's nice to get up. And [you get] so accustomed to having that kind of meal that you don't realize that it's exactly bad for you, the fat content of that grease. You learn to enjoy that food. Even now I've gone off that food, but I also seem to wander back into it ... but I always fall right back into it because it's just the smell of having that.

In both focus group studies, participants emphasized the importance of 'will power' and 'motivation,' apparently with good reason. In the home they were continuously faced with cues to resume previous (often deeply enjoyed) practices.

Occupational spaces and practices also tended to reinforce patterns of activity that contribute to cardiovascular risk. One woman who participated in an urban focus group described her working day in terms that illustrate the intimate relationship between body and place:

> In my work I really have a very sedentary job where I'm at a laptop or I'm in meetings or I'm in my car driving from one place to another, so I tend to have a very like I say, stationary kind of day in terms of being active. Once upon a time I stood up more and walked around more but now I find much longer hours … when you're fatigued. I find, when I'm under a lot of stress I get very tired and escape into sleep. Sleeping in on the weekends and all that becomes a luxury. So you tend to have less energy, you don't feel like exercising, going home and jumping on a treadmill.

She later told the group that she had lost 30 pounds while on a leave of absence from her job, but gained most of the weight back when she returned because she was unable to maintain her program of exercise in a more time-pressured context. She further attributed her increasing difficulties with weight loss to what she understood as the metabolic changes of middle years, indicating that her workplace patterns became more problematic over time:

> I find, well it's obvious, your metabolism's going down with every – is it 5 years or 10 years? So if you keep eating the same amount for the next 20 years, you're going to naturally put on weight because your metabolism's slowing down. So, you know, it's a constant battle.

Examples such as this suggest that the reversals and recidivism discussed in the previous section may result as much from contextual influences as from individual tastes and preferences. These contestations occurred in time and place, and were experienced as struggle (or a 'constant battle') to change or adhere to health-related practices. The battle involved conflicts between the practices of risk modification and situated dispositions towards forms of bodily conduct, for example, responding to deep-seated cravings for particular foods. Furthermore, habitual practices related to employment constrained the introduction of healthier repertoires of behaviour.

CHD as a Technology of Rule

To return to Teghtsoonian's observation that technologies of rule may accomplish their aims with varying degrees of success and coherence, we may understand discourses of cardiovascular risk as only one such technology, or mode of ordering (Law, 1995). The analysis here shows that designating particular individuals with coronary candidacy for CHD elicited varying responses. Some used their positioning as a coronary candidate to engage in what they considered healthier lifestyles while others did not do so. Some modified their behaviour by adhering to the established standards of practice while others did not do so. Some extended their modified behaviours because of their candidacy into their household, although not without some struggle, while others did not do so. Law (1995) explains that multiple discourses exist, and each may complicate the ways that others can be activated in practice or embodied. Although they were not always articulated, and not always clearly connected, there were a variety of discourses that the individuals in these two studies drew on to explain their engagement or non-engagement with certain practices. Of interest here in this analysis is the manner in which the discourses coexist, interact, and change in the presence of one another.

Coronary heart disease is an established medical diagnosis, the prevention of which has opened an entirely new diagnostic category: that of the coronary candidate, who is at risk of developing physical symptoms of CHD. In contrast to frequently cited cases of contested illness, laypersons instead of diagnosticians tend to reject their coronary candidacy. As coronary candidates, susceptible laypersons are expected to modify their risks by altering certain high-risk personal practices. The contestations associated with coronary candidacy are conducted at the scale of the body, and in everyday locations such as the home and the workplace. These various sites and scales constitute the terrain on which risk modification projects are formulated and pursued. This analysis shows that the individualization of such projects as the sole responsibility of coronary candidates is highly problematic and may well lead to abandonment of risk modification attempts. Influential as techno-medical rationalities may be, they do not operate unchallenged. Neoliberal subjectivities of risk may well be linked with discourse, but the practice, embodiment, and telling of risk modification is complicated by and mingled with other discourses and practicalities.

Acknowledgments

The author gratefully acknowledges funding from the Heart and Stroke Foundation of Ontario, in the form of a doctoral fellowship. This supported conduct of the study 'Home is where the heart is: Women's experiences of recovering from Coronary Artery Bypass surgery.' The author also acknowledges funding from the Ontario Ministry of Health and Long-Term Care for the focus group study, which was undertaken as part of the Community Outreach in Heart Health and Risk Reduction Trial (COHRT), led by Dr Robert P. Nolan. The focus group study team was composed of Dr Robert P. Nolan, Dr Ellen Rukholm, Dr Jan Angus, Louise Picard, and Isabelle Michel. The author gratefully acknowledges the thoughtful comments and editorial work provided by Pamela Moss and Kathy Teghtsoonian.

REFERENCES

Angus, Jan. (2001). The material and social predicaments of home: Women's experiences after aortocoronary bypass surgery. *Canadian Journal of Nursing Research, 33*(2), 27–42.

Angus, J., Evans, S., Lapum, J., Rukholm, E., St Onge, R., Nolan, R., et al. (2005). 'Sneaky disease': The body and health knowledge for people at risk for coronary heart disease. *Social Science and Medicine, 60*(9), 2117–2128.

Bartley, M., Fitzpatrick, R., Firth, D., & Marmot, M. (2000). Social distribution of cardiovascular disease risk factors: Change among men in England 1884–1993. *Journal of Epidemiology and Community Health, 54*, 806–814.

Bellg, Albert J. (2003). Maintenance of health behaviour change in preventive cardiology. *Behavior Modification, 27*(1), 103-131.

British Cardiac Society, British Hyperlipidemia Association, British Hypertension Society, & British Diabetic Association. (2000). Joint British recommendations on prevention of coronary heart disease in clinical practice: Summary. *British Medical Journal, 320*, 705–708.

Burke, L.E., Dunbar-Jacob, J.M., & Hill, M.N. (1998). Compliance with cardiovascular disease prevention strategies: A review of the research. *Annals of Behavioral Medicine, 19*(3), 239–263.

Califf, R., Armstrong, P., Carver, J., D'Agostino, R., & Strauss, W. (1996). 27th Bethesda Conference: Matching the intensity of risk factor management with the hazard for coronary disease events. *Journal of the American College of Cardiology, 27*(5), 1007–1019.

Choiniere, Robert, Lafontaine, Pierre, & Edwards, Alison C. (2000). Distribution of cardiovascular disease risk factors by socioeconomic status among Canadian adults. *Canadian Medical Association Journal, 162*(9 Suppl), S13–S24.

Davey-Smith, George. (1997). Down at heart – the meaning and implications of social inequalities in cardiovascular disease. *Journal of the Royal College of Physicians of London, 31*(4), 414–424.

Davison, Charlie, Davey Smith, George, & Frankel, Stephen. (1991). Lay epidemiology and the prevention paradox: The implications of coronary candidacy for health education. *Sociology of Health and Illness, 13*(1), 1–19.

Ebrahim, S., & Davey Smith, G. (2000). Multiple risk factor interventions for primary prevention of coronary heart disease. Cochrane Database of Systematic Reviews [computer file] (p. CD001561).

Gonzalez, Mónica Alonso, Artalejo, Fernando Rodríguez, & Calero, Juan del Rey. (1998). Relationship between socioeconomic status and ischaemic heart disease in cohort and case-control studies: 1960–1993. *International Journal of Epidemiology, 27*, 350–358.

Grover, S., Paquet, S., Levinton, C., Coupal, L., & Zowall, H. (1998). Estimating the benefits of modifying risk factors of cardiovascular disease. *Archives of Internal Medicine, 158*, 655–661.

Grundy, S.M., Balady, G.J., Criqui, M.H., Fletcher, G., Greenland, P., Hiratzka, L.F., et al. (1998). Primary prevention of coronary heart disease: Guidance from Framingham: A statement for healthcare professionals from the AHA Task Force on Risk Reduction. *Circulation, 97*(18), 1876–1887.

Heart and Stroke Foundation of Canada. (1999). *The changing face of heart disease and stroke in Canada*. Ottawa: Heart and Stroke Foundation of Canada.

Hunt, K., Emslie, C., & Watt, G. (2001). Lay constructions of a family history of heart disease: Potential for misunderstandings in the clinical encounter? *Lancet, 357*, 1168–1171.

Jaglal, Susan, Bondy, Susan J., & Slaughter, Pamela M. (1999). Risk factors for cardiovascular disease. In C. David Naylor & Pamela M. Slaughter (Eds.), *Cardiovascular health and services in Ontario: An ICES atlas* (pp. 63–82). Toronto: Institute for Clinical Evaluative Services.

Krieger, N., Chen, J., & Selby, J. (2001). Class inequalities in women's health: Combined impact of childhood and adult social class – a study of 630 US women. *Public Health, 115*, 175–185.

Law, John. (1995). *Organizing modernity*. Oxford: Blackwell.

Law, John. (2000). On the subject of the object: Narrative, technology and interpellation. *Configurations, 8*, 1–29.

Lupton, Deborah. (1999). *Risk*. New York and London: Routledge.

Orleans, C.T. (2000). Promoting the maintenance of health behaviour change: Recommendations for the next generation of research and practice. *Health Psychology, 19*(1 Suppl), 76–83.

Petersen, Alan. (1996). Risk and the regulated self: The discourse of health promotion as politics of uncertainty. *Australian and New Zealand Journal of Sociology, 32*, 44–57.

Petersen, Alan, & Lupton, Deborah. (1996). *The new public health: Health and self in the age of risk*. St Leonards, Australia: Allen and Unwin.

Potvin, Louise, Richard, Lucie, & Edwards, Alison C. (2000). Knowledge of cardiovascular disease risk factors among the Canadian population: Relationships with indicators of socioeconomic status. *Canadian Medical Association Journal, 162*(9 Suppl), S5-S11.

Preston, R.M. (1997). Ethnography: Studying the fate of health promotion in coronary families. *Journal of Advanced Nursing, 25*(3), 554–561.

Prochaska, J.O., DiClemente, C.C., Velicer, W.F., & Rossi, J.S. (1993). Standardized, individualized, interactive, and personalized self-help programs for smoking cessation. *Health Psychology, 12*(5), 399–405.

Rose, Nikolas. (1998). *Inventing our selves: Psychology, power, and personhood*. Cambridge: Cambridge University Press.

Rutlege, Thomas, Reis, Steven E., Olson, Marian, Owens, Jane, Kelsey, Sheryl F., Pepine, Carl J., et al. (2003). Socioeconomic status variables predict cardiovascular disease risk factors and prospective mortality risk among women with chest pain. The WISE study. *Behavioral Modification, 27*(1), 54–67.

Sebregts, E.H., Falger, P.R., & Bar, F.W. (2000). Risk factor modification through nonpharmacological interventions in patients with coronary heart disease. *Journal of Psychosomatic Research, 48*(4–5), 425–441.

White, Martin. (2000). Researching the changing social pattern of cardiovascular disease. *Journal of Epidemiology and Community Health, 54*, 804–805.

Wiles, Rose. (2001). Patients' understandings of heart attack: Implications for prevention of recurrence. *Patient Education and Counseling, 44*(2), 161–169.

Wing, R. (2000). Cross cutting themes in maintenance of behavior change. *Health Psychology, 19*(1[Suppl]), 84–88.

Wood, D. (1998). European and American recommendations for coronary heart disease prevention. *European Heart Journal, 19*(Suppl A), A12-A19.

6 Hepatitis C and the Dawn of Biological Citizenship: Unravelling the Policy Implications

MICHAEL ORSINI

Adriana Petryna describes biological citizenship as 'a massive demand for but selective access to a form of social welfare based on medical, scientific and legal criteria that both acknowledge biological injury and compensate for it' (2002: 6). As she explains in her examination of the aftermath of the Chernobyl disaster two decades ago, 'The damaged biology of a population has become the grounds for social membership and the basis for staking citizenship claims' (ibid.: 5). In this chapter, I discuss the implications of a shift to new forms of 'biological citizenship' for how we understand health policy and politics, using Hepatitis C as a case study. If biological citizenship is indeed becoming the grounds for new forms of collective action that take as their starting point citizens' relationships to their biological bodies, do these citizenship practices open up new spaces for contesting medical and scientific authority? Do they carry with them any emancipatory potential? Do we require a new set of analytical tools to capture these forms of citizenship and to incorporate the experiential knowledge of individual biological citizens into policy processes?

As a way of contextualizing my arguments and discussion in this chapter, I begin by providing some background on Hepatitis C itself and then discuss the notion of *biological citizenship*, focusing on how the term has been used by social scientists. I next flesh out some of these ideas in the context of a research project that examines the 'illness narratives' (see Orsini & Scala, 2006) of people living with Hepatitis C in Canada.[1] I conclude by offering some thoughts on the policy challenges associated with the emergence of biological citizenship.

Hepatitis C: A Brief History of the 'Other' Virus

The most common strains of hepatitis are A, B, and C. Hepatitis A, which is usually transmitted by the fecal-oral route, is highly infectious. Usually it is spread through contaminated water and food, and it is more common in developing countries. Unlike other strains of hepatitis, few cases of Hepatitis A virus (HAV) are transmitted by blood. Hepatitis B virus (HBV) is transmitted primarily through the use of injection drugs, sexual contact, perinatally (from mother to child), and blood transfusion. HBV symptoms are similar to HAV symptoms, but they are often more severe and longer lasting. Infection through blood transfusion was frequent during the 1980s because many asymptomatic individuals, who were unaware that they were infected, donated blood.

Hepatitis C, previously known as non-A, non-B Hepatitis, is also transmitted by blood. Like HBV, Hepatitis C can remain in the body for several years without appearing to cause infection. Once it takes up residence in the liver, the Hepatitis C virus can reproduce for many years, often without causing discernible symptoms of illness. Interferon therapy has been used commonly to treat Hepatitis C infection. Patients have seen greater success, however, with a combination therapy of interferon and ribavirin, an anti-viral drug. About 170 million people, or 3 per cent of the world's population, are estimated to be infected with Hepatitis C (World Health Organization, 2006). In Canada, about 250,000 people are said to be infected.

Scientists struggled in the 1980s to develop a test to screen for the presence of Hepatitis C (still known only at that time as non-A, non-B Hepatitis). A specific test to screen for Hepatitis C was not available and implemented in Canada until 1990, although two 'surrogate' (or substitute) tests were available to screen for non-A, non-B Hepatitis as early as 1974: one measured a liver enzyme while the other detected previous exposure to Hepatitis B. In 1986, at the same time that U.S. blood banks began using these surrogate tests, the Canadian Red Cross and the Canadian Blood Committee (the latter made up of federal and provincial government representatives) opted instead to study the tests' efficacy. The federal government and the Red Cross continued to insist that the costs of testing far outweighed any benefits. It took a highly publicized public inquiry – the Commission of Inquiry on the Blood System in Canada in 1994–95 – to put Hepatitis C on the map in Canada. The Inquiry examined the facts surrounding the contamination of the blood supply during the 1980s when more than 1,200 people were infected with HIV and more than 10,000 were infected with Hepatitis C (Orsini, 2002).

Biological Citizenship and the Body Politic

Petryna's *Life Exposed: Biological Citizens after Chernobyl* (2002) traces the features of a new 'citizenship regime' using a case study of the 1986 disaster in Ukraine, during which tens of thousands of citizens were exposed to radioactive iodine, which has been linked to deadly thyroid cancers in children and adults. In post-socialist Ukraine, she explains, 'the very idea of citizenship is now charged with the superadded burden of survival' (2002: 7). In fragile transition economies, Petryna adds, 'citizens must rely on their disease, and the knowledge they accumulate about it, as the currency through which they negotiate social, economic, and political survival' (ibid.: 9). Nikolas Rose and Carlos Novas (2005: 440) use the term *biological citizenship* 'to encompass all those citizenship projects that have linked their conceptions of citizens to beliefs about the biological existence of human beings, as individuals, as families and lineages, as communities, as population and races, and as a species.' They understand 'citizenship projects' as 'the ways that authorities thought about (some) individuals as potential citizens, and the ways they tried to act upon them' (ibid.: 439). Examples might include measures to define who is permitted to participate in public life or acts that oblige citizens to speak a common language. Previously, Rose and Novas note, many of these projects were linked to the nation state. Expanding upon Petryna's work, Rose and Novas are interested in how biological citizenship challenges, supplants, or intersects with the dominant mode of understanding citizenship as linked to a nation state or territory.

Dominant theorizing about citizenship in the social sciences often draws from T.H. Marshall's classic formulation of three types of citizenship: civil, political, and social rights, with the emphasis often placed on how the three are 'indivisible' (Lister, 2003). Framing the discussion in terms of *biological* citizenship expands the focus to consider how ill bodies become implicated in the practice of citizenship. Biological citizens are expected to be active citizens, reading their ill bodies and adjusting their behaviours in order to maximize the potential of living healthy, productive lives. This form of active biological citizenship can help raise the profile of an illness, especially when scientific knowledge might be lagging behind experiential knowledge. While it may not be novel in the Canadian context to frame health care discussions in the language of citizenship, rights, or values, biological citizenship departs somewhat from these themes by 'pioneering a new ethics of the self – a set of techniques for managing everyday life in relation to a condition, and in relation to expert knowledge' (Rose & Novas, 2005: 450). It is not sufficient, however, to focus solely on the self, as biological citizens also are expected to be other-regarding, as well. The 'new genetics,' for instance, encourages, indeed exhorts, citizens to learn more about their genetic selves and to make reproductive choices in light of what they have come to know (Petersen & Bunton, 2002). In such a universe, there may be little freedom to 'refuse to identify with this responsible community of biological citizens' (Rose & Novas, 2005: 451).

What is significant then about citizens who are increasingly framing their politics in terms of their biological status? For one, attention to biological citizenship allows us to imagine the emergence of illness as a new political cleavage, as an identity through which citizens frame their demands on the state and civil society. This new identity is linked to how we relate to our biological bodies. Waldby and her colleagues (2004: 1462) use the term *bioidentity* to describe our 'common understanding of our bodies as ours, as both supporting and being included in our social and subjective identities.' Our bodies do not speak solely for themselves; rather, they speak through and in tandem with our social and subjective selves.

Although biological citizenship is not completely new – in the nineteenth and twentieth centuries, citizens understood their allegiance and nationality partly in biological ways, in terms of race, blood lines, or ancestry – Rose and Novas (2005) nonetheless identify some novel features of biological citizenship in the current age, namely, different ideas about the role of biology in human worth, about the biological responsibility of the citizen, and about the role of technology and how it interacts with the body. Biological citizenship, they explain, is both individualizing and collectivizing. It is individualizing to the extent that individuals shape their relations with themselves in awareness of their 'somatic individuality' (ibid.: 441). Individuals are at once expected to be prudent and enterprising, actively shaping their destinies through acts of individual choice. Biological citizenship is collectivizing in the sense that it can provide the grounds for new forms of collective mobilization anchored in a 'biological conception of shared identity' (ibid.: 442). Patients may choose to press for societal and governmental recognition of their condition or illness, or focus on fighting the stigma that might accompany illnesses that are medicalized or pathologized. In other cases, they challenge 'science as industry' and 'science as procedures' (Epstein, 1991). As Steven Epstein has explained in the context of AIDS activism, in the early stages of the epidemic, activists attacked the pharmaceutical industry for its 'price gouging' of anti-AIDS drugs, but activists also insinuated themselves into the everyday practices of science when they fought for reforms to the conduct of clinical trials (Epstein, 1996). In effect, they were contesting – with differing degrees of success – the strict separation between the expert and the lay public. This form of citizenship operates also in what Rose and Novas have called 'a political economy of hope,' in which 'biology is no longer blind destiny or even a foreseen but implacable fate. It is knowable, mutable, improvable, eminently manipulable. Of course, the other side of hope is undoubtedly anxiety, fear and dread at what one's biological future … might hold' (Rose & Novas, 2005: 442).

Biological citizenship is fundamentally imbricated in processes of contestation, not least because citizenship itself is a highly contested concept. As Ruth Lister explains, the unsettled nature of this concept is related to the fact that the three elements of the citizenship equation – 'membership, identity, relationships' – are open to question (Lister, 2003: 3). For the purposes of this chapter's discussion of biological citizenship, I understand the process of contestation in three ways. First, persons with Hepatitis C may challenge the institutions of science and medicine to take Hepatitis C seriously in the first place, and to appreciate the toll it takes on a person's quality of life. Patients often do this, to varying degrees, by becoming 'citizen experts' – learning and adopting the language of science and medicine as a way to interrogate or challenge scientific knowledge from a new-found position of authority.[2] Second, patients may grapple with – and sometimes resist – the illness label, and thus refuse to embrace the identity attached to a Hepatitis C diagnosis, or, to use citizenship parlance, they may refuse membership in the Hepatitis C community. Third, contestation takes place at the collective level when individuals join forces to politicize their illness experience. This can occur when persons locate the cause of their illness, or their inability to deal with their illness effectively, in outside forces. Adopting a wide view of what constitutes collective action permits an understanding of politicization – and hence contestation – that includes the processes through which identity is constituted. For example, a support group may not appear to engage in 'political' activities, yet as a site for social interaction it serves to shape the collective identity of its members and thus has significant political effects. It is also critical to pay close attention to those instances when patients frame their individual experiences in terms of broader notions of injustice. It may be useful – and necessary – for collective actors to emphasize that harms may not arise solely from the illness itself, but may also be inflicted through inadequate professional or policy responses. Contesting these responses may form the basis of collective mobilization through which connections are forged among a disparate group of individuals united only by a medical condition. It may also provide the basis for a biologically grounded understanding of citizenship, even though this may not be sufficient to sustain the collective identity of a group.[3]

In the next section, I examine how these forms of contestation intersect in the case of people with Hepatitis C. I suggest that one's ability to contest biomedical authority as an expert in her or his own right can hinge on a willingness to identify as a person with Hepatitis C. This, in turn, has implications for whether people with Hepatitis C are able to move from identifying as individualized biological citizens concerned mainly with how Hepatitis C is affecting them in their daily lives to finding common cause with others to engage collectively in politicizing issues related to Hepatitis C. As I will argue, these processes of contestation are influenced, in direct and indirect ways, by the issues arising during diagnosis and treatment, particularly by what it means to be treated 'successfully' for Hepatitis C.

People with Hepatitis C as Biological Citizens

Although individuals may be linked by their biological existence as persons living with the Hepatitis C virus, this biological fact is not sufficient to understand experiences of living with Hepatitis C. In this section, I organize my discussion around the three forms of contestation outlined above and reflect on how contestation and biological citizenship have had both individualizing and collectivizing features. As noted earlier, persons with Hepatitis C may engage in processes of contestation by becoming well-versed in the language of science and medicine as a way of challenging these discourses, which are often dominated by medicine. For someone in the throes of illness, learning all there is to know about the illness can be an important coping mechanism during a time in which the biological body and the emotional self are being transformed. Becoming an expert in all things related to Hepatitis C may be a form of self-preservation, but it may also extend beyond the self towards helping others, many of whom are still coming to grips with their Hepatitis C status. Involvement with others who are infected with the virus may be facilitated by support groups and/or online chat rooms, as well as websites that provide up-to-date information on the latest research findings.

Although assuming the role of citizen expert can be transformative for individuals, one should be careful not to overstate its importance in the political realm. Becoming a citizen expert may not necessarily disturb existing power relations if it involves activities that are aimed solely at amassing the requisite knowledge to make informed decisions with respect to handling a Hepatitis C diagnosis. Such interventions come to be politicized when individuals use their Hepatitis C status to mount wider critiques of existing power relations, such as demonstrating the links among poverty, social exclusion, and Hepatitis C transmission. At the same time, a patient's decision to challenge a physician's counsel can be empowering, especially if that physician is willing to rethink her or his approach as a result of interactions with that patient.

The willingness to become a citizen expert rests partly on whether an individual accepts or rejects the illness label associated with being Hepatitis C positive. Understanding what has happened to oneself in the treatment process (having been 'cleared' or having been 'cured') can shape the extent to which one may align oneself with or distance oneself from the Hepatitis C community. For some patients who were treated successfully, news of 'clearing' the virus was sometimes difficult to accept, as there was anxiety about whether the 'clearing' was permanent or, instead, only a temporary blip that would be followed by the reappearance of the virus months later. Generally, patients who have cleared the virus are told that they have a 'sustained virologic response,' which refers to a situation in which the virus is undetectable in the blood 6 months or more after the completion of treatment. However, there is some dispute within the Hepatitis C community with regard to the proper nomenclature for this circumstance. Although many speak of having 'cleared' the virus, claiming to be 'cured' is contentious as there is still no known cure for Hepatitis C. As one research participant explained, 'Some will say, "Yeah, you're cured." The rest, who look at a purely cell level, they'll say, "It's still in your lymph glands." It will never leave the lymph glands, apparently … But to me the issue is, does it have the power to affect you?' (Interview, 1 December 2004).

Positioning one's post-treatment identity in terms of a discourse of curing or clearing reflects a tension between the biological and the social, that is, between the reality of biological facts that can be established under the presumably objective guise of science and the socially constructed world in which these 'facts' come to life through specific practices. Whether the virus is dormant or active is a piece of vital biological information, for example, but these biological facts themselves tell us little about how individuals will engage with or respond to this knowledge. You may be told, for instance, that the virus has been successfully treated, but there is a wide gulf between being told that you should be feeling better and actually feeling well. In fact, a round of successful treatment can actually convey a false sense of hope in persons who have undergone treatment.

What, then, is socially and politically significant about the emphasis on a discourse of clearing? As Erni (1994: 128) explains, in a study of the cultural politics of curing AIDS, it is not surprising, given the ascendancy of the life sciences, that curing would emerge as the holy grail of social and scientific discourses surrounding treatment: 'The power to invest life through and through makes curing one of the noblest pursuits of modern sciences.' Moreover, he explains, curing reflects a desire to speak in 'serialized binary' terms about the body. We contrast health with disease, disease with death, and death with life. Therefore, speaking in the language of cure, he explains, has political implications: 'Curing is no longer just a fact of social and medical endeavor; instead, it is the crucial articulator of power's intervention into the material body on the basis of a historical discourse that enables the far-reaching importance assumed by the technologies of lifesaving' (ibid.: 129).

Not unlike many people living with chronic illness, those individuals with Hepatitis C who have cleared the virus become members of the 'remission society' (Frank, 1995: 8), a place reserved for people who are feeling better but are not quite cured of the illness or condition that affected them in the first place. Although this society need not be oppressive, it can be especially frustrating for those who are desperate to move from 'the kingdom of the sick' to the 'kingdom of the well' (see Sontag, 1990). As Susan Sontag explains, 'Everyone who is born holds dual citizenship, in the kingdom of the well and in the kingdom of the sick. Although we all prefer to use only the good passport, sooner or later each of us is obliged, at least for a spell, to identify ourselves as citizens of that other place' (1990: 3; see also Prince, Chapter 2, this volume). The trouble, as Sontag points out, is that health is based on the appearance of stark opposites: either you are sick or you are well. Chronic illnesses such as Hepatitis C force us to confront the fact that there is another space that is not quite one or the other, a space in between these two kingdoms, a kingdom of the not-quite sick and the not-quite well. What is real for many individuals with Hepatitis C may not be the biological fact of a sustained virologic response, but rather a deep sense that their body and mind have not returned to their pre–Hepatitis C state. These diverse realities undoubtedly complicate efforts to mobilize a collective identity around a Hepatitis C diagnosis. Because the experience of being Hepatitis C positive may be temporary or fleeting – especially if one qualifies for and avails oneself of treatment – being officially 'in the clear' for 6 months may prompt those uncomfortable with the diagnosis to view themselves as 'cleared' and as a result to distance themselves from the Hepatitis C community. By contrast, patients who still feel that the virus has not left their body may continue to identify with, and mobilize politically on behalf of, this community.

The third form of contestation assumes a more conscious political form as individuals join forces to press for change, be it in government policy, societal attitudes, or in scientific and medical practices; it has both collectivizing and individualizing tendencies. Collectivization is linked to the first two forms of contestation I have discussed in the sense that a decision to pursue collective action is influenced by the degree to which patients embrace a Hepatitis C identity and use expert knowledge of their own ill bodies to nourish the terrain of collective action. Indeed, for many individuals, the discovery of a Hepatitis C diagnosis can be the primary precursor to political action.

However, there are a number of challenges that may undermine or deflect the impulse to politicize the experience of illness. Unlike some other forms of collective identity-building, encouraging others to 'come out' as Hepatitis C positive can be complicated by the stigma attached to the virus.[4] Regardless of how they were infected, patients encounter the shame and approbation of others who are afraid they may get Hepatitis C; this extends to children and family members of people with Hepatitis C, who are also presumed to be tainted with the virus. In addition to these socially grounded impediments, there are also serious biological barriers to becoming politically engaged. One of the most significant is intense fatigue, which is a common side effect of both treatment and the illness. This was explained by one respondent in the following way:

> I mean, people say if you're tired, why don't you just go have a nap? But it's not that you're sleepy; there's a big difference between being sleepy and being tired. This is a very invasive fatigue. It's like you wake up and your bones are tired. And it's very difficult to focus and get through the day. I had a rule at one point that I would do one thing during the day, you know, and it might be writing the shopping list. And then the next day I would try to do the shopping ... This fatigue is not understood. (Interview, 21 January 2005)

Just as we should appreciate the obstacles to collective action for individuals living with a chronic illness such as Hepatitis C, there is a need to temper any claims about the individual or political effects of an expert patient culture. Rose and Novas's notion of a 'political economy of hope' is helpful in allowing us to adopt a more nuanced view of biological citizenship practices. To be sure, as biomedical and political authorities may suggest, a Hepatitis C diagnosis may provide the occasion for individuals to re-evaluate their lives and take charge of their health, including adopting lifestyle practices that do not aggravate their condition, such as avoiding alcohol as it can harm the liver. Interestingly, this individualizing conception of biological citizenship is often mobilized from above by, for instance, pharmaceutical firms interested in creating markets for drugs. Hepatitis C is no exception. Roche, the maker of pegylated interferon, an anti–Hepatitis C medication, counsels patients: 'As you begin to accept the reality of your disease, you may be inspired to make significant changes in your relationships and be proactive about your health practices' (Hoffman-La Roche, 2007).

But the individualizing and empowering potential of biological citizenship can be limited for those who do not see their own agency, or the ability to change the circumstances of their lives. For example, for those who discover that they are infected with a strain of the virus that is difficult to treat, the initial hope afforded by the possibility of treatment is snuffed out once they discover that they are not likely to 'respond' well to treatment.[5] The language here is instructive: patients are labelled non-responders, as failing the treatment, rather than the treatment failing them. This can also affect the collectivizing potential afforded by biological citizenship. The divisions in the community between persons who contracted the virus via tainted blood and those who did so in the context of drug use can be further exacerbated by new sets of cleavages: first, between those who were treated successfully and contend that they are cured and those who have been treated and are reluctant to proclaim that they are cured; and second, between those who have undergone successful treatment and those who either did not access treatment or did not respond well to treatment.

Many of the research participants who were infected through Canada's blood system spoke as if the diagnosis – discovering they were infected – was the formative event itself. Prior to being diagnosed, they were leading 'normal' lives. In contrast, those who were infected in the course of sharing drug injection equipment spoke of the 'event' of their diagnosis in terms that could not be distinguished from their troubled lives:

INTERVIEWER: So in terms of dealing with the news were there people you needed to tell?

RESPONDENT: I called my brother and said, 'Well, at least I got a rubber stamp.' That was it. To keep this in context here I was a drug addict who was 43 years old. I'd seen it all. I'd felt it all. When you put this on top of it, it sort of … fits into the mould.

INTERVIEWER: One more thing.

RESPONDENT: One more thing. It's not something I should be surprised at because I guess I earned it. That's part of me, my drug addiction, the consequences thereof, and so on. I probably would have been far more excited if I hadn't had it …

INTERVIEWER: But you said, you 'deserve this' …

RESPONDENT: The short and sweet of it is that I was as an asshole for many, many years. A lot of people paid the price for the way I was. That I'm still alive and that whether I have hep C, that's the word 'deserve.' Guys I was running with in the street, either dead, getting transplants, in various stages of mental breakdown, and so on and so forth. I'm lucky. Because it's not affecting me. It's sort of like, it's part and parcel of the whole package. I deserved it. Hey, I was an idiot. (Interview, 21 June 2005)

Here, and in other interviews, drug users speak about their lives in ways that demonstrate a need to expand our notion of biological citizenship to challenge the presumption that biological citizens are always squarely focused on their health, and will be roused to action upon discovering that they are Hepatitis C positive. Ignoring or failing to be deeply affected by a Hepatitis C diagnosis should not be interpreted as a failure to live up to the duties of 'responsible' biological citizenship, especially given that persons with Hepatitis C often receive mixed messages about the severity of their illness. Although some are counselled to begin treatment immediately, others are told not to worry about the illness or to let it take control over their lives. Persons with Hepatitis C challenge what it means to be a responsible biological citizen, if behaving responsibly means finding out all there is to know about Hepatitis C, joining forces with others to cement a collective identity that can act as a springboard for political action, and mobilizing the expertise that has been amassed to press for policy change and to counter stigma. Some Hepatitis C patients might fit this mould, but on the whole, people with Hepatitis C do not conform to this rather narrow model of biological citizenship as proposed by Rose and Novas (2005). In addition to inviting us to reconceptualize biological citizenship, the Hepatitis C case also requires us to trouble the notion of contestation and abandon assumptions about what it means to engage in political action. People with Hepatitis C may not be marching defiantly on the streets demanding increased research funding and the like, as their predecessors in the AIDS movement have done. They have worked, however, often away from the glare of the media, to challenge popular and expert conceptions of what it is like to live with Hepatitis C.

Unravelling the Policy Implications

A shift to biological citizenship has important, as yet unexplored, implications for health policy. First, the emergence of biological citizenship requires us to probe further into how citizens construct their citizenship duties and obligations in the light of a new-found relationship to their own biological bodies. As noted, new forms of citizenship rooted in biology 'cannot merely focus upon strategies for making up citizens from above' (Rose & Novas, 2005: 441). Rather, we need to examine how citizens contest power and authority from below. How is it that they challenge prevailing discourses by targeting actors other than the state? In the case of Hepatitis C, individuals sometimes challenge the health care professionals with whom they come into contact throughout the diagnosis and treatment processes, as well as other individuals living with the illness. Indeed, for scholars interested in how collective actors contest power and authority, there is much to be gained from studying how citizens are often governed, not by the iron hand of the state, but as Nikolas Rose has argued, 'from a distance,' by a multiplicity of technologies of the self and practices of responsibilization. This is apparent in the case of Hepatitis C, where there are clear differences between the experiences of persons infected with Hepatitis C through contaminated blood and those infected through drug use. The former expressed moral outrage at their situation, while those infected through drug use appeared to internalize the blame and shame associated with being not only Hepatitis C positive but a current or former drug user as well. Persons who feel a sense of responsibility for getting infected in the first place are less likely to frame their policy interventions in the language of citizenship rights. Although biological citizenship has the potential to empower citizens to become acquainted with their biological identities and challenge the truth claims of biomedical knowledge, we need to be cautious about its emancipatory potential to reframe the role of citizens in policy processes, especially if those citizens are members of marginalized communities. In addition, if practices of contestation are confined to becoming a citizen expert, without necessarily challenging the underlying power structures that produce authorized knowledge claims, citizens may, albeit unwittingly, reinforce the privileged place of biomedicine as a form of knowledge, valorizing it as a particular way of knowing.

Second, scholars of health policy need to come to grips with how these new forms of collective mobilization occasioned by the emergence of biological citizenship will reframe policy discourses in the field of health. As Rose and Novas explain (2005: 442), the rise of 'biosocial groupings' – 'collectivities formed around a biological conception of shared identity' – forces us to ask a set of interesting questions about how common features of our biological identities are fundamentally altering conceptions of what it means to be political and to participate in the social world.[6] The fact that, in many cases, individuals who take part in these biosocial communities may interact exclusively via the Internet – what Rose and Novas term 'digital bio-citizenship' – also challenges us to rethink notions of active, civic participation and engagement in public life.

Finally, the Hepatitis C case reveals that new forms of citizenship rooted in biology require that we confront the challenge of integrating the experiential knowledge of patients into health policy-making processes. New analytical tools, including a reconstituted notion of what biological citizenship means, are needed in order to understand the important shifts under way regarding how biological citizens are made up from above, by state, medical, and scientific authorities, and from below, by and through citizens themselves. Widening the conception of biological citizenship to account for experiences in which the biological commingles with the social, and in which the biological is not synonymous with illness or disease, may provide a more realistic portrait of these new spaces of contestation that are rooted in biology.

Acknowledgments

The Canadian Institutes of Health Research provided a generous operating grant that allowed this research to take place. Doctoral candidate Michael Graydon, who conducted the interviews, provided immeasurable research assistance. Robert Johnson, Francesca Scala, Miriam Smith, Steve Kroll-Smith, and especially, the volume editors, provided useful comments and encouragement. Finally, the 101 people with Hepatitis C who participated in this research deserve a special thanks.

NOTES

1 A total of 101 persons with Hepatitis C were interviewed for this research project.
2 In the United Kingdom, the government's Expert Patient Initiative has garnered much attention. See Bury (2004).
3 Thanks to Steve Kroll-Smith for suggestions on how to reframe this discussion.
4 Körner and Treloar (2006: 16) have argued that people with Hepatitis C 'face higher degrees of stigma than those with other chronic illnesses.'
5 The latter can be affected by a person's genotype, the strain of the virus with which they are infected. Genotype 1, which is prevalent in North America, is more difficult to treat than genotypes 2 and 3 (see Orsini & Scala, 2006).
6 For a good discussion of biosociality, see Paul Rabinow, 'Artificiality and enlightenment: from sociobiology to biosociality,' in Rabinow (1996: 91–111).

REFERENCES

Bury, Mike. (2004). A Commentary. In *Perspectives on the expert patient*. Conference of the Royal Pharmaceutical Society of Great Britain (pp. 1–6). Retrieved 15 Dec. 2006, from http://www.rpsgb.org.uk/pdfs/exptpatsemrept.pdf.

Epstein, Steven. (1991). Democratic science? AIDS activism and the contested construction of knowledge. *Socialist Review*, 21(2), 35–64.

Epstein, Steven. (1996). *Impure science: AIDS, activism, and the politics of knowledge*. Berkeley: University of California Press.

Erni, John Nguyet. (1994). *Unstable frontiers: Technomedicine and the cultural politics of curing AIDS*. Minneapolis: University of Minnesota Press.

Frank, Arthur W. (1995). *The wounded storyteller: Body, illness and ethics*. Chicago and London: University of Chicago Press.

Hoffman-La Roche. (2007). The impact of Hepatitis C on your life. Retrieved 5 Jan. 2007, from http://www.pegasys.com/life-with-hcv/impact-of-hepatitis-c.aspx.

Körner, Henrike, & Treloar, Carla. (2006). Representations of people with HIV and hepatitis C in editorials of medical journals: Discourses and interdiscursive relations. *Communication and Medicine*, 3(1), 15–25.

Lister, Ruth. (2003). *Citizenship: Feminist perspectives*. New York: New York University Press.

Orsini, Michael. (2002). The politics of naming, blaming and claiming: HIV, Hepatitis C, and the emergence of blood activism in Canada. *Canadian Journal of Political Science*, 35(3), 475–498.

Orsini, Michael, & Scala, Francesca. (2006). Every virus tells a story: Toward a narrative-centred approach to health policy. *Policy and Society*, 25(2), 125–150.

Petersen, Alan, & Bunton, Robin. (2002). *The new genetics and the public's health*. New York and London: Routledge.

Petryna, Adriana. (2002). *Life exposed: Biological citizens after Chernobyl*. Princeton, NJ: Princeton University Press.

Rabinow, Paul. (1996). *Essays on the anthropology of reason*. Princeton, NJ: Princeton University Press.

Rose, Nikolas, & Novas, Carlos. (2005). Biological citizenship. In Aihwa Ong and Stephen J. Collier (Eds.), *Global assemblages: Technology, politics and ethics as anthropological problems* (pp. 439–463). London: Blackwell.

Sontag, Susan. (1990). *Illness as metaphor and AIDS and its metaphors*. New York: Anchor Books.

Waldby, Catherine, Rosengarten, Marsha, Treloar, Carla, & Fraser, Suzanne. (2004). Blood and bioidentity: Ideas about self, boundaries and risk among

blood donors and people living with Hepatitis C. *Social Science and Medicine,*
59, 1461–1471.

World Health Organization. (2006). *Fact sheet on Hepatitis C.* Retrieved 29 May
2006, from http://www.who.int/mediacentre/factsheets/fs164/en/
index.html.

7 Tracing Contours of Contestation in Narratives about Chronic Fatigue Syndrome

PIA H. BÜLOW

Throughout the past four decades, social scientists have been studying how chronic illness affects people's sense of self. The British sociologist Michael Bury (1982) described chronic illness as a *disruption of biography,* and this has become a model for conceiving crucial life events as markers dividing life history in terms of before and after.[1] This image of disruption involves the need for *re*construction. Similarly, Kathy Charmaz (1983 and 1987) writes about *loss of self* as a social consequence of chronic illness – an experience that leads to the struggle for a (new) self.

Other research about the self and illness includes a focus on stigma (Goffman, 1963) and stigmatization. According to Peter Conrad (1987), concepts like stigma force us to confront the meaning of illness – 'Why me?' and 'What have I done to be stricken with this?' These questions highlight the issue of responsibility and are important, especially in studies about *contested illness*, that is, illness that tends to be regarded as less legitimate or less 'real' in both the medical realm and in everyday life. Some illnesses become contested, in part, because of the difficulties that others may have in perceiving and understanding a set of symptoms that are impossible to confirm by medical procedures. Such symptoms are 'invisible' to medical and laypeople alike, creating challenges for diagnosis, treatment, and everyday life. Examples include Chronic Fatigue Syndrome (CFS) or Myalgic Encephalomyelitis (see Moss, Chapter 9, this volume), burnout, temporomandibular joint syndrome (TMJ), repetitive strain injury (RSI), and Fibromyalgia (see Lippel, Chapter 3, this volume). For people suffering from a contested illness, it is not the pain – or the fatigue – that seems to be stigmatic (Hilbert, 1984). It is how the symptom is communicated and the dilemma of what should be concealed and what should be openly told that people are facing when suffering from something that is 'unfamiliar as a cultural object' (ibid.: 373). Norma Ware (1992) distinguishes between two kinds of disbelief expressed by others: *trivialization* and *delegitimization*. In the former, the personal feeling of illness is rejected as a symptom of a disease; in the latter, illness is psychologized and stated to be 'all in your head.' Consequently, contested illnesses concern communication and narration in a particular way.

Drawing on the concept of disruption, Gareth Williams (1984) shows how ill people realign present, past, and self with society through what he calls a *narrative reconstruction*. Since the early 1980s, illness narratives have become an increasingly important focus for social science research (Bell, 2000; Hydén & Bülow, 2006) that explores the relationships between chronic illness, narratives, and the self (see Becker, 1997; Bell, 1999; Frank, 1995; Hydén & Bülow, 2006; Riessman, 1990). This kind of meaning-making narration does not concern the storyteller alone. In such research, personal narratives are analysed according to the concept of presentation of the self (Goffman, 1959), considered as a discursive resource used for different purposes. One example is Mary Horton-Salway's (2001) analysis of a story about CFS, co-narrated by the ill woman and her husband. The narrative is interpreted as an attributional story linked to identity since it works to construct illness as a physical disease. Another example is Gareth Williams's (1993) analysis of an elderly woman's story about her everyday life with chronic illness. Presenting herself as competent and capable, she forms a story as a pursuit of virtue. In these analyses, the self becomes something that might change because of illness, but it also alters in different contexts. Analysing the narrated self includes a moral dimension. Charmaz (1999: 367) argues that suffering is a profoundly moral status and that narratives about suffering 'reflect, redefine, or resist such moral status.'

Although much has been written about the way chronic illness affects the self and narratives about the self (see Hydén, 1997), contested illness has been studied to a lesser degree particularly from a narrative perspective. It seems reasonable to suggest that the experience of such illnesses influences people's sense of self and their stories. But in what way are the contours of contestation and the textures of living with illness discernible in stories about illness and in the way that these stories are told?

In this chapter, I trace contours of contestation in stories about CFS told by sufferers. I first present an analysis of the narrative form, exploring the meaning of contestation as it is expressed in the elements constructing the story. I then examine the moral claims made by people suffering from CFS through the telling of stories and reflect on the moral status that stories lend the narrator. I close with some insights into narrative analysis and the texture of experience.

The Study

My analysis is based on a series of interviews with 14 persons suffering from CFS. I preceded the interviews with an ethnographic study of a group activity arranged by a clinic that specializes in CFS – a so-called *patient school* (Bülow, 2004; Bülow & Hydén, 2003b). The interviewees, 10 women and four men, were all former participants in the patient school, although they came from three different cohorts. The 'school' included both lectures about CFS held by medical professionals and group talks guided by a nurse. All interviewees but one were inter-viewed twice or on three occasions. In most cases, the initial interview took place about 6 months after the school finished. The longest period to elapse between the patient school and the last interview was 2.5 years. The interviews were tape-recorded and later transcribed verbatim.

The average age of participants at the beginning of the study was 41.5 years, with a range from 30 to 60 years. The majority of the inter-viewees (12) received a diagnosis of CFS before participating in the patient school. At the beginning of the patient school, 10 of the inter-viewees had full-time sickness benefits and/or a temporary or perma-nent disability pension, two held part-time sickness benefits, and two were full-time workers. At the last interview, three persons had gone from sickness benefits to a temporary or permanent disability pension, three were receiving a lower level of sickness benefits than at the beginning of the school (one of them is now working full-time), and eight reported no changes in level and form of benefit or pension – two of these were the full-time workers at the beginning of the patient school. All names of persons, places, and other personal details have been changed. The analysis was conducted using Swedish material and later translated into English.

The Analysis

Following Mishler (1999), I use a case-centred model of analysis and consider stories as identity performances. This means that the analysis emanates from the individual stories about illness.[2] Influenced by Elliot Mishler's work on interviews (1986) and narrative identity (1999) I regard both interviews and narratives as co-produced by speaker and listener. I also consider the interviews as part of the storyteller's life story from which it is possible to pick up individual short stories about special events. As a result, I use narratives in two different ways: the entire interview (sets of interviews with one person) as a story, and specific stories about special events presented in the interviews. In the former, the interview narrative consists of different episodes as well as descriptions that form the story. In the latter, the stories are better defined and have a form that corresponds with the internal structure of spoken narratives described by William Labov and Joshua Waletzky (1967). These spoken narratives comprise different parts: an abstract and an orientation, followed by complicating actions, evaluations, and resolutions, and commonly, at the end, a coda. Since the analysis presented here is based on both kinds of narratives, single extracts will not always have the form of a story through which it is possible to discern an act and a plot.

In my analysis, I first discuss the structure of the stories in terms of their content and then the important interactive aspects of storytelling. I present the core elements in the narratives about CFS and move on to an analysis concerning different stories about the self and how the storytellers present themselves. Finally, I conclude by discussing the communicative dilemma connected to contested illness.

Core Elements in Narratives about CFS

Important elements that seem to be typical for narratives about CFS emerge from the lengthy connected stories about the time in interviewees' lives before they attended the patient school: *the pilgrimage*[3] through medical investigations, *the diagnosis*, and *the genesis of illness*. These elements did not always appear in this order in the interviews. This ordering is, rather, an analytic description of the questions the storytellers seem to have asked themselves about their experiences of illness. Thus a pattern appears in which the question 'What is wrong with me?' leads into the (usually) very long story about contacts with the health care system (and sometimes with complementary medicine), with employers, and with the social insurance office, all of which form the theme of the 'long-way story' named by one of the interviewees.

The Pilgrimage

Jill, a woman in her forties, gives a summarized version of her 'long-way story' as an 'abstract' to the whole story about her illness (cf. Labov & Waletsky, 1967):

> Eh I suppose I first got sick '94 in fact
> in fact '94 but I didn't report myself sick until '96
> in January
> And then during the years '96, '97, '98,
> '99. Four years then I was swirling around at different
> departments. As many as there were kind of looking for what
> was wrong.
> And they didn't find anything wrong actually.[4]

In its condensed version, this abstract shows several things typical for the narratives in my study. First, the *uncertainty* about onset, which was signalled in Jill's case by her vague statement about when she first got sick. Most of the interviewees spoke about fatigue as a symptom that sneaked up on them and that eventually became a problem for which they sought medical care. That Jill did not report herself sick until two years later could be a sign of the difficulty in deciding when tiredness is out of the range of normal. Another woman, Joanna, described this by saying that for a long time she blamed her tiredness on something other than illness, she just needed more sleep than others. Second, the abstract of Jill's story describes the 'long way' of *searching*, looking for explanations during a pilgrimage of suffering. This time frame, which could be rather extended, often included, as it did for Jill, encounters with many different doctors and medical specialists ('Four years then I was swirling around'). Third, and important in understanding the feeling expressed through the 'long-way' story, are the many times nothing was found. In contacts with the health care system, tests and examinations usually did not indicate any kind of disease. This experience of unanswered questions about what was wrong becomes part of the pilgrimage, and contributes to the feeling that the legitimacy of one's claims is being contested since illness is not medically confirmed by a name – a diagnosis. Several of the interviewees described this experience of being in limbo as almost as painful as the illness itself.

Although typical for the narratives in this study, the uncertainty and long period spent searching cannot alone describe the particular experience of contested illness. In fact, the same elements can be found in narratives about many chronic illnesses; Bury (2000) even describes uncertainty as a key concept in the experience of chronic illness. To understand the pilgrimage as a core element in these stories about CFS, one has to connect it with the rest of the story and how the stories are told. It is notable how interviewees whose experiences differ from this pattern emphasized the uniqueness of their story. For example, a couple of participants spoke about the exceptional luck that they had had in meeting an understanding doctor at once, or that they had been diagnosed quite soon after their first contact with the health care system. In that way they linked their personal (and different) story to the collective story of CFS.

Diagnosis

Quite a few interviewees told stories in which the long period of searching ended rather suddenly when meeting a new doctor who showed interest in their suffering and whose commitment resulted in either a diagnosis of CFS or a letter of referral to a specialist (who later confirmed the diagnosis). One participant, James, described this:

> No but then– (.) eh (.) spring '98 then. /.../ I was there
> again and complained.
> But then he didn't have time (.) Eh my family doctor
> so then I got some kind of extra doctor they had there
> who ehum (.) well he did more or less the same thing as the
> family doctor had done before but he was a bit more careful
> /.../
> And then he wrote a referral letter there [the special unit for
> CFS]
> and eh (.) well it was lucky that I met him then instead of my
> ordinary doctor.

These stories are commonly told as a turning point that made the difference between the time of the pilgrimage and the time when they had a name for their illness. Many interviewees talked about these stories as lucky coincidences, while others described this as the point when they had become tired of searching and tended to become more active agents.

The stories about getting the diagnosis are less elaborate than the stories of pilgrimage. Typically however, receiving the diagnosis of CFS was associated with the feeling of relief. Jessica, for example, said:

> But the second time when I went to X [the medical specialist]
> and got this confirmed then I felt– I felt trusted by someone
> and I became confirmed as a patient.
> And then I became happy– I actually became happy because of that.
> It sounds sort of odd but I was happy to get a diagnosis.

The account about her feelings of joy 'sounding odd' reveals the idea of a diagnosis as an unwanted answer. At the same time, it emphasizes the exculpating effect a diagnosis seems to have in contested illness. The diagnosis becomes the answer to the long-asked question, 'What is wrong with me?' Jean, another interviewee, described how before her diagnosis she could not explain her problem to others and that she felt that physicians did not really trust her. The diagnosis for her meant that 'some kind of peace spread out' and that she was able to move on. Instead of experiencing the diagnosis as a disruption, Jean saw it as an end to her history of searching.

This interpretation of the significance of getting a name for one's illness is strengthened by the way stories about *not* receiving a diagnosis are explained as misunderstandings. In one case, the interviewee explained that the communicative problem could be found within herself: 'Unfortunately I gave the wrong answers.' This woman got the diagnosis later from another doctor. Another interviewee asserted throughout the three interviews with me that the doctor had overlooked 'the missing criterion' in the illness history told at the medical interview.

The Genesis of Illness

Even if marking the end of the long-way story, the diagnosis at the same time seems to lead to new questions concerning the self and one's life: 'What kind of person am I to have this kind of illness? In what way is my illness connected to what has happened in my life before and my way of leading my life?' Trying to answer such morally loaded questions indicates the basis upon which CFS can be contested and thus catches a glimpse of the contested contours of illness.

The interviewees seemed to deal with the responsibility evoked by this kind of question by temporalizing illness in their narratives, giving it the shape of a shadow of time (Bülow & Hydén, 2003a).[5] By the way in which they told their stories, illness could become something that was unavoidable but that should have been foreseen, or something that was impossible to foresee because it was a consequence of many different and unconnected things in life for which one could not be held responsible. Illness could also be told as something that was just *one* possible outcome of a range of possibilities. Accordingly, the different ways in which the interviewees temporalized illness had consequences for the question of responsibility and implications for the further narrative reconstruction of illness. Telling a story that gives the storyteller some kind of responsibility for becoming ill seemed to force the storyteller to narratively manage the threat to her or his moral status that appears within the story.

PIA: How do you think then what was it that happened? How do you
    explain that to yourself?
    (…)
JEAN: I believe that I have been under too much stress for a much too
    long time.
    And then there during a couple of months it became acute.
    And that- (.) I don't think it's a coincidence that I became ill.
PIA: That it isn't a coincidence?
JEAN: No, no I've for sure been setting this up very carefully.
PIA: Can you tell me?

After my invitation, Jean starts to tell a very long story about the genesis of her illness, starting nine years back in time when her youngest child was born, explaining a stressful life from that time on. It is a story told chronologically, about studies at night, about a psychosocially dreadful working environment, about getting a new job and having to make a social 'restart,' about moving out and moving back home due to renovation, and – at the end – about leaving an area where she had lived most of her life and instead moving to a new house in a new town and getting another new job, and a range of difficulties due to these major changes. Jean concludes by reflecting on her sense of responsibility:

So that it has been change upon change upon change upon
change
And it has been me who's been fixing and dragging on and
nagging

Just this we're talking landlords, making contacts with real
estate agents and (..)
So of course, of course at that time I've been thinking that one
can't go on like this. That it doesn't work but just then I was in
the middle of it.
/.../
But of course I've been thinking about that many times at
which point could one have put a brake on the course so this
wouldn't have happened?
But (.) at the same time 'so what' then this happened.
And to some people it's probably unusually difficult to learn to
draw reasonable lines then.
And I was probably one of them.
But I suppose I'll have to try to learn from that then. Even if I-
Now it's like this I'll have to try to make something
constructive out of it.
I guess I'll have to try to live at a sort of slower pace.

In the beginning, Jean emphasizes her own responsibility for becoming ill. In her conclusion, though, she emphasizes how various changes piled up. This is noticeable from the different parts in the long story about different events that were putting stress on her during these years and from her repetition of the words 'change upon change.' Although most of these changes were impossible for Jean to control, or to put a stop to, she nevertheless points out her responsibility for managing the situation: 'it has been me.' She describes how she thought about how to stop this course of events but also declares that what happened did happen. The whole line of argument about stopping the process, in which she presents herself as the kind of person who has difficulties 'drawing reasonable lines' for herself, leads to the conclusion that she has to learn something from all this. This image of a responsible person willing to learn probably strengthens Jean's moral status (see Charmaz, 1999).

Narrating the Self in Stories about CFS

Even if every story can be thought of as a presentation of self, interviewees sometimes gave accounts of their sense of self in a very clear and open way. This is probably connected to CFS being a contested illness, which in every kind of situation might be challenged. As far as the interviewee knew, this might happen in the interview situation as well.

THE REAL ME

When I met Jill for the first interview, she chose to start her story by pointing at the importance of knowing who the person becoming ill 'really is' – or was:

> I believe that one has to start from the person one really is.
> 'Cause when you have CFS then you aren't really yourself.
> This is what I believe and from that eh things will happen.
> Then one becomes ill.
> And for me it took many years before I came to the patient school.

I asked Jill how many years it took, and as an answer she summarized her long-way story. However, since that seemed to me to be a potted version, I asked her to tell me more. Once more claiming that she had to start from the beginning she 'asked' for 'one minute to tell who I really am,' and then she said:

> I'm really that kind of dandelion flower[6] as they say that shouldn't
> have survived in this life
> but who did anyway because I'm terribly stubborn
> ehum (.) I have quite great inner strength so to speak (Pia: Yes),
> and, eh, have lived a rather hard life really like that
> really I have done because-
> but I'm stubborn and make up my mind about something
> and do that too. And carry out what I really want to do.
> So- so- that's me.

Jill's statement telling me who she really is opened up space for her very long story about illness and about identity. Her story was framed in two different ways: first by stating that CFS changes something about the self and, second, by categorizing herself as a weed, that is, as a kind of person who will survive even if the environment is very tough. Jill's claim of being the kind of person who always does what she decides to do was just the prelude for the storyline of the fighter and the survivor, something that she repeated throughout the interviews. Emphasizing that she had to start from the very beginning and starting her story far back in her past gave her account a temporal depth and what Charlotte Linde (1993) calls a strong form of causality. Jill's presentation of self seemed to be very important as a start to the first interview. To tell me about her illness was to take the risk of someone disputing her claims, of her self being contested. By framing her story with this kind of presentation of self, she introduced a particular way to interpret the whole story that she was going to tell.

PROVING ILLNESS

One big problem for those suffering from a contested illness such as CFS is to explain the degree of tiredness that they experience in such a way so that their illness is not thought of as merely moaning, hypochondria, or something imagined. In the interviews, there are many stories to prove illness and to illustrate how bad it is or has been. This difficulty in claiming illness sometimes became obvious in the interviews when interviewees strongly emphasized how exhausted they would be after the interview or gave examples of things they were incapable of doing because of their illness. However, the problem of explaining illness and convincing other people that the fatigue, pain, and cognitive difficulties were real was part of their everyday life with illness.

Consequently, the risk of being called into question was something that the interviewee always seemed to deal with in the interview, as well as in life in general. All of the interviewees talked about their illness as contested in some way and in some contexts. But not all of the interviewees told stories of specific instances where they were being openly distrusted. Instead, many gave more general descriptions about being doubted and having the feeling that a doctor or a relative did not really believe in their illness. Such stories were often told as dramatic scenes in which different persons appeared. Joyce, a woman in her sixties, had been ill for many years. She told several stories about being challenged in different situations:

> But she [the daughter-in-law] thinks that one should be allowed
> to call here then at 7:00 in the morning or at 11:00 at night
> and say 'Can you take care of them [the grandchildren]?'
> But I said 'that's impossible.'
> 'Why not then?' [in the 'voice' of her daughter-in-law]
> No but I can't manage.
> I can't on this short notice.
> And now she's become so mad at me she won't see me any
> more.

And I think that is something absolutely terrible.
I can- then I get furious,
and think that how can one be- how can one be like that? How
can one get angry with a person who is ill?
I don't think I've done anything. (Pia: No)
(.)
I don't think so but she thinks that it is awful to ha- that I can't
like babysit and so. [Pia: Mhm]
But that- I would of course do [that] if I could.
Then- I used to the first years when the kids when their kids
were younger when I like- before I became this ill. (Pia: Mhm)
So that such things are very hard you know to be able to handle
then.
I really don't know what I should do to make her understand
that-
yes she thinks I'm a witch of course who doesn't help them
with the kids.
Yes but everybody has his own job
and they have a tough situation and everything. I understand that
too of course
but if I can't manage so I can't.
It's not that I want to be mean.
So such things are- I think it is- it is well sad when it goes like
this.

The narrative is a mix between a story about a specific occasion and a habitual narrative (Riessman, 1993), and the dramatic scene Joyce performed lends it a sense of presence. As a listener, I could almost hear the daughter-in-law. The story, told as an illustration of what the illness has meant for Joyce, shows the difficulty in getting other persons to understand fatigue as a legitimate reason for, in this case, refusing to act as a babysitter for the grandchildren. In this way, it is a story about being contested. But the story also suggests a felt need to give an explanation, in the interview situation, for having not fulfilled the cultural expectations of a caring grandmother. In her story, Joyce emphasized that she did babysit earlier when she was not in as bad shape as she is now. She points out that she understands why her daughter-in-law thinks that she, Joyce, 'is a witch' but also notes that her refusal is not because she is unkind – she just 'cannot manage.' This act of balancing nuances the story.

But the words of others can also be used in the opposite way. Instead of displaying the experience of distrust, the words of others may become crucial for positioning the storyteller as a trustworthy person. Such stories often concern how the storyteller handled illness and proved the interviewee's moral strength in relation to illness. Jessica, a woman in her mid-thirties, told me a story about being someone who, after some time, took the initiative. Claiming that her earlier encounters with physicians had been unsuccessful, she went on to describe how, despite being 'tremendously tired,' she attended a lecture on Fibromyalgia and CFS. This 'turned into an eye-opener' for her and was an episode that appeared to be an important starting point, giving her the stamina to continue struggling for a diagnosis.

JESSICA: After that [the lecture] I called my doctor at Home Town and asked for an appointment with her.
    And then I said that 'n o w I've done some "mind-mapping" of my whole l i f e from birth up to now about how my health has been'
    /.../
    And she was- got really shocked when she saw how much I had had through the years.
    So she said 'I don't understand how you've put up with this kind of life' she said.
    'No neither do I.'
PIA: No
JESSICA: That- that is of course a sign that I'm done in I right
PIA: Hm
JESSICA: 'So I want to go to this X who is a specialist since you can- nothing else than- you only want to give me Cipramil' [SSRI antidepressant]
PIA: Mhm
JESSICA: Nothing wrong with that but I thought that this is something more so you have to get a diagnosis on it.
PIA: Mhm, and what did she say?
JESSICA: She said that she thought that my life was well very- yes I'd had a lot of health problems
    and that 'I don't really know this myself' she said. 'I'm a doctor of medicine.'
PIA: Mhm

JESSICA: 'of course when I [the doctor] see this and see how you feel
   today
   and know how you've been working and all and can put things
   together'
   Then well she realized that 'you must go to someone who has
   knowledge about those connections then so we send you right
   away' she said 'I really do think so.'
   And she thought that it was very good that I had come to a
   conclusion about that myself then.

The story is built upon both the retold dialogue between Jessica and her doctor, and her own comments concerning that particular encounter. In her narration, Jessica uses the past tense in recounting her comments but switches to the historical present when retelling the dialogue between herself and the doctor. This shift enhances the sense of authenticity of the scene, reinforcing the forthrightness of her manner vis-à-vis the doctor in spite of her illness. Jessica demonstrated *agency* by positioning herself as the more active person in her narration, as the one who asked for an appointment and who opened topics through conversation. Similarly, Jessica, in the dialogue, was the one who took the initiative and insisted that a letter of referral be sent to a specialist. Jessica demonstrates how she gained credibility with her doctor through her description of her doctor's reaction as being 'really shocked' about the details of her life, by repeating the physician's words admitting to not being an expert ('I don't really know this myself'), and by recounting the physician's decision to respond to Jessica's request to send her to someone 'who has the knowledge.' Through dialogue, she used the doctor's words, which in turn validated her own analysis and confirmed her illness. In telling her story the way she did, Jessica strengthened her moral status through her account of her struggle for a confirmation of her illness and then showing that her suffering was at last taken seriously precisely because she sought out confirmation.

Although other interviewees did not explicitly display agency, like Jessica they seemed to use the words of other people for comfort and to legitimize illness. As part of their identity work, interviewees drew on the words that doctors, husbands, wives, or friends had used in trying to convince them about the reality of their illness, representing these words in a storied form to confirm their illness. Using others' words thus seemed to function as a kind of legitimizing act conferring a higher degree of moral status on the ill person.

The Contours of Contestation

In this chapter I have shown how people use narratives (and stories within narratives) to communicate the meaning of illness and to deal with difficulties concerning responsibility and moral status. The point I intend to make from the analysis is that contours of contestation become discernible through the way these stories were told.

To explain the experience of fatigue, pain, or loss of concentration, people have to put their suffering into words. Yet telling stories about contested illness always involves a risk of becoming mistrusted. Experiencing an illness like CFS leaves sufferers in a communicative dilemma. If they do not express their experience there will be no confirmation of it. However, in communicating their experience, they run a risk of being called into question. That risk must be handled either within the story or by the way it is told. In very clear ways, these stories show that suffering, as Charmaz (1999) writes, is a profoundly moral status because the experience of illness always is personal, and thus might be challenged.

By storytelling, people narratively reconstruct their life story, pointing out significant events and connecting different parts in a meaningful way, making it comprehensible. The kind of event that is chosen as the most important in telling a story about illness provides clues as to what makes people experience a certain kind of illness in a particular way. Analysing narratives is therefore an important step in seeking to understand the experience of a contested illness as a particular aspect of suffering, and to explore what constitutes the experience of being contested. Narratives permit us to texture the experience of CFS.

My analysis shows the contouring of contestation on various levels: the experience of persons suffering from illness being challenged in different situations and contexts, and at different times in relation to illness. From the core elements of these narratives about CFS a pattern of distrust, confirmation, and self-reflecting thoughts about responsibility evolves. At first a question of self-doubt, later the contours of contestation seem to be connected to the experience of being called into question by those having the authority to legitimize illness in different ways like physicians. After the diagnosis, questions about the meaning of illness still trouble the ill person, in part because the naming of a contested illness does not provide a stabilized legitimacy compared with what diagnosis brings to illnesses for which there exist a generally accepted understanding. Therefore, stories continue to be an important resource to sustain the ill person's moral status and a key part of their identity work – which seems to never end.

Transcript Key

(.) (..) (...)	short pauses which are more extended if more dots are added
[grand children]	transcriber's comments or non-verbal activity
-	sharp cut-off
"mind-mapping"	phrase spoken in English by interviewee
.	a full stop indicates a stopping fall in tone
,	a comma indicates a 'continuing' intonation
?	a question mark indicates a rising inflection
t h e n	emphasized word or words
/... /	passage omitted

NOTES

1   The concept of *biographical disruption* has not gone unchallenged. Simon Williams, another British sociologist, criticizes the unreflective use of the concept without anchoring it in scrupulous analysis of empirical data. He argues in favour of a more nuanced use because this kind of experience cannot be presumed to be a part of every chronic illness: '*timing* and *context*, *norms* and *expectations*, alongside our *commitment* to events, anticipated or otherwise, are crucial to the experience of our lives, healthy or sick, and the meanings with which we endow it' (2000: 51–2; emphasis in original).

2   Stories concern things that happen, usually something that someone does, says, or thinks, and what happens next. Every single story is in this way constructed to have a plot. But stories are also one way to tell another person something – and to invite the listener to join the storyteller in her or his experience of another time and place (see Young, 1987). At the same time, the act of telling a story in a particular way has an impact on narration and how the story is understood. No matter what form a narrative takes, whether it is performed as a dramatic scene or just 'told,' it conveys something about the way the storyteller sees the world and about herself or himself as a person. In this way, every story also has a *storyline* – a vein of meaning that underlies the plot and by which the listener can understand the story as a certain kind of story, such as the story of the winner (Schafer, 1992). Different stories about different events told in various

ways can thus bring forth the very same storyline and tell the same kind of story throughout, for example, a whole interview.

The interviews about CFS consist of lots of stories of various lengths. Many of these seemed to play an important role as presentations of self in the interview situation. But these stories also described how the storyteller presented herself or himself in the narrated situation. The narratives are formed both by the individual experience of illness as part of a life story and by the context within which the story was told. This means that it is possible to analyse an illness narrative from various perspectives – from the content of the story told, from the way this story is told, and from a here-and-now perspective in which the interaction between the interviewee as a storyteller and the researcher as a listener becomes central.

3 I have borrowed this metaphor from a study about women's experiences with repetitive strain injury (Reid, Ewan, & Lowy, 1991).

4 See the transcript key at the end of the chapter for a guide on how to read the interview excerpts.

5 I have borrowed the notion of 'time shadows' as well as the different kinds of 'time shadowing' from Gary Saul Morson (1994).

6 In Swedish there is a phrase *maskrosbarn*, which literally means 'dandelion child' and is used to describe someone who has had a dreadful childhood but nevertheless has survived as a person. The woman called Jill uses the expression *maskrosblomma*, meaning dandelion flower. It is impossible to know if she actually meant to invoke the well-known meaning, picked the wrong word, or if she made up a phrase of her own. The interpretation made in the analysis is based on the notion of dandelion as a weed.

REFERENCES

Becker, Gay. (1997). *Disrupted lives: How people create meaning in a chaotic world.* Berkeley: University of California Press.

Bell, Susan E. (1999). Narratives and lives: Women's health politics and the diagnosis of cancer for DES daughters. *Narrative Inquiry, 9,* 347–389.

Bell, Susan E. (2000). Experiencing illness in/and narrative. In Chloe E. Bird, Peter Conrad, & Allen M. Fremont (Eds.), *Handbook of medical sociology* (5th ed.) (pp. 184–199). Upper Saddle River, NJ: Prentice-Hall.

Bury, Michael. (1982). Chronic illness as biographical disruption. *Sociology of Health and Illness, 4*(2), 167–182.

Bury, Michael. (2000). On chronic illness and disability. In Chloe E. Bird, Peter Conrad, & Allen M. Fremont (Eds.), *Handbook of medical sociology* (5th ed.) (pp. 173-183). Upper Saddle River, NJ: Prentice-Hall.

Bülow, Pia H. (2004). Sharing experiences of contested illness by storytelling. *Discourse and Society, 15*(1), 33-53.

Bülow, Pia H., & Hydén, Lars-Christer. (2003a). In dialogue with time: Identity and illness in narratives about chronic fatigue. *Narrative Inquiry, 13*(1), 71–97.

Bülow, Pia H., & Hydén, Lars-Christer. (2003b). Patient school as a way of creating meaning in contested illness: The case of CFS. *Health: An Interdisciplinary Journal for the Social Study of Health, Illness and Medicine, 7*(2), 227–249.

Charmaz, Kathy. (1983). Loss of self: A fundamental form of suffering in the chronically ill. *Sociology of Health and Illness, 5*(2), 168–195.

Charmaz, Kathy. (1987). Struggling for a self: Identity levels of the chronically ill. *Research in the Sociology of Health Care, 6*, 283-321.

Charmaz, Kathy. (1999). Stories of suffering: Subjective tales and research narratives. *Qualitative Health Research, 9*(3), 362–382.

Conrad, Peter. (1987). The experience of illness: Recent and new directions. *Research in the Sociology of Health Care, 6*, 1–31.

Frank, Arthur W. (1995). *The wounded storyteller: Body, illness, and ethics*. Chicago and London: University of Chicago Press.

Goffman, Erving. (1959). *The presentation of self in everyday life*. New York: Anchor Books.

Goffman, Erving. (1963). *Stigma*. Englewood Cliffs, NJ: Prentice-Hall.

Hilbert, Richard A. (1984). The acultural dimensions of chronic pain: Flawed reality construction and the problem of meaning. *Social Problems, 31*, 365–378.

Horton-Salway, Mary. (2001). Narrative identities and the management of personal accountability in talk about ME: A discursive psychology approach to illness narrative. *Journal of Health Psychology, 6*(2), 247–259.

Hydén, Lars-Christer, (1997). Illness and narrative. *Sociology of Health and Illness, 19*(1), 48–69.

Hydén, Lars-Christer, & Bülow, Pia H. (2006). Medical discourse, illness narratives. In *Encyclopedia of language and linguistics* (2nd ed.) (pp. 697–703). Amsterdam: Elsevier.

Labov, William, & Waletzky, Joshua. (1967). Narrative analysis: Oral versions of personal experience. In June Helm (Ed.), *Essays on the verbal and visual arts* (pp. 12–44). Seattle: University of Washington Press.

Linde, Charlotte. (1993). *Life stories: The creation of coherence*. Oxford: Oxford University Press.

Mishler, Elliot G. (1986). *Research interviewing: Context and narrative*. Cambridge, MA: Harvard University Press.

Mishler, Elliot G. (1999). *Storylines: Craft artists' narratives of identity*. Cambridge, MA: Harvard University Press.

Morson, Gary Saul. (1994). *Narrative and freedom: The shadows of time*. New Haven, CT: Yale University Press.

Reid, Janice, Ewan, Christine, & Lowy, Eva. (1991). Pilgrimage of pain. The illness experiences of women with repetition strain injury and the search for credibility. *Social Science and Medicine, 32*(5), 601–612.

Riessman, Catherine Kohler. (1990). Strategic uses of narrative in the presentation of self and illness: A research note. *Social Science and Medicine, 30*(11), 1195–1200.

Riessman, Catherine Kohler. (1993). *Narrative analysis*, vol. 30. Newbury Park: Sage.

Schafer, Roy. (1992). *Retelling a life*. New York: Basic Books.

Ware, Norma C. (1992). Suffering and the social construction of illness: The delegitimation of illness experience in chronic fatigue syndrome. *Medical Anthropology Quarterly, New Series, 6*(4), 347–361.

Williams, Gareth H. (1984). The genesis of chronic illness: Narrative reconstruction. *Sociology of Health and Illness, 6*(2), 175–200.

Williams, Gareth H. (1993). Chronic illness and the pursuit of virtue in everyday life. In Alan Radley (Ed.), *Worlds of illness: Biographical and culture perspectives on health and disease* (pp. 92–108). New York and London: Routledge.

Williams, Simon J. (2000). Chronic illness as biographical disruption or biographical disruption as chronic illness? Reflections on a core concept. *Sociology of Health and Illness, 22*(1), 40–67.

Young, Katharine. (1987). *Taleworlds and storyrealms: The phenomenology of narrative*, vol. 16. Dordrecht, Holland: Martinus Nijhoff.

8 Cancer as a Contested Illness: Seeking Help amid Treatment

MARY ELLEN PURKIS AND
CATHERINE VAN MOSSEL

Cancer is a dreaded disease. The ready availability of professionals and treatments designed to *fight cancer*[1] support its categorization as a 'legitimate' illness. So what could there be to contest about cancer?

Curious about the relationship between diagnosis and treatment for cancer and processes of identity formation, we undertook a field study of people's experiences in a cancer clinic. Although the professional literature often draws on narrative accounts to underscore how devastating a cancer diagnosis is (e.g., Bailey et al., 2005; Bradley, 2005; Mathieson & Stam, 1995), our study revealed the extensive and convoluted nature of the work people engage in as they construct their identities as persons living with cancer. When receiving a diagnosis of cancer, people are generally required to adopt an entire plan of treatment associated with that diagnosis. In our study, it became evident that neither the diagnosis nor the treatment plan is self-evident: careful work is required on the part of both the professional and the person being diagnosed to accomplish both the diagnosis and treatment plan, work that is open to significant contestation. Thus, rather than leaving unproblematized the status of 'cancer' as an obvious and uncontested illness, in this chapter we argue that the legitimacy of this diagnosis is something that is *accomplished* through a reliance on a variety of technologies – technologies that are ultimately fallible, thus creating opportunities for contestation to emerge.

With this interest in the everyday accomplishment (see Garfinkel, 1967) of cancer care in mind, we talked with people who had been through that experience in the past and others who were in the midst of it. In our analysis of these accounts, our central interest has been to investigate how the 'identity work' (Alvesson, 2001; Knights & Willmott,

1999; Munro, 1996) involved in being someone diagnosed with cancer is accomplished in relation to the sorts of technological networks (see Latour, 2005) constituting contemporary cancer care. We heard from people who felt quite certain about their identities as people diagnosed with cancer: they had *seen* the cancer in the magnetic resonance imaging (MRI) scans ordered by their physicians. They underwent surgery that removed parts of their bodies that were later identified as cancerous tissues. In these accounts, cancer comes into focus in a way that may well be all too clear.

However, these moments of clarity are fleeting. People *organized their accounts* so as to culminate in these moments of clarity. But even then, what was to be done in response to the problem was rarely, if ever, clear. Treatments had to be *negotiated* – continuously. Trajectories had to be *monitored* – continuously. Identities had to be *formed and then re-formed* – continuously. People's accounts of their encounters with the cancer care system suggested that knowledge about what was happening to them was neither clear nor complete but was always in motion, frequently being revised. This experience runs against the standard view of cancer as something that can be detected, treated, and if not cured, at least managed as a chronic disease. We argue that if the disease were understood as one that is much more contentious, people engaging in the diagnostic process might have better opportunities to question and challenge the plans that are devised for them by health care professionals.

In this chapter we explore the linkages between knowledge, decision-making, identity, and power. Specifically, we follow a promising new path opened up by Rolland Munro (2004) in which he explores 'the demanding relation.' Munro (2004: 293) understands identity as 'being *punctualized*: a "revealing" of each specified identity within the here and now; and in response to the "demand" of others.' He argues that those making demands are required to be in a position to make a specific reading on identity, something he calls a 'positioning effect' (ibid.: 294). Physicians who convey a diagnosis of cancer 'demand' that the person told this news take up a particular identity, that of a person with cancer who responds with initial disbelief and then with pleas for help and cure. But in addition to this positioning effect, Munro argues that there is also a 'timing effect,' an effect that he claims is less understood. Here 'the "call" for a specific identity demands a display that annuls other "calls" – principally by overtaking these in the here and now' (ibid.). We suggest that, in the cancer centre, faced with a professional giving a diagnosis, patients must put aside all previous knowledge to respond to what the doctor has just said. This is the demanding relation. We draw on this concept to help explain the contentiousness of the diagnostic and treatment processes of cancer.

Using the accounts of the people with whom we spoke, we show how the work of cancer care is accomplished as if the diagnosis and treatment were straightforward and incontestable and also how negotiating treatment, monitoring trajectories, and forming and re-forming identities proceed as patients manage the many contested spaces they encounter. We then theorize these accounts as forms of identity work fuelled by *desires* about living a life, desires that are sculpted by skilled judgments of the *risks* associated with obtaining treatment for cancer.

Negotiating Treatment

People's stories of being diagnosed with cancer shared a basic structure. The story most often begins when either they or their physicians notice something out of the ordinary. Health care professionals offer reassurances: 'It's likely nothing at all but we should just check to rule anything out.' Then a series of often very confused, unhelpful encounters occur, usually involving numerous, often disconnected tests, many of which are painful. Finally, people experience an encounter where they receive news about the cancer.

Although the initial, well-rehearsed story is told in such a way that the person's agency in the events is diminished, people begin to re-tell the story, now with their agency much more evident. One of our participants, Debbie, said:

> I went in there fully expecting to be told it wasn't cancer, right, because nobody could find it. It was a shock, for sure. But I was fine, you know. I talked to the doctor for a couple of minutes, and realized that he honestly didn't have the kind of information that I needed.

Debbie's account underlines the manner in which her 'call' to the physician for information was perhaps annulled by other calls on his time – or his interests. She describes realizing within 'a couple of minutes' that she was not going to be able to get the sort of information she required from this physician.

Debbie's account illustrates how her identity is handed over to her. This handover happens, we argue, because the questions that Debbie has are not the sort the physician can, or wants to, answer. Debbie described knowing very precisely what she needed at that moment:

> What I wanted to know right at the point that he told me it was cancer is, 'What happens next and how long is it going to take? What kind of time frame is involved here?'

As we will see later, these questions persisted for Debbie throughout her treatment trajectory. They were never answered by health professionals. She had to generate her own answers to them on a moment-to-moment and treatment-to-treatment basis.

Diagnosis positions people to turn towards the professional ranks for advice, leading to advice-seeking encounters that people describe as very disappointing. Any interpretation of symptoms that might be generated by the patient and his or her family and friends (including interpretations that would set a very different course for living with cancer, for instance, living with it and not seeking treatment) are set aside in that moment of being 'called' to listen to what the physician says. Yet the questions that this information calls from the person diagnosed do not have the same demand on the physician. The physician does not, apparently, have to have answers to the questions that the person asks, questions such as: 'What's going to happen to me? How long will it take? What will it be like?' Within the cancer centre, the physician's task is not to answer such questions but rather to get the person on a treatment pathway.

This unexplicated division of labour is a source of great distress for people who are diagnosed with cancer. Debbie's account illustrates that, in her case, the oncologist was able to establish the demanding relation – positioning her to make a decision about treatment:

DEBBIE: I had to make a choice at that point. And I got as much information as I could about the sentinel node biopsy as opposed to the axillary dissection. And in the end, I chose to have the sentinel biopsy.

INTERVIEWER: Based on what?

DEBBIE: Based on, again, what I was being told by my health care professionals, about the size of the tumour, the type of the cancer that they felt it was and that in the end it would affect me less physically. And that's what I was looking at. I was trying, at that point, to look past the cancer to the outcome, right? 'Teeny, tiny little cancer, gonna be OK.' That's what I kept telling myself. That's what kept being affirmed. So I wanted ... I was looking past all of it and saying, 'OK, when it's all over and done with, I want to be back to my normal life as much as possible.' And again, like I said, I'm a very physical person. So I wanted to have as little physical involvement as possible.

Debbie described the basis of her decision to select one form of treatment over another. She was weighing up her risks (selecting a less invasive treatment to avoid long-term disability) against her desires (to return to a healthy life). At this early stage, she was moving forward on the basis of an anticipated short-term treatment regime. She relied on the information affirmed by the professionals: the cancer was very tiny, hardly perceptible at all.

Other people described their decision-making experience with professionals similarly – as though it was a strategy used by health care professionals to lock patients into the demanding relation imposed through the technologies of cancer treatment protocols. For instance, Melanie described having 'choices' set out in front of her regarding her treatment:

> I had a choice of two different ones [treatments], the CEF [a type of che-motherapy] and one other one. And the other one I believe was more of a newer one. And it would have, I think it would have been a shorter period. It was 4 months instead of the 6 months. And we went home, and we just didn't know what we were going to do. And both of them, you're going to lose your hair. Yeah, right. I just couldn't picture myself with no hair. And the CEF, you know, with every drug there's side effects. It's possible you'll have heart problems and possible of you getting, I think, leukaemia. Or something. But we chose to take it anyway because it was tried and true, and it was something that was going to work, and the other one I felt was more of a herbal thing. But I'm not sure. I can't remember exactly what it was. But in my mind, it wasn't strong enough to get rid of the cancer.

This excerpt illustrates how 'negotiation' operates in the cancer centre. Negotiation is not conducted between Melanie and her health care professional; instead treatment information is given to her at the cancer centre in the form of options, presented in relative terms: 'You can either take treatment A or treatment B. Treatment A will result in these things. Treatment B will result in these other things. Both are equally effective.' In the cancer centre, the choices made by patients when confronted with these sort of options are called 'decisions.' But that does not seem to adequately reflect what is going on. While treatments A and B are different, the results are the same. Apparently, it makes no difference which drug Melanie 'chooses.'

However, some negotiation does take place. Because *to her*, it does make a difference. The negotiation occurs with oneself and within the context of one's relationships, particularly personal relationships. In this instance, Melanie described taking home the information given to her by the doctor and, with her partner, working through the pros and cons of each treatment. For example, both drugs are going to involve a loss of hair. Even though she could not picture herself without hair, that item ended up being non-negotiable. Instead, for Melanie, it came down to a decision based on assessments of strength: her impression was that one of the drugs was 'a herbal thing,' and she did not believe it would be strong enough to get rid of the cancer. So, despite the fact that the CEF chemotherapy might cause heart problems and result in significant blood diseases (perhaps the very signs she was reading as signalling strength as a property of the treatment she chose), the strength of the CEF chemotherapy is a risk worth taking. She negotiated on the basis of potency and decided to accept the CEF treatment.

Both Debbie and Melanie based their negotiations on their desires – to maintain their physical strengths and abilities and to 'get rid of the cancer.' Both were confident that they were making their own decisions accordingly. Catherine Belsey (2002: 124) argues that 'a decision is prompted by circumstances.' Belsey reflects on the manner in which it can be said that in making decisions, individuals are positioned to take responsibility, that is, how responsibility is demanded of them: 'The decision is not in practice the outcome of the thought that led up to it, but it is always a matter of urgency … does it follow that decisions are properly, appropriately, or inevitably irresponsible? On the contrary, but they always involve a risk. To take responsibility is always to take a risk, precisely because a stance that is no more than the outcome of a prior knowledge cannot be seen as our own responsibility' (ibid.: 124–5).

It is interesting to note that neither Melanie nor Debbie took up the opportunity to make a decision about whether or not to believe the oncologist about where their part in the decision-making process lay: that is, choosing between treatment A and treatment B. Instead, Melanie and Debbie were positioned by the diagnosis to make so-called decisions about drugs that are 'the outcome of a prior knowledge' (Belsey, 2002: 125) for which they cannot take responsibility. The accounts of people who had experienced this situation suggest that they were positioned to make decisions about treatment without having 'all' of the information that they would have liked to have had – or indeed, could have had – to make a good decision. And the scope of their decision-making was often limited to 'choosing' one treatment over another. In the absence of 'all' the information, are the decisions made by these people irresponsible? We would argue they are not.

Negotiating treatment in this context demands responsibility of people diagnosed with cancer. But it would be incorrect to think that their responsibility is in relation to the 'choices' that they make. In engaging in these decision-making practices people are being made responsible for the risks associated with treatment. There is no security in any of these treatments – there is only the willingness of people to take responsibility for the risk of what is offered by the professionals.

In these small moments we see opportunities to contest the purely scientific, professional version of cancer care espoused at the cancer centre. In so doing, we need to consider the relationships operating between decisions and identity. At the cancer centre, the risks (see Douglas, 1992; van Loon, 2002) entailed by positioning oneself to respond to the demand to make decisions arise through everyday professional practice that supports the enrolment of people into patient identities. A large part of this identity is that patients will make decisions about treatments that place them at significant risk.

Monitoring Trajectories

Debbie structured her story in such a way that a more menacing outcome always seemed to be just around the corner. She wanted as little 'physical involvement' as possible so she could get back to her 'normal life.' She recalled making her decision about treatment based on the size of the tumour, the type of cancer they felt it was, and the physical effects of the options – all information given to her by her health care professionals. However, in Debbie's account, there was already a foreshadowing of new, conflicting information that would arise later, and indeed, it did. Debbie explained:

> [The doctor] told my family that they thought they'd got it all. That it was quite a lot bigger than they thought. There were actually two tumours side by side. One was what's called VCIS [a type of breast cancer] which is inside a milk duct and fairly contained. It was 5 centimetres. Then there

was another one beside it that was 2.5 centimetres. And it was an invasive cancer. So they removed that, he took it … so that's quite a sizeable piece of tissue that he took out. But he took out a 1.5 centimetre margin around both of them and sent it off to pathology and told my family that as far as he could tell he'd got everything.

We previously noted that Debbie described making 'good' decisions based on the information that was given to her at the time. In light of this new information, it may not have been such a good idea to have had the localized surgery. Having gone in to remove one 'teeny' tumour, the surgeon was apparently confronted with two tumours. One was larger than what was anticipated but was 'contained'; the other was only half as big, but 'an invasive cancer.' Again the story foreshadows more bad news ahead: 'he took out a 1.5 centimetre margin around both of them and sent it off to pathology and told my family that as far as he could tell, he'd got everything.'

Within a week the pathology report came back and indeed the edges of the tissue were not clear of cancerous tissue. More surgery would be required. Unlike before, the surgeon now became more directive: she 'was very firm this time on having the axillary dissection with the tumours being the size they were.' It seems that under these circumstances, Debbie no longer gets to 'choose' her treatment. Now the treatment decisions are removed from her and taken over by the oncologist. We speculate that, having responded to the demand to 'choose' at the time of initial diagnosis, people are now sufficiently implicated in these outcomes that it is no longer necessary for professionals to demand that they continue to make further decisions. They are already committed to the treatment pathway. Hooking people onto this treatment pathway seems the more compelling reason to demand that they become involved in decision-making.

Despite the demands to accept the flow of treatment as it is shaped by the powerful interests fuelling treatment pathways at the cancer centre, Debbie continued to frame her experience as being manageable within discrete periods of time. She said:

Each part of my treatment was to say, it's temporary. OK. This is how long this is going to take, right? Chemotherapy is going to take me 4 months. OK, I might be horribly ill for 4 months, but it's only 4 months. I can do that. If I have to I can put it on a calendar and mark it off day by day. If that's what I have to do. But I can do 4 months. This isn't something that's going to be for the rest of my life. I have a friend with Parkinson's disease. She's going to have that for the rest of her life. She's going to get progressively worse for the rest of her life. That's not happening to me. What's happening to me is I'm going to be horribly ill for 4 months. Four months, OK, I can do 4 months.

Debbie started out negotiating her treatment against the long-term outcome she desired: a return to normal strength and agility. However, at this stage in her treatment, her horizon has shortened considerably. Now she is just seeking to get through the next 4 months. She may be 'horribly ill' for 4 months but she expresses her belief that she is not going to get progressively worse as is her friend who has been diagnosed with Parkinson's disease.

This shortening of horizons is significant. For us, it signals the work Debbie engaged in as she created her own answers to the questions she asked of the oncologist who gave her the diagnosis in the first place. Her interest in knowing how long all this was going to take and what it was going to be like for her had still not been answered. And they were clearly still very important to her as she negotiated the uncertainty and risks that treatment represented to her.

The lack of certainty introduced through the diagnostic process was simply too much to enable Debbie to sustain a long-term vision of the integrity of the self. As Debbie's account suggests, integrity of the self can be sustained for the duration of a regime of chemotherapy. If the chemotherapy is going to last 4 months, the marker of success becomes 'doing 4 months.' She searched for a terrain that is solid on which to locate herself and plan her life – for the short term, since the long term had been proven unpredictable. Debbie landed on terrain that *she* rendered less disputable, more predictable, if even for just a short period of time.

Despite being surrounded by professionals, drugs, machines, laboratory tests, and so on, being a cancer patient is ultimately a solitary experience. The technologies of tests and their interpreted results position people to confront a new version of themselves – as a self with cancer – and before they can take time to understand what that might mean, they are invited to make 'choices' that set them onto a treatment pathway that concretizes their relationship with health care providers in such a way that any contestation over the meaning of the diagnosis is deflected, deferred, set aside.

At this juncture, we return for a moment to Munro's (2004) interest in both the positioning and the timing effects of the demanding relation. It is our argument that the cancer diagnosis has a *positioning effect* which means that the person turns towards the cancer specialists for help. But there are *timing effects* here, too. The cancer specialists are able to deflect all questions regarding what the patient can expect – either in terms of long-range planning or in terms of immediate advice about how to proceed. The patient is not able to deflect the need to have these questions answered. As long as the person/ patient is 'hooked' on and by the diagnosis, she or he will continue to heed the call of the cancer experts, taking up the identity of a 'lucky' cancer patient one moment (i.e., one who has a small, contained cancer that is easily removed) and then changing stride by becoming the 'unlucky' cancer patient next (i.e., one who, upon further evidence, now must heed the demands of an invasive cancer). None of this is routine. Programs cannot be designed to ease the person's transition through the treatment pathway. What can be acknowledged, however, are the *demanding relations* within which people diagnosed with cancer operate – and the implications, in terms of identity work, necessitated by these particular forms of professional practice.

Identities Forming – and Re-forming

Cancer is uncertain and ever-changing. Experiences with the cancer clinic and its array of technologies that seek to pin the cancer down illustrate that this task is much more elusive than official narratives would suggest. It is left to patients to create certainty and, in so doing, to continuously re-form their identity as individuals living with (a form of) cancer. For instance, one of our interviewees, Gerry, described the process of being diagnosed as feeling as though a wall had come down – perhaps a reference to the drawing in of the horizon within which she was going to do her thinking and planning for a life beyond cancer:

> I was doing it on my own. Absolutely on my own. And, and … how I did it I think I just … a wall down, a sort of wall came down the minute I found out I had cancer. And I said, 'Okay. You're now in a fight for your life. Everything else has just got to go to the side and you had better just be focused.'

Gerry recalled coming across a note she had written years earlier to a friend diagnosed with cancer in which she had said to her friend that if she, Gerry, was ever diagnosed with cancer, she would refuse treatment. She expressed some surprise to realize that when she was actually faced with the situation, she responded quite differently than she had predicted. As noted above, Gerry conceived of herself as being in a 'fight for [her] life.' Even as she progressed through a number of treatments including surgery, chemotherapy, and radiation therapy, and especially as each of those came to have very particular meaning for her, she maintained the 'focus' she described above. She said:

> The more I understood what oncology, what chemo meant, what radiation ... the more I realized I really was going to be fried. And virtually butchered. But, I thought 'I've got to do this. I've got to survive.'

It became clear to us that after people had committed to a negotiated regime of treatment, their expectations about their ability to move past the cancer narrowed radically. Rather than continuing to rely on a vision of a future free of cancer, people began thinking in terms of just getting through treatment. Here, the length of time for chemotherapy or radiation becomes important in terms of stabilizing the time frame within which a form of 'survival' has to be monitored and maintained. The expectation within each of these treatment trajectories is that at the end of it, the person can again begin to anticipate a future without cancer. But as we have seen, just as the edges of a tumour may not be clean, neither may the edges of these treatment trajectories be all that clean. Second rounds of chemotherapy are ordered on the basis of the 'failure' of the person to respond to the treatment as expected. Experiences of extreme exhaustion following a round of radiation therapy pull people who seek release from the disease and its treatment down into fatigue from which they wonder if they will ever recover. Debbie's account reveals an ever-changing diagnosis requiring ever-changing treatment that caused her to adapt constantly to a new reality with different expectations. Rather than the cancer demanding a response, the cancer patient experiences the demands of professionals and treatments – each of which demands a revised identity.

Another participant, Sherry, described a similarly difficult process of diagnosis and treatment – but with very different results. For Sherry, an initial biopsy had shown evidence of cancer. A decision was made that she would have a lumpectomy. The pathology report from that initial surgical event revealed that only normal breast tissue had been removed – no cancerous tissue was found. She described her reaction:

> I read it and it says that they've removed normal breast tissue, healthy normal breast tissue. And I never read pathology reports before but I thought, 'Well that's strange. What happened to this cancer that was in me?'

This event left Sherry very confused. In an effort to gain resolution relating to her identity as a person with cancer, she agreed to have a second lumpectomy. This procedure, too, resulted in a second pathology report of 'normal breast tissue.' Interestingly, at the time we spoke with her, her medical treatment team were urging her to continue with radiation and chemotherapy *as though* she were a person with breast cancer.

INTERVIEWER: You mentioned something about radiation. So are you going, did you go for radiation?

SHERRY: Well, the protocol was always once the tissue was removed then they can test it for ER, estrogen receptors, and all these wonderful things, and to find out what your protocol was. But if they don't have the tissue, if they don't have the carcinoma in the tissue, then you're again left in limbo. And that's where I've been all this time because they haven't had the pathology that meets the diagnosis ... I'm no farther ahead. Like, what am I supposed to be doing? ... The [neighbouring city] group are saying for me to just go straight on to Tamoxifen, and the oncologist here is saying I should have radiation. And I said, 'Well, what are we radiating? If you can't take the tissue out, if the tumour isn't out, what are we, you know, is it in there, is it not in there?' And he just, he says, 'It's protocol with a lumpectomy.'

The advice given to Sherry was founded on a research-based protocol outlining the recommended treatment for an ideal outcome. Presumably based on evidence, the protocol clearly states that radiation follows a lumpectomy. Having taken the initial decision, the responsibility and risk of having the first lumpectomy, her identity was now tied in a demanding relation to her treatment. Although the diagnosis was not clear, she felt that demand. She took steps to form an identity of a cancer patient for whom a protocol must be followed. The reliance on a 'protocol' in the absence of evidence of cancer was as disconcerting to her as it might well be to many who would take the objectivist claims of science to heart. Sherry described being left 'in limbo.' Her identity as a cancer patient remained open and all too questionable.

The risks involved in this account are multiple and layered. Presumably, the protocol is intended to reduce the risk of cancer returning; if Sherry does not follow standard procedure, is she taking a risk? If she does not follow the advice of many well-researched studies by experts, is she taking another kind if risk? Is she taking a risk by following the advice of these experts?

Sherry's reluctance to follow the advice of the medical experts arose out of an assessment of the risks of proceeding with treatment. The risks here are not just those associated with choosing properly – although, given the range of options, one could be forgiven for thinking that patients actually have a choice. The risks are also about getting hooked into the demanding relation and thereby becoming subject to the regimes implied by a cancer diagnosis.

As with so many of the people we spoke with, Sherry lived her life as though she were in control of her decisions – until such time as technology, in the form of a biopsy, intervened and she received a diagnosis of cancer. From that moment, she was 'on call' to be a cancer patient and one who, despite evidence to the contrary, was asked to open herself to a wide array of additional cancer treatment technologies that can be demanded by this newly transformed 'doctor-patient relationship.' Munro (2004: 297) argues that it is within the effects of technology to change the scope and nature of the demand. Not just any response will do: 'Technology is a revealing that "orders" as it expedites' (ibid.). The transformation of Sherry's identity from that of a healthy woman to that of a cancer patient was swift. The technologies of professional knowledge, biopsies, surgeries, and pathology reports all contributed to the transformation. With each deployment of technology, Sherry's identity underwent an ordering that evidence to the contrary (i.e., clean pathology reports) could not disrupt. Instead, a more persuasive technology, that of 'the protocol,' had already established a path that demanded Sherry's action.

Reflecting on Risk and Desire

Having negotiated treatment against a preferred future, the people we spoke with then described a need to draw in and closely monitor treatment trajectories, all the while seeking ways of forming and re-forming their identity as individuals who would get through the physical and emotional assaults inherent in cancer treatment. It is our contention that 'successful' cancer care is achieved by enrolling (Latour, 1987) people at a particular point in the illness trajectory – namely, at the outset when their *desire* to turn this situation around is very strong – to take responsibility for their decisions. Taking such responsibility always involves risk (Belsey, 2002). Positioned in this way, people are ready to respond to the demanding relations of cancer care.

One of the things that surprised us most in our research was that, despite reservations about its potential effectiveness or appropriateness, people agreed to undergo – or returned to – recommended treatment and then, in the face of the effects[2] of that treatment, continued with it. Many people remembered the diagnosis phase as a time of con-siderable shock, a terrible event that set in motion a series of meetings with professionals. The discussions at these meetings were often described as being well out of step with the enormity of what the per-son was feeling and experiencing.

When a person becomes suspicious that a lump may be cancerous, or is told during a routine check-up that something asymptomatic may be cancerous, the desire is to seek the security of knowledge in those locations where experts reside and, in doing so, the person enters the risk-laden system of cancer treatment. Once people have entered the cancer treatment 'system,' they discover *limitations* to the questions that can be raised about choices. The demanding relation (Munro, 2004) positions them to fulfil the requirements of the protocol rather than question it, or even ask questions about it.

Because the *diagnosis* of cancer organizes and expedites a series of events that generates its own risks that cannot be controlled or ordered by oneself, and are quite apart from those embedded in cancer as a dis-ease process, it is risky. People negotiate treatments through a compli-cated set of calculations about how they desire to live their lives. These negotiations rely on information from professionals about the nature of the cancer as well as the number and type of treatments available. They are also made in the context of life now with – but also outside of – cancer: Can I imagine myself without hair? Am I prepared to risk developing heart disease? If I take this treatment, will the cancer go away? If that one doesn't work, will this next one work?

Some people described receiving clear information but the rele-vance of that information kept changing. As a result, they felt that their good decisions about treatment – negotiated within the terms of their expectations about their life, as it would now be expected to proceed – were being undermined by the shifting context for deci-sion-making. Others described being cast adrift by professionals who conveyed information but failed to connect that information with implications for living through the diagnosis and treatment and, in fact, beyond. This gap left people grasping for information from those they deemed to be expert in other ways, to help negotiate their way through decisions about treatments that were being demanded of them at times of great uncertainty.

Our analysis in this chapter raises important questions about the ethics of conventional understandings of 'successful cancer care.' The analysis arises out of typical accounts of cancer care. Most surprising to us was that, despite a range of different experiences, there was a consistency in the accounts of people responding to the relation demanded of them by institutionalized processes of cancer treatment. In light of what turns out to be a much more contentious disease process than what most professionals acknowledge, we would like to suggest that ethical practice might create more, rather than fewer, opportunities during the treatment trajectory for people to re-assess their commitment to the forms of treatment on offer. We recognize the challenge this poses for forms of 'advanced' health care such as cancer treatment. So much emphasis, and indeed hope, is placed on the technologies of testing, diagnosis, and treatment. Our analysis illustrates how difficult it is to raise questions about any of this when the pathway already organizes and expedites ahead of itself.

But the questions do not disappear. Rather, people are left to answer these questions largely on their own, and often at a time when making 'alternative' choices has to be done in opposition to conventional advice – rather than at the outset when concern for the person might be better demonstrated by coming along beside and walking through the uncertainty together.

Acknowledgments

Our first thank you goes to the women and men who participated so generously in our study. We acknowledge the Social Sciences and Humanities Research Council for funding the Capacity and Continuity in Cancer Care Research Project. Maxime Alfort, Carl May, Kathy Teghtsoonian and Pamela Moss for the opportunity to put these thoughts into words and for their judicious feedback on this chapter.

NOTES

1 We use this language intentionally. As Susan Sontag (1978) noted in her classic work, *Illness as Metaphor*, cancer represents the quintessential case of an illness that has been bound up in militaristic metaphor. Those who succumb to the disease are said to have 'lost their battle,' often 'after a long struggle' with cancer. Those who undergo treatment are said to have 'fought back' against the cancer. Interestingly, given our interest in the events surrounding diagnosis, military metaphors were heard less frequently in our interviews. Rather, as will be revealed, people created understandings about their illness through use of spatial metaphors: a disease that was 'right in their face,' or accepting treatment in order to keep the 'horizon' of good health (their health prior to diagnosis) in sight.

2 Many of the participants in this study described the treatments for cancer as being worse than the disease itself. Of course, to the extent that treatment alters the course of the disease, this is a challenging statement for practitioners (and researchers) to respond to. We believe that practitioners do have access to information about how a range of patients have responded to various treatments and we would advocate that much more explicit descriptions be offered to patients as part of the process of obtaining 'informed consent.'

REFERENCES

Alvesson, Mats. (2001). Knowledge work: Ambiguity, image and identity. *Human Relations, 54*, 863-886.

Bailey, R.K., Geyen, D.J., Scott-Gurnell, K., Hipolito, M.M.S., Bailey, T.A., & Beal, J.M. (2005). Understanding and treating depression among cancer patients. *International Journal of Gynecological Cancer, 15*, 203-208.

Belsey, Catherine. (2002). *Critical practice* (2nd ed.). New York and London: Routledge.

Bradley, Patricia. (2005). The delay and worry experience of African American women with breast cancer. *Oncology Nursing Forum, 32*, 243-249.

Douglas, Mary. (1992). *Risk and blame: Essays in cultural theory.* New York and London: Routledge.

Garfinkel, Harold. (1967). *Studies in ethnomethodology.* Englewood Cliffs, NJ: Prentice-Hall.

Knights, David, & Willmott, Hugh. (1999). *Management lives: Power and identity in work organizations.* London: Sage.

Latour, Bruno. (1987). *Science in action: How to follow scientists and engineers through society.* Milton Keynes, U.K.: Open University Press.

Latour, Bruno. (2005). *Reassembling the social: An introduction to actor-network theory.* New York and Oxford: Oxford University Press.

Mathieson, Cynthia, & Stam, Henderikus. (1995). Renegotiating identity: Cancer narratives. *Sociology of Health and Illness, 17*, 283-306.

Munro, Rolland. (1996). Alignment and identity work: The study of accounts and accountability. In Rolland Munro & Jan Mouritsen (Eds.), *Accountability: Power, ethos and the technologies of managing* (pp. 1–19). London: Thomson International Business Press.

Munro, Rolland. (2004). Punctualizing identity: Time and the demanding relation. *Sociology, 38*, 293-311.

Sontag, Susan. (1978). *Illness as metaphor.* Toronto: McGraw-Hill Ryerson.

van Loon, Joost. (2002). *Risk and technological culture: Towards a sociology of virulence.* New York and London: Routledge.

9 Edging Embodiment and Embodying Categories: Reading Bodies Marked with Myalgic Encephalomyelitis as a Contested Illness

PAMELA MOSS

Arguably the most compelling mechanism for defining ill bodies within biomedical practice is diagnosis. Despite attempts to put into place practices that are reproducible over time and across space by professionals working within a biomedicine paradigm, the practice of diagnosis is greatly influenced – to the extent of being constituted – by the social relations embedded within the relationships of those engaging with medicalized knowledge. The people and practices comprising sites of health care provision, health and medical financing, workplaces, and home environments use various and multiple discourses to make sense of medicalized knowledge, expressed in a diagnosis, to describe an ill body. In this sense, diagnosis is, in itself, a social construct, a category full of meaning derived from multiple practices within biomedicine including, for example, observation, self-report, clinical tests, and interpretation.

Interpretation is by far the most flexible aspect of diagnosis, and it is also the most sensitive to shifts in cultural and social understandings of medicalized knowledge. Interpretation within diagnosis is my entry point in attempting to understand how to read bodies that have been marked with contested illness. Because of their precision in delineating a specific set of symptoms that respond to a prescribed range of particular treatments, some diagnoses have settled understandings as conventional, straightforward, regular, and even 'normal,' and are widely accepted as legitimate illness. Other diagnoses, especially those rooted in varying sets of diffuse, roaming, fluctuating, and migratory symptoms, are unsettled and contested within both biomedicine and social relationships.

Most literatures addressing individual and collective experiences of disease processes differentiate between disease and illness, noting that disease is the material, physiological, or pathological process affecting material bodies and illness is the experience of these symptoms by individuals (e.g., Kleinman, 1988). However, I conflate the boundary between the two purposefully, to get at the interpretive aspect of the constitution of illness. In no way do I want to perpetuate the notion that disease is solely located within the *materiality* of the body, just as I do not want to suggest that illness is merely the *experience* of the material body. The premise upon which I offer this reading is that the discursive and the material are entwined and can only be usefully distinguished conceptually. I use 'ill bodies' as a way to challenge the pervasiveness of medicalized knowledge in determining categories of disease and illness and in the words used to describe pain, fatigue, and other bodily sensations that come to be known as symptoms. Interpretation is a practice located squarely within multiple sets of social relations, and is itself constituted by and constitutive of what and how ill bodies are read, experienced, and defined.

In this chapter, I offer a reading of ill bodies marked with a specific contested illness: Myalgic Encephalomyelitis (ME). I draw on feminist theories of embodiment to make my case that diagnosis as a construct, as currently understood, carries with it both material and discursive effects of ill bodies, and that embodiment as a concept can be re-edged to think through the connections between diagnosis and ill bodies. I then turn to stories of diagnosis as told to me by women who are ill with constellations of symptoms that have variously come to be known as ME in both Ireland and British Columbia, Canada, and the corresponding sets of criteria used to diagnose ME. I close with a short discussion as to why reading ill bodies matters in the context of understanding contested illness.

Siting Medicalized Knowledge in Ill Bodies

Myalgic Encephalomyelitis is but one diagnostic category used to describe ill bodies. ME is claimed to be a disease by some support groups, court decisions, and research groups; and it is constitutive of ill bodies in particular places (see Bülow, Chapter 7, this volume). Several working definitions and diagnostic protocols exist that define ME as a category of disease – some complementary, some contradictory. Because both the identifying features of the constellation of symptoms forming an ill body with ME and the parameters of the distinguishing characteristics defining ME in the practice of diagnosis fluctuate, the interpretations of the illness, disease, and ill body are up for grabs. The uncertainty of both the ill body and the diagnostic category provides ample terrain upon which cultural and social groups and institutions can struggle over medicalized knowledge that informs debates over ME, whether within or outside biomedicine. For example, the World Health Organization in their international classification of disease (1996) categorizes Benign Myalgic Encephalomyelitis (a term not often used since the 1970s) under the general heading of 'Disorders of the Nervous System' (G00-99), the sub-heading 'Other Disorders of the Brain' (G93), and under the specific heading of 'Post-viral Fatigue Syndrome' (G93.3), a more contemporary term used to describe long-lasting fatigue after a viral infection. Chronic Fatigue Syndrome (CFS), a term often used interchangeably with ME in research, clinical, and vernacular settings, is categorized under the heading of 'Symptoms, Signs and Abnormal Clinical and Laboratory Findings, Not Elsewhere Classified' (R00-R99), the sub-heading of 'General Symptoms and Signs' (R50-R69), and under the specific heading of 'Chronic Fatigue, Unspecified' (R53.82).[1] In Canada, one of the arenas within which the debate over defining ME has emerged is through court cases involving persons claiming disability benefits from long-term disability insurance underwriters through the workplace.[2] There are also groups that deal directly with medical and health research. For example, Co-Cure: ME/CFS and Fibromyalgia maintains an archive of research articles relating to ME and Fibromyalgia, and acts as a national U.S. support and advocacy group.[3] MERGE (Myalgic Encephalomyelitis Research Group for Education and Support) is a charity that raises funds to support biomedical research on ME. One of MERGE's central goals is to further refine ME as a diagnostic category so as to differentiate the disease process of ME from other syndromes with similar sets of symptoms.[4] In Ireland and the United Kingdom, several support and advocacy groups exist that have divergent views as to what ME is and how it is to be treated.[5] Within these milieus, ill bodies with ME emerge, take on, and carry with them the specifics of these struggles and debates. The multiple framings of ME as a diagnostic category in these various venues create opportunities to both challenge and support the authority of medicalized knowledge as it is drawn upon to assign diagnoses, firm up boundaries of disease categories, and 'fix' ill bodies through treatment regimes.

Edging Embodiment

Embodiment as a concept is a popular way to incorporate fleshed ways of being, knowing, and acting into theories of gender, sexual difference, and subjectivity (e.g., Butler, 1993; Diprose, 1994; McLaren, 2002). Within feminist engagements of the body, embodiment takes several meanings, ranging from descriptions of processes through which selves become lived bodies (e.g., Benhabib, 1992; Eckermann, 1997; Grosz, 1994), through explanations of the constitution of knowledge and its applications (e.g., Birke, 2000; Sawicki, 1991), to accounts of how sets of activities that people engage in are carried out through bodies themselves (e.g., Baylis, Downie, & Sherwin, 1999; Leslie & Butz, 1998), sometimes literally (Scheper-Hughes, 2005). The extensive and ongoing work about embodiment in various contexts speaks to the copious possibilities that such a concept offers to understandings of society, polity, and culture (e.g., on social movements, see Brown et al., 2004; Zavestoski, McCormick, & Brown, 2004; on citizenship, see Bacchi & Beasley, 2002; on sexual difference, see Braidotti, 2003). In most of these accounts, the authors use embodiment in order to make sense of the body (or some aspect of the body) as a *discursive construction* (e.g., Conboy, Medina, & Stanbury, 1997), its *materiality* (e.g., Shildrick & Price, 1998), or some combination of both (e.g., Williams & Bendelow, 1998).

Such a multipronged and comprehensive conceptual scene for embodiment facilitates its usefulness in finding a way to read bodies marked with ME as a contested illness. Working with a concept of embodiment that addresses both discourse and materiality makes sense given that ME is both discursive (with competing definitions, diagnostic protocols, and treatment regimes) and material (uncertainty over the presence of an ill body in light of fluctuating, migratory, and sometimes fleeting bodily sensations). I understand embodiment as 'those *lived* spaces where bodies are located conceptually and corporeally, metaphorically and concretely, discursively and materially, being simultaneously part of bodily forms and their social constructions' (Moss & Dyck, 2002: 49). These spaces are where the *specifics* of any one body or sets of bodies are momentarily *fixed* as bodies, replete with identities, subjectivities, and power as well as senses, content, and expression.[6] Here, embodiment denotes a particular arrangement and deployment of social relations constitutive, discursively and materially, of that which is experience, fixed long enough and strong enough to be able to claim some *specificity* (or at least the illusion of specificity) as a context-dependent sensation, feeling, or act.

Because embodiment deals with the *specificity* of bodies, the relationship between the body and any particular topic under investigation is usually problematized.[7] Even so, the flesh of bodies is still paramount in either the overarching goal of the project or the topic matter (see Bray & Colebrook, 1998; Breckenridge & Vogler, 2001; Davidson, 2003; Duden, 1991; Shildrick & Price, 1996). Other types of problematizations are important because they point to the fraying of the edges bounding embodiment directly to bodies. In discussions about embodiment, for example, Michel Foucault, in both *Discipline and Punish* (1979) and *The History of Sexuality, Volume 1* (1990), maintains that the body is the condition of subjectivity, not its site. Judith Butler (1990) argues that gender as a differentiating category comes alive and is sustained through repetitive acts of bodies that constitute and define what that differentiation is. And Seyla Benhabib (1992), in her discussion of the generalized and the concrete Other, notes that a mode of one's being in a body feeds an identity based on sexual difference, and it is through negotiating the spaces between inscriptions that concrete identities emerge. But what if embodiment addressed things that are not bodies? What if embodiment were re-edged so as to risk critical engagement with discursive constructs and material entities other than the body – in an embodied way?

Diagnosis may offer terrain on which to take up such a project. As an obvious link between the fleshed body and biomedical discourse, diagnosis appears to be an excellent example of embodiment. As practice, diagnosis entails a physician assigning a name to a constellation of symptoms, thereby identifying a disease process. To be sure, diagnosis is a complicated process of matching up new information about a particular body with already observed empirical patterns of experience of symptoms and of numerical representations of bodily functions. As inscription, diagnosis marks a concrete body with an idealized notion of a specific type of ill body. A body in turn carries this inscription as a marker of a *specific* illness or disease – sometimes knowingly through dialogue or types of interaction, sometimes unknowingly through the actions (and inactions) of others. As descriptor, diagnosis captures a particular depiction of a body, or a group of bodies, that appear to be ill or that respond to treatment and interventions in the same or similar ways.[8] Yet this rendition of diagnosis does not readily fit my notion of embodiment as lived spaces. Although based on material aspects of the body, diagnosis in these readings actually eclipses the materialized ill body because once attached to a specific body, the category itself becomes more important in defining the body as ill than the ill body (Moss & Dyck, 1999). The extensive utilization of the diagnostic category in other authoritative contexts (e.g., benefits assessment, return to work policies) normalizes particular features of the defining criteria, which may or may not coincide with medical uses of a specific diagnostic category, that then gives rise to yet another idealized ill body. As a result, it seems that conceptually I cannot access those lived spaces unless I go directly through *specific* materialized ill bodies. I wonder, however, if there is a way to edge embodiment so that I can. Two strategies jump immediately to mind. The first involves employing body concepts that do not necessarily address bodies per se. The second draws on attempts to reconceptualize a notion or idea while stripping it of the contexts within which it arose.

First, a concept that does not refer only and necessarily to bodies is Gilles Deleuze's and Félix Guatarri's (1987: 149–156) notion of *body without organs* (BwO). A BwO can be contrasted to an organized body, one that is structured, disciplined, and regulated into conformity, orthodoxy, and normativity. A BwO is one that is non-stratified, fuelled by desire, and unruly in such a way as to be self-destructive without being suicidal, meaningless without being nihilistic, and undifferentiated without being formless. A BwO is, in effect, a limit, a limit of dismantling that which holds an organism together. As examples of BwO, Deleuze and Guattari (1987) describe a hypochondriac body that sloughs off organs into non-existence and a masochist body that desires pain. As a description of a set of social relations, BwO could be used to describe political groups that could either be totalitarian or egalitarian, hierarchical or democratic, tightly controlled or loosely affiliated. In the context of diagnosis, BwO could be used to make sense of how biomedical interpretations of bodies (via empirical observations) get organized without having to use experience of illness as a starting point for analysis. So, to access embodiment as lived spaces, it might be useful to figure out what characterizations of ill bodies biomedical researchers are dumping into the diagnostic category of ME and then map where these characterizations emerge and how they shift over time.

Second, Jana Sawicki (2004) offers a reconceptualization of queer politics. She reads Foucault's work as an attempt to re-site queer politics away from integrating individual expressions of homosexuality into the legal fabric of society, towards re-articulating the body in ways that challenge the predominant regime of sexuality, one that reduces sexuality to innate desire. She argues that by creating new cultural forms that challenge dominant cultural understandings of sexuality, other aspects of queerness can be highlighted including, for example, new forms of erotic and intimate relationships (2004: 171), self-understanding as a sexual being (ibid.: 178), and form of life (ibid.: 179). By taking a concept out of the context within which it emerges, Sawicki's desexualization of queer politics opens up possibilities of self-making and community formation. Her arguments are interesting when applied within the context of reading bodies marked with contested illness because they place into question the necessity of directly dealing with bodies when using the concept of embodiment.[9]

Untying the truth-correspondence between the materiality of the body and the application of a specific discursive category to an ill body frees one up to: (1) examine the internal links between the material aspects of ill bodies and their representation without being forced to look only at the resonant equivalence between a discursive category and its object (i.e., binding diagnostic criteria to a disease process), and (2) discuss stories about diagnosis without being forced to make the claim that women are not being diagnosed properly (i.e., matching up a disease process with an ill body). Practically, this may not be a good choice because the health care system relies almost exclusively on diagnosis. Politically, this may not be a good choice because many ME activist and support groups locate themselves as watchdogs and advocates for people diagnosed with ME. Conceptually, however, this is a good choice because one can (re-)enter the discussion about diagnosis free of the encumbrances of the need for correlation between diagnostic description and bodily sensations, or between diagnosis and ill bodies, and still remain embodied. Dispensing with these encumbrances does not counter the claim that embodiment is simultaneously discursive and material; rather, loosening the conceptual stitching between the particular use of a discursive category and its application to specific ill bodies makes room for more clarity around how discourse and materiality exist and how they are called upon to define ill bodies.

Data from Two Studies

To be able to work with this re-edged notion of embodiment in an empirical context, I draw on two data sets: a handful of personal histories of women diagnosed with ME, and four sets of diagnostic and treatment protocols for ME. The first data set includes interviews with women in Ireland and British Columbia, Canada. The interviews in both places were similarly structured, focusing on diagnosis and everyday life while living with ME. Interviews included 19 women from Ireland and 25 women from British Columbia in two different time periods.[10] For this chapter, I present stories from four interviews – Elizabeth and Siobhan from Ireland, and Erin and Sandra from British Columbia. Although I present these stories as backdrops to my reading of bodies marked with contested illness, these stories are central to my understanding of how embodiment actually works in everyday life.

The second data set includes four sets of defining criteria for ME that came into play for the women I talked with in Ireland and British Columbia: the Ramsay definition (Ramsay, 1988), the London Criteria (Dowset et al., 1994), the Centers for Disease Control and Prevention (CDC) definition (Fukuda et al., 1994; see also CDC, 2006), and the Canadian Criteria (Carruthers et al., 2003); see Table 9.1 for a brief description of each set of criteria. In Ireland, physicians primarily used the Ramsay definition and the London Criteria to render a diagnosis of ME during the time of my interviews. On a few occasions, the Irish women in my study mentioned the CDC definition being used in their own diagnosis. In British Columbia, the CDC definition was the only set of criteria consistently used for diagnosis. I include a discussion of the Canadian Criteria, although published several years after my interviews with women in British Columbia, because the women were part of the same context within which the working clinical definition of these criteria emerged.[11]

Living from Experience

At the onset of symptoms, Elizabeth, in her late 20s, was incredibly fit and active in a wide range of athletic activities – tennis, cricket, hockey, orienteering, badminton, canoeing. She had established herself in her job and was in a stable relationship. She pinpointed onset to a hamstring injury: 'But it is just when I pulled my hamstring I knew instinctively that I had pulled something way up through my body, I knew it wasn't just my hamstring.' After the injury, she was never able to concentrate quite right, her energy was off, she wasn't up to walking; after work she would sit at home in a chair immobilized, and she started getting sick in different ways with stomach problems and bad headaches. She felt isolated and disconnected. She was diagnosed fairly quickly, but, as she put it, made a mistake by not reading up on ME for

Table 9.1
Four sets of defining criteria for Myalgic Encephalomyelitis

Defining criteria	Primary manifestations	Other manifestations used as part of diagnosis	Other defining criteria
Ramsay (Ramsay, 1988)	• Muscular phenomena • Circulatory impairment • Cerebral dysfunction		• Using the wrong words • Alteration to sleep rhythm or vivid dreams • Frequency of micturition • Hyperacuisis • Episodic sweating • Orthostatic tachycardia
London Criteria (Dowset et al., 1994)	• Exercise-induced fatigue after trivially small exertion • Memory impairment and loss of concentration with other neurological and psychological disturbances • Fluctuation of symptoms	• Usually follows an infection	
CDC http://www.cdc.gov/ncidod/diseases/cfs/about/what.htm (Fukada et al., 1994, as an update to Holmes et al., 1988)	• Severe fatigue for 6 months or longer	Four of the following: • Short-term memory or concentration impairment • Sore throat • Tender lymph nodes • Muscle pain • Multi-joint pain without redness or swelling • Headaches of new type, pattern, or severity • Unrefreshing sleep • Post-exertional malaise lasting more than 24 hours	

Table 9.1
Four sets of defining criteria for Myalgic Encephalomyelitis *(Continued)*

Canadian Criteria (Carruthers et al., 2003)	• Fatigue • Post-exertional malaise and/or fatigue • Sleep dysfunction • Pain	• Two symptoms of neurological/ cognitive manifestations • One symptom from two of three categories: – Autonomic – Neuroendocrine – Immune	• Onset usually sudden, but can be gradual • 6 months of illness for adults and 3 months for children

her own information. She continued to work 5 days a week. After a few weeks, she collapsed. When she was feeling a bit better after several months, she was able to organize her paid work from home and now works the equivalent of about 3 days a week. In addition to forms of body and energy work, she exclusively uses alternative remedies for self-treatment.

Siobhan lived across the country, away from her family, when she became quite ill. Her doctor diagnosed depression and treated her with antidepressants, but her symptoms persisted. She would feel better, and then get sick all over again. She worked for a while and then had to quit. She moved back to her home town, with family support, and now lives on her own in a one-room flat. She pursued alternative remedies in hopes of finding a way to regulate her sleep patterns, relieve her menstrual pain, and settle her stomach. Fatigue, exhaustion, and inability to concentrate were the symptoms that were for her the most debilitating. Siobhan's experiences led her to think about ME. Unlike all the other women described here, she has never been formally diagnosed with ME, at least to her satisfaction. She is well versed on the 'biomedical research' (her words) on ME and would like to see if she actually *has* ME. She feels her diagnosis was based on the exclusion of other possibilities, rather than on actively diagnosing ME as a clinical entity.

Diagnosis of ME for Erin came after dealing with Fibromyalgia for over a decade. She worked at several types of jobs – government, service, and most recently, retail – but it was always difficult to get the next job because of the extreme muscle pain and stomach problems. 'A Dr X, and he was very angry with me, he got very verbally abusive and would yell at me. "Why aren't you better?" I finally quit him because nobody deserves that kind of treatment.' It was only when she changed physicians that the doctor mentioned in a 'by the way' tone that she also had ME. What such a diagnosis meant for Erin is that her ongoing exhaustion, extreme fatigue after walking only a block, inability to concentrate in conversations, and chest pain had some physical, disease-based legitimacy. Up until that point, she had been dismissed as a whiner and malingerer by physicians, and even doubted her own bodily sensations.

Prior to the onset of symptoms, Sandra was fit and participating in a wide range of physical activities. Onset was abrupt. She had been water-skiing, and as she came out of the water, her legs weren't 'working well,' reminiscent of a flu she had had 6 months earlier. 'And then [a bit later] I was sitting there talking to a friend and apparently I went white as a sheet. I thought I was going to pass out. And they got me some sugar and stuff, and I felt horribly ill – for the rest of the weekend I couldn't – I kept falling over.' Sandra's inability to control her legs prompted physicians to consider Multiple Sclerosis as a possible diagnosis. Headaches, adrenaline rushes, nausea, and fatigue plagued her for a couple of years during the diagnosis process. When tests proved inconclusive, she saw the neurologist again. He talked with her, did some more basic neurological tests, and then diagnosed her with ME. Since that time she has been able to return to work on a part-time basis and sustains her recovery by closely monitoring her energy and cognitive abilities.

Competing Diagnostic Categories

The Ramsay definition is one of the oldest definitions that ME practitioners have drawn on for both research and diagnosis.[12] Ramsay based his definition on his long-time interest in ME after he first observed an outbreak at the Royal Free Hospital in London, England (see Ramsay, 1973; Ramsay et al., 1977). His definition focuses on three groups of symptoms: muscle phenomena, circulatory impairment, and cerebral dysfunction. The key diagnostic criterion is severe fatigue after little exertion followed by a long (up to 3 days) recovery period.

A U.K. National Task Force developed the London Criteria. Researchers drew up a set of selection parameters for participants in research projects. The three primary criteria included were the following: exercise-induced fatigue after trivially small exertion, short-term memory and/or concentration impairment, and fluctuation of symptoms. Although this set of criteria notes that ME usually follows an infection, evidence of a viral infection is not a prerequisite for diagnosis. One aspect that differentiates the London Criteria from the Ramsay definition is that mental exertion was added as a specific category under 'Exertion.' Another aspect differentiating the two was the addition of a 6-month period of severe and ongoing fatigue prior to diagnosis.

The CDC definition builds on previous definitions from both the United Kingdom and the United States. The distinguishing characteristics for CFS[13] include 6 months of severe and ongoing fatigue and at least four of eight other symptoms (see Table 9.1). Additional symptoms are listed as being reported by individuals diagnosed with CFS, but are not part of the diagnosis. These include abdominal pain, alcohol intolerance, bloating, chest pain, chronic cough, diarrhea, dizziness, dry eyes or mouth, earaches, irregular heartbeat, jaw pain, morning stiffness, nausea, night sweats, psychological problems (depression, irritability, anxiety, panic attacks), shortness of breath, skin sensations, tingling sensations, and weight loss.[14] These criteria have been influential outside the United States, and are still used in Denmark, Germany, and New Zealand.[15]

The Canadian Criteria differ from previous definitions in that, rather than being primarily for research purposes, they are one of three clinically based sets of guidelines for both diagnosis and treatment.[16] They also differ in that there are four primary sets of symptoms used to diagnose ME/CFS: fatigue, post-exertional malaise, sleep dysfunction, and pain, each with a specific description of the symptoms experienced. These criteria are used in conjunction with additional clusters of symptoms. For a diagnosis, a person must have two neurological/cognitive manifestations, and one from each of two of the following three clusters: autonomic manifestations, neuroendocrine manifestations, and immune manifestations.

Embodying Categories

Experiences of the defining criteria for ME for the women in Ireland and British Columbia vary. Depression was a common diagnosis at the onset of symptoms prior to an ME diagnosis for women in both Ireland and British Columbia. Like Siobhan, the women in Ireland tended to be initially diagnosed with depression by physicians. The second most common initial diagnosis was glandular fever (as set out in the London Criteria).[17] It was only when the woman sought out a physician conversant with ME as an illness, as Elizabeth did, that a physician would diagnose ME within the first year or so of illness. In British Columbia, Myelodysplasia and Hepatitis were the only additional diagnoses mentioned at the onset of symptoms that were not present with the Irish women. Erin's diagnosis of Fibromyalgia, and later of ME, reflects the tendency in North America to link the two illnesses. Only two Irish women mentioned that Fibromyalgia was a possible diagnosis, and only one of them was diagnosed with Fibromyalgia, whereas in British Columbia five women mentioned that they were diagnosed with Fibromyalgia first, and ME afterwards.[18] The persistence to obtain an ME diagnosis was strong in all the women, none of whom was satisfied with any diagnosis until they came to be diagnosed with ME. Sandra's experience was relatively rare in that she remained in paid employment after having only been off work for just less than 2 years. Yet her experience illustrates the limited range of possibilities for recovery that the women faced: Only when an ME diagnosis was present were the women likely to develop a treatment regime relevant and appropriate to their particular set of bodily sensations and material circumstances, including in most instances application for disability benefits and in some cases the possibility of paid work.

The resonance the women felt with the diagnostic category of ME is curious. The variation in the combinations of symptoms that they experienced was so vast, I wondered how any one set of criteria could capture the complexity and diversity of the bodily sensations of all these women, the range of which is demonstrated by Elizabeth, Siobhan, Erin, and Sandra. Granted, as time wore on, the women without a formal diagnosis of ME became more concerned about the possible treatment of their symptoms, rather than about ensuring a specific match between their bodily sensations and the symptoms listed as part of diagnostic criteria (except Siobhan who is still pursuing an ME diagnosis). At the same time, however, when these same women came across the description of ME, they were able to point to ME and say, 'Yes, this is what I have.' Yet the correspondence between a discursive category and an ill body is not the correspondence a diagnostician seeks; rather, a diagnostician relates a discursive category to a disease process. This dissonance accounts for the lengthy time periods that the majority of women ill with ME in both Ireland and British Columbia endure before obtaining a diagnosis of ME. Resonance with a diagnostic category via the virtue of being an ill body does not permit diagnosis; diagnosis as a practice remains within the realm of professionals steeped in biomedicine.

The comprehensiveness of the four sets of defining criteria for ME vary. Ramsay's was the earliest definition and the most useful for practitioners diagnosing ME. What was unique about his definition was the descriptive nature of the criteria (as opposed to elaborating the genesis of a symptom). For example, he described, as a primary feature of ME relating to circulatory impairment, an 'ashen grey facial pallor, 20 to 30 minutes before patient complains of being ill' (Ramsay, 1988: n.p.).[19] Other symptoms identified as part of the criteria were similar in that they were descriptions of the ill body rather than of the disease process.

In the London Criteria, circulatory impairment as a primary set of symptoms was dropped, and a theory of the genesis of symptoms was introduced: 'typically follows an infection, usually a viral illness' (Dowset, Goudsmit, MacIntyre, & Shepherd, 1994; quoted from M.E. International, 2006). Although set up as criteria for inclusion in research projects, elements of the criteria were used in clinical diagnosis, particularly when onset occurred after viral infection. For example, discussion of viral infection, with a link to glandular fever, was present in all of the Irish women's stories about diagnosis as a singular cause of ME. The other key element in the London Criteria was the introduction of the descriptor 'fluctuation of symptoms' as a defining feature. Thus, a notion of *uncertainty* was integrated into the core of a category to be used to define a disease process. The significance of integrating uncertainty into a stable category should not be downplayed by framing it as simply another way to describe episodes. Fluctuation in itself is uncertainty, which then feeds into the contestation of both the material aspects of the body (with consequences for the materialized ill bodies) and the concreteness of the discursive category (by introducing flux as integral to its content).

The CDC definition, developed as guidelines for both clinical diagnosis and research, includes a more extensive list of possible symptoms, and more choice with regard to figuring out which symptoms are primary. Some leeway with respect to what types of symptoms actually define the syndrome remains central in linking long-lasting fatigue (with exclusions of known medical conditions after clinical diagnosis) to a sub-set of symptoms. This arrangement forestalled coming to a definitive answer as to whether ME is an immunological disorder or a disorder of the central nervous system.[20] Where the London Criteria introduced uncertainty into the definition of ME, the CDC definition introduced *flexibility.* The eight symptoms included were drawn from a wider list of symptoms reported by persons with CFS and were recognized as distinguishing features of the illness. This flexibility in the category to account for the variation of symptoms in ill bodies is note-worthy. Because there can be several versions of CFS as an illness, the CDC definition remains popular (and dominant) among practitioners and persons ill with ME in the Western world.

Of the four sets of criteria, the Canadian Criteria probably represent most extensively the number and range of symptoms that the women talked about in all of the interviews. The Canadian Criteria were devel-oped for clinical diagnosis and treatment, making them unique in pre-sentation and content. The text itself is 110 pages, with 30 pages of discussion of the definition of ME/CFS, 32 pages of treatment protocols for specific symptoms, 14 pages of research review and suggested direc-tions for further research, and 34 pages of acknowledgments and refer-ences. Content-wise, these criteria bring together *description*, *uncertainty*, and *flexibility* in a way that captures the materiality of the body without focusing solely on the disease process. For example, the four primary conditions of ME/CFS include fatigue that substantially reduces activity level (this is a description in addition to a 6-month criterion for adults and an additional defining characteristic of a reduced 3-month period of fatigue for children); post-exertional malaise and/or fatigue of at least 24 hours (note the shorter time period than in the London Criteria); sleep dysfunction (resisting attempts to define the specific quality or quantity of sleep, e.g., lack of sleep or excessive sleep that is present in depressive disorders); and pain (pain here includes joint and muscle; cf. Ramsay's definition). The emphasis on pain and sleep dysfunction as central to the syndrome could be related to the historical linkages, medi-ated through research, diagnosis, and activism in North America, with and between ME and Fibromyalgia. Also unique about the Canadian Criteria is the creation of a different kind of path to make sense of the 'other' symptoms present. Designating as necessary two or more symp-toms having to do with neurological and/or cognitive symptoms is less restrictive than requiring the presence of specific symptoms such as short-term memory problems or poor concentration. In addition to the set of primary symptoms and the more specific categorization of cogni-tive impairments, there is to be a manifestation of at least one symptom in two of three different categories of body systems – autonomic, neu-roendocrine, immune – symptoms that have been presented as defining criteria in other guidelines (e.g., circulatory and immune deficiency). Although the categories are more extensive and the 'rules' of diagnosis more detailed in the Canadian Criteria, they are not necessarily as restrictive as other criteria. For example, a new symptom included in the neurological and cognitive category, one that most persons with ME can articulate as a distinctive experience of ME, is the 'crash.' The Canadian Criteria define 'crashing' as part of an 'overload' of processing cognitive, sensory, and/or emotional information. Among the women in British Columbia, 'crashing' was part of the colloquial way to describe the experience of ME, especially to others who have ME! That this notion was integrated into the criteria without being subject to biomedical terms such as anxiety, depression, episodic relapse, etc., is interesting conceptually: ME as a diagnostic category is shifting away from capturing a disease process and moving towards depicting an ill body.

Reading Bodies Marked with ME as a Contested Illness

The two themes brought out in the discussion in this chapter – experiencing the initial application of a diagnostic category of ME and capturing the materiality of an ill body – depict the topography of contestation within the discursive category of ME. Contestation of a diagnostic category takes place not only within the primary discourse defining the illness, biomedicine in this case, but also within the social practices that clinicians and ill bodies engage in, for example, interpreting symptoms and describing bodily sensations. Of equal importance is the attempt in defining ME as a diagnostic category to capture the materiality of the ill body – in terms of both the disease process (exemplified by suggesting clinical tests that will distinguish ME from other illnesses) and the description of the body while ill (demonstrated by the inclusion of 'crashes' in the defining criteria of ME). In this reading of a body marked with ME, it appears that the diagnostic label applied to an ill body depends on the historically situated constitutive processes that link ill bodies and their descriptions, the specific processes through which ill bodies present symptoms to physicians for scrutiny, and the particular place where one lives. Together these context-dependent conditions set the scene for both the diagnosis *as* ill bodies and the experience *of* ill bodies.

Conceptually, this reading supports the re-edging of the notion of embodiment. This reading shows that diagnosis as a discursive construct is actually less discursive and more material than expected. ME becomes an example of where the seemingly fixed discursive category has moved away from its original conception (as a category linked to a disease process) towards a more materially informed discursive category corresponding to the experience of the ill body. In this sense, ME is an example of an embodied construct that is both material and discursive. But not in the same way that it was intended to be, that is, as a representation of an ill body. Instead, what seems to be happening over a relatively short period of time is a mutual constitution of both diagnostic categories and ill bodies, simultaneously being discursive and material, existing in those lived (imagined and real) spaces of everyday life.

Reading bodies marked with a diagnosis of contested illness is a departure point for understanding how materialized ill bodies come to be articulated as ill bodies discursively, and how ill bodies are both discursive and material at the same time. Taking advantage of interpretation as a key component of diagnosis as a practice permits a less medically authoritative and more embodied notion of diagnosis to emerge so that *bodies* of women like Elizabeth, Siobhan, Erin, and Sandra can come to be understood as ill – materially and discursively. Practically, this may be a difficult task to undertake because of the abundance of diagnostic categories within contested illness that need to be overhauled. Politically, it may be a difficult strategy to sustain because of the pressing need to engage in other crucial struggles including those against privatization and corporatization of health care. Conceptually, however, if this new notion of diagnosis can be supported in *specific* social practices that engage medicalized knowledge, then ill bodies can begin to embody diagnostic categories.

Acknowledgments

Thanks to the women in the studies! Funding for the Irish study came from the National Institute for Regional and Spatial Analysis, National University of Ireland, Maynooth. Funding for the B.C. study came from the Social Sciences and Humanities Research Council of Canada, grant nos. 410-95-0267 and 410-2005-1152. I appreciate comments from my colleague Kathy Teghtsoonian on earlier versions of this chapter.

NOTES

1   WHO (1996) also categorizes Fatigue Syndrome, conceivably a term synonymous with Chronic Fatigue Syndrome (CFS), under the general heading of 'Mental and Behavioural Disorders' (F00-F99), the sub-heading of 'Neurotic, Stress-related and Somatoform Disorders' (F40-F48), and under the specific heading of 'Neurasthenia' (F48).

2 Two Canadian cases considered to be landmark cases in terms of the struggle by ME activists to get institutions to define ME as a physical disease instead of a psychological disease are: *Baillie v. Crown Life Insurance Co* and *Eddie v. Unum Life Insurance Company of America.*

3 See http://www.co-cure.org/ and http://listserv.nodak.edu/archives/co-cure.html. In North America, research on CFS is often associated with Fibromyalgia because of the overlap in key diagnostic criteria, including pain and cognitive impairment.

4 Publications can be found at http://www.meresearch.org.uk/information/publications/index.html. For an overview, see esp. the presentation by Spence (2005).

5 Groups in Ireland include: The Irish ME Trust, http://www.imet.ie/ and the Irish ME/CFS Support Group, PO Box 3075, Dublin 2, Ireland. Groups in the United Kingdom include: MEActionUK, http://www.meactionuk.org.uk/; MEACH Trust, http://www.meach.org/; Search ME, http://www.search-me.org.uk/index.html; Support ME, http://www.supportme.co.uk/definitions.htm; The 25% ME Group, http://www.25megroup.org/; The ME Association of the UK, http://www.meassociation.org.uk/; and Tymes Trust, http://www.tymestrust.org/.

6 On content and expression, see Deleuze & Guattari (1987: 89).

7 Even with the extensive conceptualizations of embodiment in feminism and in non-feminist works, there still exist many uses of the term *embodiment* that refer to a simplistic, anthropomorphic notion of personification or, perhaps a little more complexly, incarnation.

8 See Åsbring & Närvärnen (2004) for a discussion as to how women with ill bodies deal with the uncertainty of how the illness plays out.

9 Sawicki's (2004) argument could also be read as a rationale for demedicalizing diagnosis.

10 I conducted all of the Irish interviews and half of the B.C. interviews. I interviewed women in Ireland in late spring 2003. We completed the interviews in British Columbia in 1997 (see Moss & Dyck, 2002, for a detailed presentation of the full study).

11 Given that the Canadian Criteria emerged from over 20,000 case histories and Dr Bruce Carruthers (the lead author and member of the panel) served the area in which the women I interviewed lived, some of the women's case histories may have been directly included. I am not saying that any or all of the women I interviewed in British Columbia comprised any of the clinical case histories upon which the diagnostic and treatment protocols for the Canadian Criteria were based. Rather, I am saying that the context within which these

women sought treatment for their symptoms was the same one within which some of the participants on the panel were enmeshed.

12 Though formalized in 1988 through the ME Association of Essex, U.K. (http://www.meactionuk.org.uk/definition.html), physicians and researchers worked with this definition throughout the 1980s.

13 The CDC has always used CFS as the descriptor of this syndrome. In Ireland and the United Kingdom, the preferred term is Myalgic Encephalomyelitis, but Myalgic Encephalopathy is gaining popularity. In Canada, both ME and CFS are used, mostly interchangeably.

14 There has been discussion regarding changing the definition among members of study groups that the CDC supports (see Reeves et al., 2003). In these discussions, researchers suggest ways of refining the definition of CFS in order to make research selection of participants more consistent between studies.

15 See the following websites: http://www.anzmes.org.nz/what_is_me.htm; http://www.fatigatio.de/2?PHPSESSID=182d1930d39332f6b54500fd93bb 186c; and http://www.me-cfs.dk/Sygdommen/diagnose.html.

16 The others are in Britain (Royal College of Physicians, 1996) and Australia (Royal Australasian College of Physicians, 2002). A general practitioners' handbook was published after the Australian guidelines in 2004 (South Australian Department of Human Services, 2004), and follow closely the Canadian Criteria.

17 Glandular fever in Ireland is roughly equivalent to mononucleosis in British Columbia.

18 See note 3.

19 A racialized body is present here. Presumably the 'ashen grey pallor' refers to persons with white and light-coloured skin.

20 In British Columbia, the women talked about infection as only one of a series of possible causes, and only one woman was diagnosed with mononucleosis, whereas five were diagnosed with Fibromyalgia with a focus on pain and cognitive impairment.

REFERENCES

Åsbring, Pia, & Närvärnen, Anna-Liisa. (2004). Patient power and control: A study of women with uncertain illness trajectories. *Qualitative Health Research, 14*(2), 226–240.

Bacchi, Carol Lee, & Beasley, Chris. (2002). Citizen bodies: Is embodied citizenship a contradiction in terms? *Critical Social Policy, 22*(2), 324–352.

Baillie v *Crown Life Insurance Co.* (1998). Alberta Court of Queen's Bench, 235. 9303–22591. Justice C. Philip Clarke.

Baylis, Françoise, Downie, Jocelyn, & Sherwin, Susan. (1999). Women and health research: From theory, to practice, to policy. In Anne Donchin & Laura M. Purdy (Eds.), *Embodying bioethics: Recent feminist advances* (pp. 253-268). Lanham, MA: Rowman and Littlefield.

Benhabib, Seyla. (1992). *Situating the self: Gender, community and postmodernism in contemporary ethics.* New York and London: Routledge.

Birke, Lynda. (2000). *Feminism and the biological body.* New Brunswick, NJ: Rutgers University Press.

Braidotti, Rosi. (2003). Becoming woman: Sexual difference revisited. *Theory, Culture and Society, 20*(3), 43-64.

Bray, Abigail, & Colebrook, Claire. (1998). The haunted flesh: Corporeal feminism and the politics of (dis)embodiment. *Signs, 24*(1), 35–67.

Breckenridge, Carol A., & Vogler, Candace. (2001). The critical limits of embodiment: Disability's criticism. *Public Culture, 13*(3), 349–357.

Brown, Phil, Zavestoski, Stephen, McCormick, Sabrina, Mayer, Brian, Morello-Frosch, Rachel, & Gasior Altman, Rebecca. (2004). Embodied health movements: Uncharted territory in social movement research. *Sociology of Health and Illness, 26*(1), 1–31.

Butler, Judith. (1990). *Gender trouble: Feminism and the subversion of identity.* New York and London: Routledge.

Butler, Judith. (1993). *Bodies that matter: On the discursive limits of 'sex.'* New York and London: Routledge.

Carruthers, Bruce M., Jain, Anil K., De Meirleir, Kenny L., Peterson, Daniel L., Klimas, Nancy G., Lerner, A. Martin, et al. (2003). Myalgic Encephalomyelitis/Chronic Fatigue Syndrome: Clinical working case definition, diagnostic and treatment protocols. *Journal of Chronic Fatigue Syndrome, 11*(1), 7–115.

Centers for Disease Control and Prevention (CDC). (2006). Definition of Chronic Fatigue Syndrome. Centers for Disease Control and Prevention, Atlanta, Georgia. Retrieved 1 May 2006, from http://www.cdc.gov/ncidod/diseases/cfs/about/what.htm (last updated 11 May 2005).

Conboy, Katie, Medina, Nadia, & Stanbury, Sarah. (Eds.). (1997). *Writing on the body: Female embodiment and feminist theory.* New York: Columbia University Press.

Davidson, Joyce. (2003). *Phobic geographies: The phenomenology and spatiality of identity.* Aldershot, UK: Ashgate.

Deleuze, Gilles, & Guattari, Félix. (1987). *A thousand plateaus.* Minneapolis: University of Minnesota Press.

Diprose, Rosalyn. (1994). *The bodies of women: Ethics, embodiment and sexual difference.* New York and London: Routledge.

Dowset, E.G., Goudsmit, Ellen, MacIntyre, A., & Shepherd, C. (1994). London Criteria for M.E., *Report from The National Task Force on Chronic Fatigue Syndrome (CFS), Post Viral Fatigue Syndrome (PVFS), Myalgic Encephalomyelitis (ME)* (pp. 96–98). London: Westcare.

Duden, Barbara. (1991). *The woman beneath the skin: A doctor's patients in eighteenth-century Germany.* Cambridge, MA: Harvard University Press.

Eckermann, Liz. (1997). Foucault, embodiment and gendered subjectivities: The case of voluntary self-starvation. In Alan Petersen & Robin Bunton (Eds.), *Foucault, health and medicine* (pp. 151–169). New York and London: Routledge.

Eddie v Unum Life Insurance Company of America. (1999). Court of Appeal for British Columbia, 507. CA024740. Justices Jo-Ann A. Prowse, Mary V. Newbury, & John E. Hall.

Foucault, Michel. (1979). *Discipline and punish: The birth of the prison.* New York: Vintage Books.

Foucault, Michel. (1990). *The history of sexuality, volume 1: An introduction.* (Robert Hurley, Trans.). New York: Vintage Books. (Original work published in 1978.)

Fukuda, K., Straus, S.E., Hickie, I., Sharpe, M.C., Dobbins, J.G., Komaroff, A., & the International Chronic Fatigue Syndrome Study Group. (1994). Chronic Fatigue Syndrome: A comprehensive approach to its definition and study. *Annals of Internal Medicine, 121,* 953-959.

Grosz, Elizabeth. (1994). *Volatile bodies: Toward a corporeal feminism.* Bloomington & Indianapolis: Indiana University Press.

Holmes, G.P., Kaplan, J.E., Gantz, N.M., Komaroff, A.L., Schonberger, L.B., Straus, S.E., et al. (1988). Chronic Fatigue Syndrome: A working case definition. *Annals of Internal Medicine, 108,* 387–389.

Kleinman, Arthur. (1988). *The illness narratives: Suffering, healing, and the human condition.* New York: Basic Books.

Leslie, Deborah, & Butz, David. (1998). 'GM suicide': Flexibility, space, and the injured body. *Economic Geography, 74,* 360–378.

M.E. International. (2006). London Criteria for M.E. *M.E. International.* Available online, http://uk.geocities.com/me_not_cfs/Myalgic-Encephalomyelitis-London-Criteria-V2.html: n.p. (accessed 15 May 2007).

McLaren, Margaret A. (2002). *Feminism, Foucault, and embodied subjectivity.* Albany: State University of New York Press.

Moss, Pamela, & Dyck, Isabel. (1999). Body, corporeal space and legitimating chronic illness: Women diagnosed with ME. *Antipode, 31,* 372–397.

Moss, Pamela, & Dyck, Isabel. (2002). *Women, body, illness: Space and identity in the everyday lives of women with chronic illness*. Lanham, MA: Rowman and Littlefield.

Ramsay, A. Melvin. (1973). Benign Myalgic Encephalomyelitis. *British Journal of Psychiatry, 122*, 618–619.

Ramsay, A. Melvin. (1988). *Myalgic Encephalomyelitis and postviral fatigue states: The saga of Royal Free Disease*. Essex, England: M.E. Association. Available online, http://www.meactionuk.org.uk/definition.html (accessed 15 May 2007).

Ramsay, A. Melvin, Dowsett, E.G., Dadswell, J.V., Lyle, W.H., & Parish, J.G. (1977). Icelandic Disease (Benign Myalgic Encephalomyelitis or Royal Free Disease). *British Medical Journal, 21*(1), 1350.

Reeves, William C., Lloyd, Andrew, Vernon, Suzanne D., Klimas, Nancy, Jason, Leonard A., Bleijenberg, Gijs, et al. (2003). Identification of ambiguities in the 1994 Chronic Fatigue Syndrome research case definition and recommendations for resolution. *BMC Health Services Research, 3*(25). Available online, http://www.biomedcentral.com/1472-6963/3/25 (accessed 15 May 2007).

Royal Australasian College of Physicians. (2002). *Chronic Fatigue Syndrome: Clinical practice guidelines – 2002*. Sydney, Australia: Author, Health Policy Unit.

Royal College of Physicians, London. (1996, Oct.). *Chronic Fatigue Syndrome. Report of a joint working group of the Royal Colleges of Physicians, Psychiatrists and General Practitioners*. London: Author.

Sawicki, Jana. (1991). *Disciplining Foucault: Feminism, power, and the body*. New York and London: Routledge.

Sawicki, Jana. (2004). Foucault's pleasures: Desexualizing queer politics. In Dianna Taylor & Karen Vintages (Eds.), *Feminism and the final Foucault* (pp. 163-182). Urbana-Champaign: University of Illinois Press.

Scheper-Hughes, Nancy. (2005). The last commodity: Post-human ethics and the global traffic in 'fresh' organs. In Aihwa Ong & Stephen J. Collier (Eds.), *Global assemblages: Technology, politics, and ethics as anthropological problems* (pp. 145–167). London: Blackwell.

Shildrick, Margrit, & Price, Janet. (1996). Breaking the boundaries of the broken body. *Body and Society, 2*(4), 93-113.

Shildrick, Margrit, & Price, Janet (Eds.). (1998). *Vital signs: Feminist reconfigurations of the bio/logical body*. Edinburgh: Edinburgh University Press.

South Australian Department of Human Services. (2004). *Myalgic Encephalopathy (ME) and Chronic Fatigue Syndrome (CFS): Management guidelines for general practitioners*. Primary Health Care Branch. Adelaide, South Australia: Author.

Spence, Vance. (2005). *Biomedical research in ME/CFS: Issues and challenges*. Presentation at Cross Party Group on ME, Reception, Scottish Parliament.

Retrieved 10 Oct. 2005, from http://www.meresearch.org.uk/information/publications/parliament/parliamentpres1.html.

Williams, Simon J., & Bendelow, Gillian A. (1998). *The lived body: Sociological themes, embodied issues*. New York and London: Routledge.

World Health Organization. (1996). *International statistical classification of disease and related health problems* (10th rev., 2nd ed.). Geneva: Author.

Zavestoski, Stephen, McCormick, Sabrina, & Brown, Phil. (2004). Gender, embodiment, and disease: Environmental breast cancer activists' challenges to science, the biomedical model, and policy. *Science as Culture, 13*(4), 563-586.

10 Managing the Monstrous Feminine: The Role of Premenstrual Syndrome in the Subjectification of Women

JANE M. USSHER

Throughout history, and across cultures, the reproductive body of woman has provoked fascination and fear. It is a body deemed dangerous and defiled, the myth of the monstrous feminine made flesh, yet also a body that provokes adoration and desire, and enthralment with the mysteries within. We see this ambivalent relationship played out in mythological, literary, and artistic representations of the feminine, where woman is positioned as powerful, impure, and corrupt, a source of moral and physical contamination; or as sacred, asexual, and nourishing, a phantasmic signifier of threat extinguished. Evidence of this dread is present in representations of the dangers of the menstruating woman, whose 'touch could blast the fruits of the field, sour wine, cloud mirrors, rust iron, and blunt the edges of knives' (Walker, 1983: 643), or in the belief that the world's most feared poison, moon-dew, made by Thessalian witches, came from girls' first menstrual blood (Graves, 1966: 166).

Mythology, because of its rich symbolism, and its exaggerated lore, is easy to dismiss – at least by those of us who live in a secular, scientific, modern (if not postmodern) age. However, as Michel Foucault (1990) argued in *The History of Sexuality, Volume 1,* contemporary medical surveillance of the reproductive body transforms the taboos and rituals that positioned the menstruating woman as polluted, dangerous, and abject, into medical, legal, or scientific truths. Surveillance of the fecund body starts at menarche, with menstrual blood positioned as sign of contamination, requiring careful concealment and adherence to hygiene rules, and menstruation as cause of debilitation, leading to women being seen as weak, erratic, and unreliable, and management of the fecund body, in shameful silence, woman's unquestioned recourse.

In the case of Premenstrual Syndrome (PMS), the problem is located within: The monster in the machine of femininity positioned as endocrine or neurotransmitter dysfunction, or 'female sex hormones,' a pathology within the woman, outside of her control (but within the control of medical experts, we are assured). Indeed, fecundity is positioned as so detrimental to women's mental health that it is blamed for women reporting higher rates of depression than men, the 'sex hormone,' estrogen, positioned as the cause (Studd, 1997).

This may appear to be an improvement on cultural or mythological representations of woman as inherently monstrous – here it is her faulty hormones that are the problem, easily resolved by medical intervention. However, it is not a positive position to take: created through a process of consultation and concurrence on the part of medical and psychological experts, the reproductive syndromes have become catch-all diagnostic categories that conveniently attribute female distress and deviance to the reproductive body, legitimating medical management of the reproductive excess, and implicitly, of the monstrous feminine. This has significant implications for the ways in which we, as women, inhabit our bodies and for knowledge about what our bodies are, and what they are meant to do. It also materializes in our experience of our fecund flesh, and more broadly, in the development of our subjectivity, our sense of ourselves as women, as we see below.

In this chapter I contest reductionist models of Premenstrual Syndrome through critically examining the construction, regulation, and experience of the premenstrual body, and the positioning of transgression from ideals of hegemonic femininity as embodied illness, which acts to maintain fears of the monstrous feminine within. Drawing on interdisciplinary theory and interviews conducted with women in the United Kingdom and in Australia, I examine hegemonic truths that define premenstrual distress as embodied pathology to illustrate how women are regulated through a process of subjectification. However, this does not negate women's experience of premenstrual distress. I argue that the emergence of premenstrual distress as well as women's self-positioning as PMS sufferers are connected to the self-policing practices of self-silencing, self-surveillance, over-responsibility, self-blame, and self-sacrifice, all of which are closely associated with hegemonic constructions of femininity. Premenstrually, a rupture in self-silencing occurs, yet this is followed by increased self-surveillance, leading to guilt, shame, and blaming of the body. Identifying these self-policing practices allows women to develop more empowering strategies for reducing or preventing premenstrual distress, developing an ethic of care for the self, and no longer blaming the body for premenstrual anger or depression.

PMS: Regulating the Reproductive Body

Since discussions of premenstrual symptoms first appeared, contemporaneously in the medical and psychoanalytic literature, in 1931, this has been a research field dogged by controversy and disagreement. Initially described as 'premenstrual tension' and attributed to either hormonal imbalances (Frank, 1931) or to intrapsychic conflict exacerbated by women's social role (Horney, 1931), it was renamed 'Premenstrual Syndrome,' in 1953; Late Luteal Phase Dysphoric Disorder in the *Diagnostic and Statistical Manual of Mental Disorders* (DSM III-R) of the American Psychiatric Association, in 1987, and Premenstrual Dysphoric Disorder (PMDD) in the DSM-IV-TR in 2000. Estimates of prevalence range from 10 to 95 per cent of women, depending on the definition used. Regardless of the diagnostic classification adopted, the divide between biomedical and psychological explanations continues to this day, with a range of competing theories associating PMS with a single causal factor (Bancroft, 1993; Ussher, 1992) and a range of competing treatments being proposed. Recent medical literature advocates serotonin reuptake inhibitors (SSRIs) to correct serotonin imbalance (Rapkin, 2003), and the psychology literature suggests cognitive-behaviour therapy (Blake, Salkovskis, Gath, Day, & Garrod, 1998).

However, for the many feminist critics who vociferously argued against the inclusion of PMDD in the DSM (Figert, 1996), PMS has been positioned as merely the latest in a line of diagnostic categories acting to pathologize the reproductive body and legitimate the attribution of distress or deviance to factors within the woman (Nash & Chrisler, 1997; Ussher, 1996 and 2006). This view draws on broader postmodern debates in critical psychology and psychiatry where the very concept of mental illness or madness is contested, being positioned as a social construction that regulates subjectivity and produces disciplinary practices that police the population through pathologization (Fee, 2000). The psy-professions are seen to define what is normal and what is pathological, providing the means by which people can inspect, regulate, and improve the self, invariably finding themselves wanting.

These feminist and postmodern critiques stand in direct opposition to the biomedical and psychological accounts of PMS which position the woman as a rational unitary subject and premenstrual change as a sign of pathology, explained within an essentialist framework – be it biological or psychological. Yet in emphasizing the regulatory power of discourse, postmodernism can be read as negating agency, and failing to recognize the existence of distress (Burr & Butt, 2000). It can also be seen to negate embodied or psychological change across the menstrual cycle, or other material aspects of women's existence that may be associated with their distress. This is problematic, as a substantial proportion of women *do* experience change during the premenstrual phase of the cycle, of that there is no doubt (Hardie, 1997). However, this change, whether it is experienced at a psychological or physical level, or both, is not pure, somehow beyond culture, beyond discourse; it is not simply *caused* by the reproductive body, by a syndrome called PMS. And it is not inevitably experienced, or positioned, as distressing or problematic. 'PMS sufferer' is a position that women take up (or a position that they are put in by others). And, it is a position that women can contest.

The process by which women take up the position of abjection personified, where premenstrual change is pathologized, and the fecund body is positioned as *cause* of distress, can be described as a process of subjectification. Drawing on Foucault, Nikolas Rose describes subjectification as 'regimes of knowledge through which human beings have come to recognise themselves as certain kinds of creatures, the strategies of regulation and tactics of action to which these regimes of knowledge have been connected, and the correlative relations that human beings have established within themselves, in taking themselves as subjects' (1996: 11). It is the regimes of knowledge circulating within medicine, science, and law that are reproduced in self-help texts and the media (Chrisler, 2002), that provide the discursive framework within which women come to recognize themselves as PMS sufferers, positioning premenstrual deviations from ideals of femininity as manifestations of the monstrous feminine, with self-surveillance and self-policing the only means of ensuring containment of feminine excess.

To illustrate the ways in which this process of subjectification operates, I take two interconnected truths within the regimes of knowledge that construct and regulate PMS, and draw on interviews conducted with British and Australian women who position themselves as PMS sufferers, to demonstrate the ways in which these truths impact upon women's experience of premenstrual change (Ussher, 2003b and 2004a).

The two truths are: (1) PMS is a static thing that can be objectively defined and measured, and (2) PMS is a pathology to be eradicated. If we critically examine these truths, we can see the ways in which they insinuate themselves into women's experience and management of the fecund body, making it almost inevitable that premenstrual change will be positioned as PMS.

Details of the Interviews

Thirty-six women from the United Kingdom who reported a 30 per cent increase in premenstrual 'symptoms,' as measured by prospective diaries over a 3-month period, and who met DSM-IV diagnostic criteria for PMDD took part in in-depth narrative interviews, the aim being to examine women's subjective experience of PMS and what PMS meant to each individual woman. The women were randomly selected from a larger group, who were taking part in a randomized controlled trial comparing medical and psychological interventions for moderate-to-severe premenstrual symptoms (Hunter et al., 2002b). Thirty-four women from Australia, who were taking part in an evaluation of a self-help intervention for PMS (Ussher & Perz, 2006a) and who met the diagnostic criteria outlined above, were also interviewed. This chapter draws on the pre-intervention interviews for both groups.

Regimes of Knowledge that Construct and Regulate PMS

PMS IS A STATIC THING THAT CAN BE OBJECTIVELY DEFINED AND MEASURED

> We *live* with it but we're distraught about it and, and it's 'My God, you know, is this *the sort of a thing* we've got to live with?'

> I wake up one day and I'm feeling a bit grotty and I think, 'Oh, what's this?' and I, you know, I count the days and I think, 'Oh yeah. Of course! *That again*!'

PMS is described as 'a thing we've got to live with,' a 'thing' that women have or do not have, in women's talk, as we can see from the quotes above. These accounts reflect the truths we are told by experts, where PMS is conceptualized as an identifiable *thing* that can be objectively defined and measured. This is evidenced by the way in which women are dichotomously categorized as PMS sufferers, or as non-sufferers, in epidemiological surveys and in individual clinical examinations – implying that they either *have* or *do not have* this 'thing' PMS, with standardized symptom checklists being used to ascertain accurate and objective diagnosis (Bancroft, 1993; Walker, 1995).

When women were asked in an open-ended questionnaire, 'describe your PMS,' they did reproduce the key symptoms found in these checklists, reporting tiredness, depression, anxiety, anger, loss of control, pain, bloating, cravings, and skin problems. One simple explanation of this is that these *are* the symptoms that women experience. However, when given an opportunity to present their own interpretations of premenstrual experiences within the open-ended narrative interview, the same women presented a much richer and more contextualized picture of their 'symptomatology.' They talked spontaneously of issues such as problems in relationships, problems at work, needing time to themselves, feelings of overwhelming responsibility, and failing to cope and be in control at all times as constituting 'PMS.' This demonstrates that the framework provided by the experts will significantly influence the way in which women understand and experience premenstrual change. However, if women are given a different framework – one that allows for the description of premenstrual experiences in a more complex way, a different picture emerges.

Equally, positioning PMS as a 'thing' implies that it is a static entity that suddenly emerges – or is treated, and disappears – that serves to position women as passive and docile in relation to the arrival of their monthly affliction, with expert intervention positioned as the only hope of cure. This also leads to anticipatory anxiety on the part of many women, as they await the morning when they wake to find they they've 'got' PMS, or are 'taken over,' as we see in the interview extracts above. However, when we talk to women about the development and course of their experience of premenstrual change, it is clear that the taking up of the position of a PMS sufferer is not a static process, and women are not passive or lacking in agency in relation to their suffering from this *thing*, PMS. Women experience embodied or psychological changes premenstrually, to varying degrees; they become aware of these changes (or are made aware by others) – or ignore them; they experience distress – or accept and tolerate premenstrual change; they evaluate these changes as PMS – or resist this diagnosis; and they cope in a range of different ways – including repression or expression of feelings, avoidance of others, self-care, or presentation to experts for help (Ussher, 2002). Thus, taking up the position of a PMS sufferer is a complex and fluid process, which can be disrupted, or the woman can be offered support, or alternative ways of understanding her premenstrual change, at any point: PMS is not simply a static entity that emerges, fully formed, a pathology with clear boundaries that is the same for all women, regardless of what the experts tell us.

PMS IS A PATHOLOGY TO BE ERADICATED

> I think because I react differently. I might be more intolerant with him or shorter or abrupt … There, there's a *change* in me.

> I find that particular time of the month very difficult, and I'm sure everybody else around me finds it very difficult. There's a *big change in me*, and it makes me feel as if I'm not in control.

This representation of premenstrual psychological change as pathology is the most pervasive truth about PMS, taken for granted in both popular and medical accounts (Markens, 1996). Premenstrual experiences are positioned as pathology, as PMS, because for 3 weeks of the month women say that they don't experience these 'symptoms.' However, the notion that subjectivity, mood, and bodily experience *should* be consistent is a social construction – a product of the regimes of knowledge that currently dominate Western conceptualizations of mental health. It reflects a modernist position that conceptualizes identity as unitary, and the individual as rational and consistent, with deviation from the norm as a sign of illness. A postmodern approach would contest this, seeing subjectivity as pluralistic, made up of contradictory and shifting subject positions; there is no core self, and change is expected, not pathologized.

Postmodernism is not alone in adopting this stance. Eastern approaches to mental health, such as that which underpins Buddhist mindfulness meditation, directly confront the illusion of a core consistent 'me' who is always positive and good. Change is accepted, rather than being positioned as a sign of pathology, and mindfulness practice leads to an appreciation of the temporally based dimension of self, through paying attention to bodily based experiences and sensations *as they occur* (Epstein, 1995). Within this Buddhist framework, premenstrual changes would not be pathologized, would not merit 'diagnosis,' for it would be accepted that difficult feelings and thoughts arise in the normal course of life, and that if we try to repress or deny them, this will only be a temporary solution, as they will invariably come out at times when we are vulnerable or under pressure – the premenstrual phase of the cycle being such a time for some women.

PMS: A Material-Discursive-Intrapsychic Experience

Yet 'PMS' is not simply a rhetorical construction, a fiction framed as fact created by self-proclaimed experts. Many women *do* feel anger, or feel depressed, or have a desperate need to be alone at this time of the month. There are many complex reasons why these feelings emerge at this time. There is convincing evidence from previous research that many women experience increased vulnerability and sensitivity to emotion or external stress during the premenstrual phase of the cycle (Sabin, Farrell, & Slade, 1999; Ussher & Wilding, 1992), resulting from a combination of hormonal or endocrine changes (Parry, 1994), sensitivity to premenstrual increases in autonomic arousal (Kuczmierczyk & Adams, 1986; Ussher, 1987), and differential perceptions of stress (Woods et al., 1998). Experimental research has demonstrated that dual or multiple task performance is more difficult premenstrually (Slade & Jenner, 1980), and while women can compensate with increased effort, this can result in increased levels of anxiety (Ussher & Wilding, 1991). It is thus not surprising that many women report reacting to the stresses and strains of daily life with decreased tolerance premenstrually, particularly when they carry multiple responsibilities – indeed, in one study, career women with child-rearing responsibilities were found to report the highest levels of premenstrual distress (Coughlin, 1990). This is the one time in the month that women cannot live up to internalized idealized expectations of femininity, with increased vulnerability or reduced tolerance leading to a rupture in self-silencing in the face of over-responsibility – anger or distress being positioned as PMS. Examining the practices of the self-policing that leads to this self-silencing and self-surveillance thus provides us with an explanation for women's experience of uncontrollable distress or anger premenstrually, dethroning those who would position the abject body as being a culprit to blame (Ussher, 2004b).

Women's Self-policing: Regulation from Within

PMS AS OVER-RESPONSIBILITY: WOMEN AS EMOTIONAL CARERS AND
NURTURERS OF OTHERS AND THE NECESSITY OF SELF-RENUNCIATION
The positioning of women as emotional nurturers of others, in particular men and children, necessitating women's self-renunciation in order
to legitimate their taking disproportionate responsibility for caring, is
central to constructions of idealized femininity (O'Grady, 2005). When
asked to talk about their 'PMS,' women positioned their major 'symptoms' as not wanting or not being able to provide unconditional care
and support for others while premenstrual, and spoke of wishing to
divest themselves of overwhelming responsibility:

> All I ever do is clean and cook and look after the kids, and all I ever do is
> run around and clean up after everybody. And I think, like I said, for
> 3 weeks of the month it doesn't bother me 'cause I'm sure I'm doing it
> every week, but it just seems the week before my period I, I just don't
> cope with that so well. I don't want to do that anymore [laughs]. I want
> someone to look after me.

In positioning the desire to attend to her own needs as a sign of internal pathology, PMS, the participant quoted just above is exhibiting
self-policing, judging her own desires or needs in relation to hegemonic discursive constructions of woman as responsible and emotionally nurturing, always able to offer unlimited care and attention to
others. At the same time, 'PMS' also stands for the anger, depression,
or frustration that many women experience in response to the unre-
lenting expectations placed upon them:

> You know, I mean there are some days when I think, 'Oh. I don't really
> want to get out of bed today.' You know, I can't, I can't stand the thought
> [laughs] of having to get up and clear up after everybody and you know.
> Um [clicks tongue] and it may, it may be the depression starts first but I'm
> not really aware of it and then later comes the anger when you're, you
> know, you're *low* anyway and then people start making demands on you
> that you don't like or just happen to hit a raw nerve! [laughs] And then
> you *fly* into this *rage* [laughs].

Rather than being a symptom of 'PMS,' a problem tied to the body,
this 'depression' could be conceptualized as an emergence of emotions

that are repressed during the majority of the month, and their outward expression through anger as a rupture in the self-silencing that is central to women's self-renunciation (Ussher & Perz, 2006b). Self-silencing, the presentation of one image to the world in an attempt to be a 'good woman,' with the containment of feelings within, is a pattern of behaviour that has been found to be common in women who are depressed (Duarte & Thompson, 1999; Jack, 1991). The rupture in self-silencing that occurs premenstrually appears to function to allow the expression of both day-to-day frustrations and anger associated with more substantial issues, which are normally repressed as women attempt to be 'good' in order to live up to idealized representations of femininity (Ussher, 2002 and 2003b). For without exception, when women were asked to characterize their experience of 'PMS,' they used a 'short-fuse' metaphor to describe incidents that were viewed as annoying, or even as catastrophic premenstrually, while being tolerated or dismissed at other points in the cycle:

> The funny thing is the week before they could have been twice as bad and really horrible and you've put up with it and you've let them get away with it. You know. But then when they do something really little, and you'll go bananas over it.

At the same time, a 'pressure cooker' metaphor was used to describe emotions building up during the month, and then overflowing during the premenstrual phase of the cycle, as is illustrated in this example:

> There's a few days of the month where I feel I'm not *myself*, or there's you know, anger or tension that builds up and then I release it at that point. And others around me suffer the consequences! Of that build up. Whatever it is.

Both of these women are describing self-silencing for 3 weeks of the month over minor irritations or more substantial relationship issues, which they 'cope with' or 'don't pay attention to,' a self-silencing that is broken premenstrually, as the frustration or irritation becomes overwhelming, or the woman feels that she's had enough, as her own needs come to the fore, or she cannot (or does not want to) 'cope' anymore (Ussher, 2003a). However, rather than the frustrations being heeded by the woman or her partner, and the problems or inequities being addressed, her feelings are positioned as irrational, as symptoms of 'PMS,' and thus the woman is pathologized and dismissed.

THE ERUPTION OF THE MONSTROUS FEMININE PREMENSTRUALLY: THE JUXTAPOSITION OF THE GOOD AND BAD WOMAN

> Dr Jekyll to Mr Hyde. Horrible, bitchy, vicious, violent and depressed.

> I'm just stressed and anxious – not a pleasant person to be around. It's like Dr Jekyll and Mr Hyde.

The juxtaposition of the good and bad woman is central to women's positioning of themselves as having PMS – where the premenstrual self epitomizes the monstrous feminine made flesh, and women using metaphors such as 'Dr Jekyll and Mr Hyde' to describe the premenstrual self, as is illustrated above. Women position the premenstrual phase of the cycle as a time when they are not themselves, instead, they are a woman possessed:

> Um, I become increasingly, um, *irritable* and have absolutely no tolerance for anybody or anything, and I feel terrible that I'm being so terrible. But it's just like there's an, another person inside of me so that, um the slightest thing I'll get cross about, upset about, irritated about.

When emotions or behaviours are split off as 'not me,' as symptoms of PMS, women foster a sense of alienation or distance from themselves. Implicit within these self-judgments are notions of the standards of behaviour that women aspire to, and are judged against: an idealized version of femininity that is hyper-responsible, able to cope, and always in control, reflecting hegemonic representations of the good woman juxtaposed with the bad: self-sacrifice, care, coping, and calmness contrasted with aggression, impatience, and anxiety (Ussher, 1997).

A number of PMS/non-PMS contrasts appeared throughout the interviews: bad versus good; introversion versus extroversion; out of control versus in control; irresponsible versus responsible; failing versus coping; angry versus calm; anxious versus relaxed; depressed versus happy; irrational versus rational; intolerant versus tolerant; vulnerable versus strong; irritable versus placid; frustrated versus accepting (Ussher, 2002). There is no room for transgression here – the standards against which women are judged, and against which we judge ourselves, are impossibly high. Thus the 'PMS-self' is condemned, both by others, and most significantly, by the woman herself:

This wasn't anger, this was sort of the real depression and just feeling *completely* lost. I find I *loathe* myself, I really hate myself you know.
I look sometimes at myself when I'm pre-menstrual and I think ... that I don't ... I don't like myself. I don't like what I've become.
But *rationally* I think, 'Well, it's not *me*.' It's not me.

In her analysis of anorexia, Hilda Bruch (1978: 55–6) argues that the 'secret but powerful part of the self, the monster in the machine of anorexia, is experienced as a personification of everything [women] have tried to hide or deny as not approved of by themselves.' The same could be said of PMS. The discursive construction of the premenstrual body as object to blame functions to exonerate women from responsibility for this part of the self, as it is positioned as a 'symptom' of pathology, disassociating it from a woman's sense of self. It is not *her* that is the monster, it is 'PMS,' and an unruly body that must be constrained and contained.

PMS AS LOSS OF CONTROL: WOMAN'S SUBJECTIVITY IS TIED TO AN UNRULY BODY, NECESSITATING DISCIPLINE AND CONTAINMENT
In discussing representations of woman as monster in Greek mythology and contemporary Hollywood horror films, Rachel Gear comments, 'The monstrous woman is represented as out of control, threatening, and all-consuming' (2001: 321). The positioning of PMS as lack of control, attributed by the woman, and in many cases also by her partner, to the body, thus reflects hegemonic representations of woman as monstrous, closer to nature, with excess emotion or lack of control attributed to corporeality. If women see themselves as being at the mercy of their raging hormones, they position themselves as being attacked from within. The body thus becomes objectified, alien to the woman, something that is acting against her in an out-of-control manner, as is illustrated in the extract below.

INTERVIEWER: What are you feeling when you get this sort of tension and pressure?
INTERVIEWEE: What am I feeling? I guess annoyed at myself, I want to stop the way I am but I can't ... I get quite frustrated by my body, 'cause, I know I'm doing it, and I know there's no reason for me to do it, but I can't stop. And that's very difficult. Very, very difficult.

Sandra Bartky (1990: 20) has argued that 'a variety of cultural discourses have brought it about that [women] inhabit an "inferiorized body.''' Women, she goes on to say, experience their bodies as the enemy: 'I am defective not just for others, but for myself: I inhabit this body, yet I live at a distance from it as its judge, its monitor, its commandant' (ibid.: 21). This blaming of the body may appear to function to exonerate the woman from judgments that attack her sense of self, as her transgressions are split off and projected onto a pathological condition over which she has no control. Yet, as the focus of this projection is the reproductive body, which is implicitly positioned as disordered, unruly, and deviant, the outcome of this self-policing is a direct assault on the woman's corporeality. Michael White (1991: 34–35) describes women with eating disorders as 'collaborating in the subjugation of their own lives and the objectification of their own bodies' and, as a result, becoming '"willing" participants in the disciplining of, or policing of their own lives.' In positioning premenstrual anger, distress, or need for solitude as symptoms of a disorder, 'PMS,' which is caused by an unruly body and necessitates regulation of that body, the women interviewed here are doing the same.

Contesting PMS – Acknowledging Premenstrual Distress

Individuals do not experience the body in a sociocultural vacuum. The bodily functions that we understand as signs of 'illness' vary across cultures and across time. Women's interpretation of physiological and hormonal changes as being 'symptoms' of PMS, rooted in the reproductive body, cannot be understood outside of the social and historical context within which they live, influenced by the *meaning* ascribed to these changes by Western medicalized discourses. Premenstrual changes in state or reactivity are positioned as 'PMS' because of hegemonic constructions of the premenstrual phase of the cycle as negative and debilitating (Rittenhouse, 1991; Ussher, 2003b), which impact upon women's appraisal and negotiation of premenstrual changes in affect or sensitivity (Ussher, 2002). At an individual level, this appraisal is also influenced by factors such as a woman's previous history of abuse or neglect (Golding, Taylor, Menard, & King, 2000), her current relationship context and the attributions family and friends make for premenstrual changes (Jones, Theodos, Canar, Sher, & Young, 2000; Ussher, 2003a), and the ways in which menstruation and embodied change were dealt with in her family of origin, particularly by her mother. Reinforcing the importance of cultural context, there is much evidence of differences across cultures in both women's reporting of premenstrual changes and their perception of these changes as signs of 'PMS' (Dan & Mongale, 1994). In cultures where PMS does not circulate as a discursive category, women do not attribute psychological distress to the premenstrual body, and they do not position premenstrual change as pathology (Chrisler & Caplan, 2002).

Identifying and naming specific forms of self-policing is the first step to exposing and resisting the regulatory practices that subjugate women; to contesting PMS as a pathological diagnosis. Naming self-policing practices can happen at the level of public discourse – feminist self-help texts, Web-based information, newspaper and magazine articles, or books. But it also needs to happen at an individual level, as the regimes of knowledge that frame our experiences are so taken for granted that we often cannot see them for what they are. They are effective *because* of the fact we position them as truths, rather than positioning them as simply one narrative that can explain our experiences, leading to particular subject positions that are not inevitable or unchangeable. Psychological interventions based within a narrative or constructivist framework are one means of supporting women to identify and understand self-policing, facilitating the process of the development of more agentic subject positions. This is a suggestion that might seem antithetical to a postmodern or feminist analysis of fecundity, as it may seem to smack of expert management and control, further regulation of the woman and her unruly body. But it does not have to be this way.

To this end, I was involved in the development of a women-centred psychological intervention (Ussher, Hunter, & Carris, 2002) that addressed the complex interconnection between the material, discursive, and intrapsychic factors that contribute to women's premenstrual distress (Ussher, 1999), and facilitated women's re-authoring of their experience of PMS through exploring alternative narratives. The intervention was primarily situated within a narrative re-authoring framework (White & Epston, 1990), yet it also drew on cognitive behavioural models of PMS (Blake, 1995; Morse, Bernard, & Dennerstein, 1989; Slade, 1989), in order to increase women's control of the present, as well as psychodynamic models, in order to facilitate the process of deconstructive questioning, thus allowing women to broaden their understanding of the past and its impact on the present (McQuaide, 1999: 345). The aims of the intervention were the following: to valorize women's knowledge and expertise regarding premenstrual experiences; to provide a non-pathologizing space for women to tell their story of PMS; to examine cognitions and narrative constructions of

PMS, relational issues, perceptions of stress and of premenstrual symptoms, self-silencing, and cultural constructions of femininity and PMS and how they impact upon women's premenstrual symptoms; to develop coping strategies for dealing with symptoms; to encourage assertiveness and self-care throughout the cycle; and to allow for reflexivity on the part of the therapist. In a randomized control trial conducted in the United Kingdom (Hunter et al., 2002a and 2002b), where women were either given SSRIs or they took part in this psychological intervention over eight weekly one-to-one sessions, narrative re-authoring was found to be as effective as SSRIs in reducing premenstrual distress over a 6-month period, and more effective at 1-year follow-up. In a study conducted with Australian women, a self-help package based on the intervention was found to reduce premenstrual distress and anxiety and to increase coping abilities (Ussher & Perz, 2006a).

The post-intervention changes in both studies can be summarized as women taking up a position of greater agency, not pathologizing themselves in relation to difficulties in relationships or in relation to life in general, and moving away from a position of self-sacrifice and over-responsibility. Women still experienced premenstrual change, but they no longer felt anxious in their anticipation of the premenstrual phase of the cycle, and they no longer positioned premenstrual change as an illness that was out of their control. Women were less likely to engage in self-surveillance and self-judgment, becoming more accepting of who they were, and of embodied or psychological changes that took place across the menstrual cycle. The premenstrual phase of the cycle was reframed as a time when women needed to attend to their own needs and to ask for support, rather than a time when women fail or are ill (Ussher, 2006). This is a position that previous researchers have found was also adopted by women who reported positive experiences of the menstrual cycle (Lee, 2002: 31). Thus when women can move away from the position of self-sacrificing femininity, which leads to self-castigation for not living up to impossible ideals of perfect womanhood and the pathologization of distress, they are more able to tolerate premenstrual changes in ability to cope, or ability to care for others before themselves. This does not mean that premenstrual changes are dismissed, however. Indeed, part of the function of this approach is to legitimate women's experience of premenstrual distress, while providing a means of understanding this distress that does not position the woman as 'mad,' or her experience as unimportant because it is 'PMS' – the position women were previously in.

What this illustrates is that women can be supported in the process of contesting PMS as an illness, allowing them to shift from a disempowering, pathologizing subject position, where distress is blamed on the reproductive body, and where bodily changes are split off as pathology, to a position where distress is experienced as an understandable reaction to the circumstances of women's lives, and where women are not positioned as failing or as bad, for being angry, unhappy, or anxious – or for sometimes feeling that *they* need support, that they cannot look after everybody else's needs at the cost of their own. This shift in positioning can have a significant effect on women's experience of distress, through facilitating the development of self-care, and through their experiencing the fecund body as part of their subjectivity, not as an unruly force that is Other to them, and feared because it is out of control. Thus the position of pathological femininity is effectively contested, and the medicalized version of the monstrous feminine is exposed as misogynistic myth.

Acknowledgments

This research was funded by a grant from the North Thames Regional Health Authority (United Kingdom), and a University of Western Sydney Research Partnership Scheme grant, in conjunction with FPA Health (Australia). Full ethics approval was granted by University College London and University of Western Sydney. The interviews were conducted by Jane Ussher, Susannah Browne, and Sue Stuart. Thanks are extended to Janette Perz for discussion of the ideas in this chapter. An extended version of the arguments in this chapter appears in *Managing the Monstrous Feminine: Regulating the Reproductive Body* (chapters 1 and 2).

REFERENCES

American Psychiatric Association. (1987). *Diagnostic and statistical manual of mental disorders* (3rd ed. – revised). Washington: Author.
American Psychiatric Association. (2000). *Diagnostic and statistical manual of mental disorders* (4th ed. – Text Revision). Washington: Author.
Bancroft, John. (1993). The Premenstrual Syndrome: A reappraisal of the concept and the evidence. *Psychological Medicine* (Suppl.), *241*, 1–47.
Bartky, Sandra. (1990). *Femininity and domination: Studies in the phenomenology of oppression*. New York and London: Routledge.

Blake, Fiona. (1995). Cognitive therapy for Premenstrual Syndrome. *Cognitive and Behavioral Practice, 2*(1), 167–185.

Blake, Fiona, Salkovskis, Paul, Gath, Dennis, Day, Ann, & Garrod, Adrienne. (1998). Cognitive therapy for Premenstrual Syndrome: A controlled trial. *Journal of Psychosomatic Research, 45*(4), 307–318.

Bruch, Hilda. (1978). *The golden cage: The enigma of anorexia nervosa.* New York: Vintage Books.

Burr, Vivian, & Butt, Trevor. (2000). Psychological distress and postmodern thought. In Dwight Fee (Ed.), *Pathology and the postmodern: Mental illness as discourse and experience* (pp. 186–206). London: Sage.

Chrisler, Joan C. (2002). Hormone hostages: The cultural legacy of PMS as a legal defence. In Lynn H. Collins & Michelle R. Dunlap (Eds.), *Charting a new course for feminist psychology* (pp. 238–252). Westport, CT: Praeger.

Chrisler, Joan C., & Caplan, Paula. (2002). The strange case of Dr. Jekyll and Ms. Hyde: How PMS became a cultural phenomenon and a psychiatric disorder. *Annual Review of Sex Research, 13,* 274–306.

Coughlin, Patricia C. (1990). Premenstrual syndrome: How marital satisfaction and role choice affect symptom severity. *Social Work, 35*(4), 351–355.

Dan, Alice J., & Mongale, Lisa. (1994). Socio-cultural influences on women's experiences of perimenstrual symptoms. In Judith H. Gold & Sally K. Severino (Eds.), *Premenstrual dysphoria: Myths and realities* (pp. 201–212). London: American Psychiatric Press.

Duarte, Linda M., & Thompson, Janice M. (1999). Sex-differences in self-silencing. *Psychological Reports, 85,* 145–161.

Epstein, Mark. (1995). *Thoughts without a thinker: Psychotherapy from a Buddhist perspective.* New York: Basic Books.

Fee, Dwight. (Ed.). (2000). *Pathology and the postmodern: Mental illness as discourse and experience.* London: Sage.

Figert, Anne E. (1996). *Women and the ownership of PMS: The structuring of a psychiatric disorder.* Hawthorne, NY: Aldine de Gruyter.

Foucault, Michel. (1990). *The history of sexuality, volume 1: An introduction.* (Robert Hurley, Trans.). London: Penguin. (Original work published in 1978.)

Frank, Robert. (1931). The hormonal causes of premenstrual tension. *Archives of Neurological Psychiatry, 26,* 1053.

Gear, Rachel. (2001). All those nasty womanly things: Woman artists, technology and the monstrous-feminine. *Women's Studies International Forum, 24*(3/4), 321–333.

Golding, J.M., Taylor, D.L., Menard, L., & King, M.J. (2000). Prevalence of sexual abuse history in a sample of women seeking treatment for premenstrual syndrome. *Journal of Psychosomatic Obstetrics and Gynaecology, 21*(2), 69–80.

Graves, Robert. (1966). *The white goddess*. New York: Farrar, Straus, and Giroux.

Hardie, Elizabeth A. (1997). Prevalence and predictors of cyclic and noncyclic affective change. *Psychology of Women Quarterly, 21*(2), 299–314.

Horney, Karen. (1931). Die Pramenstruellen Verstimmungen [The premenstrual debate]. *Zeitschrift für Psychoanalytische Padagogik, 5*, 1–17.

Hunter, Myra S., Ussher, Jane M., Browne, Susannah, Cariss, Margaret, Jelley, Rosanna, & Katz, Maurice. (2002a). A randomised comparison of psychological (cognitive behaviour therapy), medical (fluoxetine) and combined treatment for women with Premenstrual Dysphoric Disorder. *Journal of Psychosomatic Obstetrics and Gynaecology, 23*, 193-199.

Hunter, Myra S., Ussher, Jane M., Cariss, Margaret, Browne, Susannah, Jelley, Rosanne, & Katz, Maurice. (2002b). Medical (fluoxetine) and psychological (cognitive-behavioural) treatment for premenstrual dysphoric disorder: A study of treatment process. *Journal of Psychosomatic Research, 53*, 811–817.

Jack, Dana C. (1991). *Silencing the self: Women and depression*. Cambridge, MA: Harvard University Press.

Jones, Andrew, Theodos, Violet, Canar, W. Jeffrey, Sher, Tamara Goldman, & Young, Michael. (2000). Couples and premenstrual syndrome: Partners as moderators of symptoms? In Karen B. Schmaling & Tamara Goldman Sher (Eds.), *The psychology of couples and illness: Theory, research, and practice* (pp. 217–239). Washington: American Psychological Association.

Kuczmierczyk, Andrzej R., & Adams, Henry E. (1986). Autonomic arousal and pain sensitivity in women with premenstrual syndrome at different phases of the menstrual cycle. *Journal of Psychosomatic Research, 30*(4), 421–428.

Lee, Shirley. (2002). Health and sickness: The meaning of menstruation and premenstrual syndrome in women's lives. *Sex Roles, 46*(1–2), 25–35.

Markens, Susan. (1996). The problematic of 'experience': A political and cultural critique of PMS. *Gender and Society, 10*(1), 42–58.

McQuaide, Sharon. (1999). Using psychodynamic, cognitive-behavioral, and solution-focused questioning to co-construct a new narrative. *Clinical Social Work Journal, 27*(4), 339–353.

Morse, Carol, Bernard, Michael E., & Dennerstein, Lorraine. (1989). The effects of rational-emotive therapy and relaxation training on premenstrual syndrome: A preliminary study. *Journal of Rational Emotive and Cognitive Behavior Therapy, 7*(2), 98–110.

Nash, Heather C., & Chrisler, Joan C. (1997). Is a little (psychiatric) knowledge a dangerous thing? The impact of premenstrual dysphoric disorder on perceptions of premenstrual women. *Psychology of Women Quarterly, 21*(2), 315–322.

O'Grady, Helen. (2005). *Woman's relationship with herself: Gender, Foucault and therapy*. New York and London: Routledge.

Parry, Barbara. (1994). Biological correlates of premenstrual complaints. In Judith H. Gold & Sally K. Severino (Eds.), *Premenstrual dysphoria: Myths and realities* (pp. 47–66). London: American Psychiatric Press.

Rapkin, Andrea. (2003). A review of treatment of premenstrual syndrome and premenstrual dysphoric disorder. *Psychoneuroendocrinology, 28* (Suppl. 3), 39–53.

Rittenhouse, C. Amanda. (1991). The emergence of premenstrual syndrome as a social problem. *Social Problems, 38*(3), 412–425.

Rose, Nikolas. (1996). *Inventing ourselves: Psychology, power and personhood.* Cambridge: Cambridge University Press.

Sabin Farrell, Rachel, & Slade, Pauline. (1999). Reconceptualizing premenstrual emotional symptoms as phasic differential responsiveness to stressors. *Journal of Reproductive and Infant Psychology, 17*(4), 381–390.

Slade, Pauline. (1989). Psychological therapy for premenstrual emotional symptoms. *Behavioural Psychotherapy, 17,* 135–150.

Slade, Pauline, & Jenner, F.A. (1980). Performance tests in different phases of the menstrual cycle. *Journal of Psychosomatic Research, 24,* 5–8.

Studd, John. (1997). Depression and the menopause. *British Medical Journal, 314,* 977.

Ussher, Jane M. (1987). *The relationship between cognitive performance and physiological change across the menstrual cycle.* Unpublished doctoral dissertation, University of London, London.

Ussher, Jane M. (1992). The demise of dissent and the rise of cognition in menstrual cycle research. In John T.E. Richardson (Ed.), *Cognition and the menstrual cycle* (pp. 132–173). New York: Springer-Verlag.

Ussher, Jane M. (1996). Premenstrual syndrome: Reconciling disciplinary divides through the adoption of a material-discursive epistemological standpoint. *Annual Review of Sex Research, 7,* 218–251.

Ussher, Jane M. (1997). *Fantasies of femininity: Reframing the boundaries of sex.* London: Penguin.

Ussher, Jane M. (1999). Premenstrual Syndrome: Reconciling disciplinary divides through the adoption of a material-discursive-intrapsychic approach. In Annemarie Kolk, Marrie Bekker, & Katja Van Vliet (Eds.), *Advances in women and health research* (pp. 47–64). Amsterdam: Tilberg University Press.

Ussher, Jane M. (2002). Processes of appraisal and coping in the development and maintenance of Premenstrual Dysphoric Disorder. *Journal of Community and Applied Social Psychology, 12,* 1–14.

Ussher, Jane M. (2003a). The ongoing silencing of women in families: An analysis and rethinking of premenstrual syndrome and therapy. *Journal of Family Therapy, 25,* 388–405.

Ussher, Jane M. (2003b). The role of premenstrual dysphoric disorder in the subjectification of women. *Journal of Medical Humanities, 24*(1/2), 131–146.

Ussher, Jane M. (2004a). Blaming the body for distress: Premenstrual Dysphoric Disorder and the subjectification of women. In Annie Potts, Nicola Gavey, & Ann Wetherall (Eds.), *Sex and the body* (pp. 183–202). Palmerstone North, NZ: Dunmore Press.

Ussher, Jane M. (2004b). Premenstrual syndrome and self-policing: Ruptures in self-silencing leading to increased self-surveillance and blaming of the body. *Social Theory and Health, 2*(3), 254–272.

Ussher, Jane M. (2006). *Managing the monstrous feminine: Regulating the reproductive body.* New York and London: Routledge.

Ussher, Jane M., Hunter, Myra, & Carris, Margaret. (2002). A woman-centred psychological intervention for premenstrual symptoms, drawing on cognitive-behavioural and narrative therapy. *Clinical Psychology and Psychotherapy, 9,* 319–331.

Ussher, Jane M., & Perz, Janette. (2006a). Evaluating the relative efficacy of a self-help and minimal psycho-educational intervention for moderate premenstrual distress conducted from a critical realist standpoint. *Journal of Reproductive and Infant Psychology,* 24(2), 347–362.

Ussher, Jane M., & Perz, Janette. (2006b). Women's experience of premenstrual change: A case of silencing the self. *Journal of Reproductive and Infant Psychology,* 24(4), 289–303.

Ussher, Jane M., & Wilding, John. M. (1991). Performance and state changes during the menstrual cycle, conceptualised within a broad band testing framework. *Social Science and Medicine, 32*(5), 525–534.

Ussher, Jane M., & Wilding, John, M. (1992). Interactions between stress and performance during the menstrual cycle in relation to the premenstrual syndrome. *Journal of Reproductive and Infant Psychology, 10*(2), 83-101.

Walker, Anne. (1995). Theory and methodology in Premenstrual Syndrome research. *Social Science and Medicine, 41*(6), 793-800.

Walker, Barbara G. (1983). *The women's encyclopedia of myths and secrets.* San Francisco: Harper and Row.

White, Michael. (1991). Deconstruction and therapy. In *Dulwich Centre Newsletter* (pp. 21–40). Adelaide: Dulwich Centre Publications.

White, Michael, & Epston, David. (1990). *Narrative means to therapeutic ends.* Adelaide: Dulwich Centre Publications.

Woods, Nancy Fugate, Lentz, Martha Jane, Mitchell, Ellen Sullivan, Heitkemper, Margaret, Shaver, Joan, & Henker, Richard. (1998). Perceived stress, physiologic stress arousal, and premenstrual symptoms: Group differences and intra-individual patterns. *Research in Nursing and Health, 21*(6), 511–523.

11 Resisting an Illness Label: Disability, Impairment, and Illness

SHARON DALE STONE

Particularly in academic texts devoted to explaining the scope of the sociology of health and illness, the terms *illness* and *disability* are often used in the same breath (e.g., Freund, McGuire, & Podhurst, 2003; Weitz, 2004). Even though such texts usually point out that the two terms are not coterminous and that there are different issues involved in understanding the experience of illness and the experience of disability, the very fact that the terms are discussed together creates the impression that disability is a particular kind of illness.[1] This is not to say that the conflation of disability and illness is sustained only by their juxtaposition in academic texts. Indeed, many features of contemporary society work to focus attention on disability as a health issue requiring medical intervention,[2] while deflecting attention away from the ways in which disability is not a question of health. The World Health Organization (WHO), for example, is influential in this regard. An understanding of disability in terms of illness is shored up in a variety of ways.

In this chapter I examine some troublesome ramifications of the conflation of disability with illness, while commenting on issues that need consideration in attempts to delineate the borders between illness and disability. For example, the conflation of disability with illness is an important reason (but by no means the only reason) why it can be difficult to appreciate that people who have impairments are not necessarily suffering[3] or in need of medical attention. I illustrate the point that impairment does not imply suffering or the need for medical surveillance by drawing on the experiences of young women I interviewed about living with the consequences of hemorrhagic stroke. My discussion of their experiences highlights that, although they are typically understood by medical experts and others primarily in terms of having suffered a trag-edy, their own bodily experiences lead them to a different self-under-standing. Biomedicine, which so far seems uninterested in the self-understandings of these young women, regards them objectively as 'stroke victims' or 'stroke sufferers.' The concepts of suffering or victim-hood, however, do not resonate with the stories that these stroke *survivors* had to tell me. Clearly, there is a need to appreciate the importance of lived bodily experience as a source of authoritative expertise.

Towards a Delineation of Borders: A Perspective from Disability Studies

From the perspective of disability studies, one thing is clear: disability is not a property (characteristic, feature) of an individual body, but is socially created through practices that deny the ubiquity of impairment, that is, cognitive or physical difference. Impairment may or may not be experienced as troublesome, and impairment is not inherently dis-abling. Thus, someone with an impairment such as one-sided weakness is not disabled because of an inability to control one side of the body, but is disabled in situations where the expectation is that someone has full control over all parts of the body. From this perspective, disability is an oppression that is imposed on people with impairments. Disability is, therefore, always contextual, and it is not something to be treated through medical surveillance. Neither disability nor impairment are inherently tragic and neither imply suffering. Treating disability and impairment as tragic typically contributes to the experience of disable-ment (which is, lamentably, what causes suffering).

Illness, in contrast, is not socially created in the same way. Rather, ill-ness is an experience that is usually conceptualized as flowing from dis-ease, but which can also be conceptualized as flowing from impairment or flowing from environmental conditions. Regardless of the cause, ill-ness is something that an individual subjectively feels, and it implies suffering on some level. Thus, one who experiences illness is typically (but not always) motivated to find ways to lessen suffering or even to eradicate the underlying illness. However, reflecting the hegemony of biomedicine, people who feel ill typically seek medical intervention to treat their illnesses, and medical intervention can often (but not always) successfully ameliorate symptoms. For example, antibiotics may coun-teract an infection, antidepressants may dissipate feelings of depres-sion, or anti-seizure medication may prevent epileptic episodes. This is not to say that medical intervention is necessarily appropriate for eradicating the cause of illness. The focus of medical intervention on the individual can sometimes allow the individual to feel better, but biomedicine cannot address oppression.

The borders between disability and illness are clearest when discussing acute (i.e., temporary) illness. They are murkiest when discussing chronic (i.e., long-lasting, even permanent) illness. This is because chronic illness, by definition, will not 'go away' with medical intervention. Thus, the experience of chronic illness can often resemble the experience of disability.[4] That is, regardless of whether someone has either a chronic illness or a disabling impairment, that person is commonly understood to be suffering and in need of medical intervention. Moreover, not everyone who is diagnosed as having a chronic illness or an impairment necessarily accepts that the diagnosis requires medical attention and surveillance. I conceptualize this as *resisting an illness label*, by which I mean resisting both the idea that suffering is inherently 'bad' and resisting the social imperative to submit to medical surveillance.

The practice of resisting an illness label can be illustrated with an example from my own life. I have been diagnosed with osteoarthritis – biomedically understood as a chronic illness – but I regard it less as an illness and more as something that prevents me from doing all that I might otherwise do. On a day-to-day basis, I do not 'feel' that my osteoarthritis is an illness so much as an attribute of my body, much the way other impairments that I live with are attributes of my body. The pain that arthritis can cause is something I would be happy to live without, but this does not mean that I am unhappy to live with pain. Yet the idea of having an impairment caused by arthritis resonates with my experience. Rather than experiencing my arthritic knee in terms of suffering, I experience it in terms of (permanent) bodily impairment. As such, it is neither good nor bad, it just *is*. Although there are disabling consequences in this ableist society, I feel no need to subject myself to medical surveillance to 'treat' my arthritis.[5] In this way, I personally resist an illness label.

Disability According to the World Health Organization

Outside disability studies, there is little to support a distinction between disability and illness. Indeed, disability seems to be regarded as a type of illness by the World Health Organization, an organization widely understood as having legitimate authority to pronounce on matters related to disease, illness, and disability. The WHO is responsible for creating the well-known International Classification of Impairments, Disability and Handicap (ICIDH), and the more recent International Classification of Functioning, Disability and Health (ICF). In creating the latter document, the WHO says:

> ICF is named as it is because of its stress is [*sic*] on health and functioning, rather than on disability. Previously, disability began where health ended; once you were disabled, you where [*sic*] in a separate category. We want to get away from this kind of thinking.
>
> ICF puts the notions of 'health' and 'disability' in a new light. It acknowledges that *every human being can experience a decrement in health and thereby experience some disability*. This is not something that happens to only a minority of humanity. ICF thus 'mainstreams' the experience of disability and recognises it as a universal human experience. By shifting the focus from cause to impact it places all health conditions on an equal footing allowing them to be compared using a common metric – the ruler of health and disability. (2002: 3, emphasis added)

Here, with disability regarded as 'a decrement in health' it is implicitly defined as coterminous with illness, and as a property of individuals. In this document, there is no border to distinguish illness from disability, and there is no interest in establishing such a border. This in itself is a problem, but much more insidious is the WHO's complicity in creating the concept of the 'disability-adjusted life year' (DALY) which promotes the idea that disability is inimical to health and long life. As Melanie Rock (2000: 408) explains: 'The DALY was developed for the World Bank and the World Health Organisation under the leadership of Christopher Murray of the Harvard School of Public Health. It has quickly gained prominence as a health indicator. In measuring health, the DALY regards disability as pathology – as disease in need of elimination. The DALY does not, therefore, measure social, economic or individual resources that may affect the impact of bodily circumstances. It deems time lived with a disability as having less worth than time spent in "perfect health."'

The DALY has been vociferously criticized by disability studies scholars as a concept that pretends it is possible to objectively determine the impact of disability on a life. Robert Metts (2001: 451), for example, argues that 'the DALY system of disability severity weightings embodies the false assumption that any given disabling condition always results in a disability of a certain severity, regardless of the context in which it occurs.' More disturbing, as Rock (2000) points out, is that the assumptions embedded in the use of the DALY can serve in the minds of many to justify murder, as happened when Tracy Latimer, who had a severe form of cerebral palsy, was murdered by her father.

For my purposes here, the DALY is significant for two reasons. First, it consolidates an understanding of disability as a bodily attribute,[6] and second, it assumes 'that living with a disability represents a net drain on society' (Groce, Chamie, & Me, 1999: n.p.). The DALY was created to measure 'the global burden of disease' (World Bank, 1993); thus, it regards disability in terms of burdensome pathology requiring elimination.[7] This medicalization of disability is deeply problematic. With powerful authorities promoting use of the DALY, and with the measurement's popularity in countries around the world, it can be difficult indeed to maintain that disability per se is neither coterminous with illness nor a threat to living a long and healthy life. As Patricia de Wolfe points out (2002: 259), 'the characterisation of a bodily problem as an illness or disease, places it, more or less by definition in Western society, under the auspices of medical practitioners and researchers who aspire not only to improve quality of life, but to rectify or prevent what is construed as a disorder.'

Resisting Medicalization

Both the disability rights movement and disability studies scholars challenge the medicalization of disability. Briefly, the primary challenge arises from a social model of disability, which makes a fundamental distinction between impairment (a bodily attribute) and disability (a socially created disadvantage that oppresses people with impairments). Increasingly, however, feminist disability scholars such as Jenny Morris (1991), Liz Crow (1996), and Carol Thomas (1999) are criticizing the social model for ignoring experiences of bodily distress. As Bill Hughes and Kevin Paterson (1997: 326) articulate the problem, the social model 'actually concedes the body to medicine and understands impairment in terms of medical discourse.' Shelley Tremain (2002) goes further in her criticism and argues against maintaining the distinction between impairment and disability. All these scholars maintain that we need to develop a social theory of impairment, to not only recognize the ways in which impairments are socially created, but also to get out from under the oppressive hegemony of the medicalization of impairment.

The disability rights movement is working to wrest ownership of the definition of disability away from biomedicine; the same needs to be done for the concept of impairment.

To effectively resist an illness label, there is an equally pressing need to oppose the medicalization of illness. As Arthur Kleinman argues (1988: 8–10), biomedicine is dangerous for the chronically ill. Certainly, there is nothing troublesome about people who understand themselves as chronically ill using the services offered by biomedicine, provided that they do so with a critical awareness of the potentially harmful effects of biomedical advice.[8] There is more to illness, however, than having medically defined cognitive and/or bodily problems.

At the same time, it is currently far more difficult to resist the medicalization of either impairment or illness than it is to resist the medicalization of disability. To be clear, I am not interested in rejecting *all* biomedical knowledge about illness, and I certainly do not reject the ephemeral ability of medical professionals to alleviate suffering. I am happy, for example, that anti-inflammatory drugs and even knee replacements are available to address my arthritic pain and permanent damage. Yet, I cherish the right to decide, on an ongoing basis, whether to use such interventions. I reject the medical profession's authoritative claim that it has the right to make pronouncements not only about the state of the body and what to do about it, but also about the person who lives with that body.[9] Resisting the medicalization of either impairment or illness minimally entails recognizing the crucial importance of lived, bodily experience as a source of authoritative expertise.

To resist an illness label, then, is to resist the hegemonic belief that those who are ill do not have the authority to know and care for their own bodies, but require medical surveillance. It is also to resist an understanding of illness as an unmitigated tragedy that causes nothing but pain and suffering. Regarding this latter point, Susan Wendell (2001: 30–1) draws on her own experiences with Myalgic Encephalomyelitis (ME) to point out that 'it is difficult to say that one is glad to have been ill and be believed, despite the fact that many people who are or have been ill testify that it has changed them for the better … living with pain, fatigue, nausea, unpredictable abilities, and/or the imminent threat of death creates different ways of being that give valuable perspectives on life and the world. Thus, although most of us want to avoid suffering if possible, suffering is part of some valuable ways of being.'

Notwithstanding recent challenges to the biomedical dominance of health care, mainstream Western society has not moved beyond a naive belief that those who are ill are duty-bound to take up the Parsonian 'sick role.' In particular, when sick or ill, we are still expected to seek treatment from a physician and follow the prescribed treatment plan. Currently, 'patients' sometimes have a certain latitude to question their physicians or negotiate with them about how to proceed, but it remains the case that the physician is widely regarded as the ultimate authority. It is incumbent upon the 'good citizen' (Marc Renaud, cited in Herzlich & Pierret, 1987: 231–2) to subject herself or himself to medical surveillance. It seems that those who are ill are not, after all, allowed to take charge of their own bodies.

Given the authority of physicians in contemporary society to pass judgment on who is or is not ill and make pronouncements on what to do about it (Wendell, 1996), it is hard to imagine that someone with a seriously debilitating illness has never consulted a physician. It is in the medical encounter, after all, that one finds out in the first place that there is a name for disconcerting bodily experiences. Thus, it does not actually make sense to say that someone who has never seen a physician has a chronic illness. Susan Greenhalgh (2001: 3) notes:

> In a culture that worships science it is to scientific (or conventional) medicine that we first turn for help. Women desperate for someone to acknowledge and alleviate their suffering go to their doctors to name and ease their new pains. Professionally obligated to heal and motivated by humanitarian impulses, our doctors try to live up to our expectations ... Research scientists develop diagnostic criteria for a new syndrome, clinical scientists work out treatment protocols, and a new group of specialists emerges with a guaranteed stable of patients for life. Before long, a bona fide new disease has entered the medical and cultural mainstream. In this way, distress is transformed into disease, and the 'diseasing' of social life moves ineluctably forward.

This is not to say that all those who have been diagnosed with a chronic illness necessarily accept the label; there are all sorts of reasons why someone might want to challenge the diagnosis. Not least of those reasons would be feeling healthy: 'Definition and experience of chronic illness dialectically affect each other. A view of oneself as only having a minor ailment or occasional bouts of serious illness can last if the illness is episodic. At those points, illness comes to the foreground, but otherwise it remains in the background' (Charmaz, 1991: 20).

What it means to feel healthy is the subject of numerous investigations (e.g., Hughner & Kleine, 2004; Saltonstall, 1993; Wakewich, 2000). Suffice it to say that objective, biomedical definitions do not always correspond neatly with subjective experience. This is another reason why there are similarities between the experiences of chronic illness, impairment, and disability, and why medicalization needs to be resisted.

Impairment and Lived Bodily Experience

Whatever similarities exist between chronic illness and disability, it is nevertheless the case that many disabled people resist being seen as ill or in need of medical surveillance (e.g., Clare, 1999). To illustrate this point, I turn now to discussing young women's experiences of surviving hemorrhagic stroke. I intend my discussion to illustrate that, despite their residual impairments, these survivors do not understand themselves as tragic victims in need of medical surveillance.

The three stories that follow are selected from among 28 interviews I conducted with a diverse group of young women about their experiences of surviving hemorrhagic stroke.[10] Like many stroke survivors, we[11] have been left with permanent and intrusive impairments on the cognitive, physical, and/or emotional levels, which are variously invisible, visible, or sometimes both. Perhaps it is because of these impairments that stroke survivors are sometimes included in the literature on experiencing chronic illness (e.g., Olsson et al., 2003; Thorne et al., 2002). Regardless, illness is not a concept that any of the women I interviewed used to characterize their post-stroke experiences. Rather, our lives have been transformed, often in unexpected and welcome ways. Contrary to what popular wisdom and medical opinion lead us to expect, our post-stroke experiences have taught us that there is high-quality life beyond stroke.

The theme of positive transformation was found in many of the interviews, but three women were particularly clear in explaining how they benefited from their stroke-related experiences. Two women, Cindy Davis[12] and Vicky Evans, told me that the stroke was literally the best thing that ever happened to them. A third, Ornella Marsico, did not say this in so many words, but she did say that the good definitely outweighed the bad.

Cindy Davis

Cindy was only 4 years post-stroke at the time of the interview, and in addition to clumsiness due to right-sided weakness, she was dealing with significant cognitive disabilities. She went from living a busy, high-stress life, to not being able to deal with any level of stress, and having communication problems. One thing that particularly angers her is that others do not acknowledge the difficulties she now has:

> Because, because I don't walk with a stick, because I'm able to speak, and because I'm intelligent. And therefore I can articulate most of what I want to say … and when I say I have problems with language, people say, 'Well, you can speak *fine*.' 'No, I *can't*.' *I* know I can't do what I used to be able to do. You know, um – and it is, it's like banging your head against a wall, that. 'Cause, *yes*, people don't recognize that I've got problems.

When Cindy was discharged from the hospital, she moved in with her mother, but not long after that, her mother died. This left Cindy bereft of all family. She tried to return to her former employment, which involved interviewing people, but she lost the job when it became clear that she could no longer cope with the work. At one point in the interview I asked her if she had ever been depressed about her losses. She replied that she had never gone through a period of depression.

A mere 2 years after her stroke, Cindy decided that she needed to make drastic changes in her life. She had always loved a rural part of England by the sea, and no longer having any ties to her former home, she decided to move. With her mother's legacy, she bought herself a little house and set about getting to know people by working part-time in a local shop and being friendly. Then she realized that she could develop her own business teaching people how to use computers. This was where she was in her life when we met for an interview. In her words, after she had the stroke:

> I sort of came out the other end of it and thought, 'Oh! I'm fed up with this!' Um, and, and then my mom died and I thought, right, OK. At that stage you either – well, *my* thoughts are, you either go off and kill yourself, which I don't think, I need, I don't – not interested in that. *Or* you make a new life … In some ways, it was the best thing that ever happened to me, it made me stop and think about meself. And me life and, and

what's important to my life. And that's why I came down here ... it's given me direction. Um, it's allowed me to think about life and, you know, all that *deep* stuff. Um, and the, the few disabilities that I've got, I've got used to them now and I'm stuck with them.

Cindy readily acknowledges that she can at times get frustrated with not being able to do what she thinks she ought to be able to do, but she would rather work within her limits to accomplish what she can. Her ability to focus on what she has rather than what she has lost, provides strong evidence that learning to negotiate life with impairments can be transformative in positive ways.

Vicky Evans

The other woman who told me that the stroke is the best thing that ever happened to her is Vicky Evans. At age 31, Vicky was an up-and-coming media publicist for a large corporation. She was feeling proud of herself and her advancement in the business world. As she said laughingly, 'You know, I was not doing bad for not having a university education!' She was so focused on progression in her career that she did not always take care of herself, and often got by just on adrenalin. Her stroke, however, put an end to her busy lifestyle.

Like Cindy, Vicky's residual impairments are not immediately apparent. At 3 years post-stroke, Vicky mostly felt disabled by some left-sided weakness, difficulty dealing with crowds, and fatigue. The physical consequences of her stroke, however, pale in comparison with the psychological consequences. Vicky was deeply changed from who she had been before the stroke. She was exceptionally thoughtful in the interview, and even though she sometimes had trouble expressing what she wanted to say, I would like to quote Vicky at length. Her many long pauses, I think, are indicative of the thought she put into trying to express herself, and the way she often threw a colloquial 'you know' into her speech is indicative of the difficulty she had with fully articulating the strength of her feelings.[13]

When I went back to work I remember thinking [long pause] thinking 'this is all shit. This doesn't mean anything. We're not doing anything constructive here!' Like just feeling really [long pause] not negative but just like [long pause] you know 'what's it all about?' Like how can I go from such a life/death experience ... to pedalling entertainment again!

You know! And telling people to come to concerts and it was like talking to the media and it was like, you know? This is so, this is so much bullshit I just don't [long pause] I don't [long pause] I, I, couldn't see, I couldn't see, I couldn't see me ever wanting to do it ever again.

Later in the interview she reinforced these points and added:

And you know, going back to [work] was important for me because I had to prove to myself that I could do the job. And that I wasn't weak. Which is really, sick, because [long pause] why did I need to prove anything to, you know; and I also felt I was trying to prove something to [the people] who worked there when I was there and, you know. And I didn't need to prove anything. But I had to figure that out for myself. And I went to [work] and it was like, 'these people are sick.' [laughs] 'I don't, I don't like this. I don't need to do this. I don't, this is not important to me!' And, and so then I quit of my own volition … They wanted me to stay, but I knew I wasn't up to snuff. That I just didn't have the, have the energy. And you know what? Maybe I don't. I don't honestly know, to tell you the truth. I don't really know if I have the stamina to do what I did before. I know I certainly don't have it in my heart. But I don't think I have the physical stamina. And that's okay.

Vicky went on to talk about her post-stroke move to a rural area, and how surprised she was at finding that she enjoyed being away from the hustle and bustle of the big city. She said she is 'positive' that the 'move would never have happened if I did not have the stroke.' She also talked about the stroke having changed her relationship with her partner 'for the better.' Although 'it was a good relationship to begin with,' she said:

But I think it made it deeper. It made me realize, it made me realize what – that whole idea of forever? You know? I'd never really [long pause] understood it. Like I'd always, you know I'd always taken for granted that we were together … But I never really [long pause] un-, I never really appreciated that whole idea of loving forever until I was sick.

Summing up her experience, Vicky said:

I don't want anyone, like I don't – no one needs to say, 'Poor Vicky.' Or, 'What a horrible thing.' 'Cause it wasn't. It's actually been a – one of the best things that's ever happened to me. Ironically.

Ornella Marsico

Ornella Marsico was 19 when she had an aneurysm rupture, and 10 years post-stroke when I interviewed her. Ornella is from a working-class, non-English-speaking, immigrant family. At the time of the stroke, she was living with her parents, working two part-time jobs, and attending business college. She had to quit school because of the stroke. At the time of the interview, Ornella was working full time and had occasional seizures. Other than two seizures that were bad enough that she lost her driver's licence for a time, her seizures have been very mild. She knows she's having one when she starts to stutter or has problems finding words. She experiences this as more of a minor annoyance than as a significant disability. Indeed, when interviewed, she said that the only continuing problems she noticed on a daily basis were a very poor memory, both short term and long term, and becoming easily fatigued. She found her memory difficulties particularly troublesome, and was worried about forgetting things and events that were important to her. Ornella told me:

> I used to have a very, very, very strong memory. And all of a sudden I didn't remember, I didn't know anything anymore, I didn't remember anything anymore. And it, and it was a problem for me. It interfered a lot with my work. And just, um, just knowing that at one time – they used to call me a walking telephone book because you – they would say, 'What's her number?' and I, I'd memorized it and I'd know what it was, and that's her number, they didn't even have to look through a telephone book, so not being able to do that anymore was something that bothered me because it was something I was able to do. And it was like one of my talents, I would say, and it wasn't anymore.

Nevertheless, Ornella wanted to make it quite clear that she was not sorry that she had had a stroke. She said:

> I've got nothing, nothing negative about this experience at all. Nothing at all. Everything has been positive … Because this happened I feel like I've achieved so much, I, I feel like nothing can, can knock me down.

Outlining the transformation of her attitude towards life, Ornella said:

> It's changed my life. I really don't care about what the future holds for me. I'm not a career-oriented person where at one point I was. Now I'm,

now I'm not. I don't care if I'm going to be at this company for the next 5 years. I'd rather have a family and stay at home and be a mom. Those are the important things to me now in life, not the extra 40,000, 50,000 a year that can buy me a, maybe a boat that's going to help me retire.

Transformations

As noted above, the theme of positive transformation ran through many of the stories of women I interviewed. In the interviews, I was struck with the intensity of emotion expressed on this issue, and I detect a sense of joy that they had not only survived a life-threatening illness, but also that they can live a full life with impairments. No one said this about impairment or disability in so many words, but interspersed with complaints about difficulties with doing things were lengthy comments about how genuinely happy they were to have what amounted to a new chance at life – a chance to do things differently. The stories of Cindy, Vicky, and Ornella are illustrative of this. Each, in her own way, implicitly contests the idea that she is a victim who has suffered a tragedy.

Looking in from the outside, some might be tempted to observe that their impairments are not especially severe. Yet invisible impairments are in some ways more troublesome than those that are immediately obvious (Stone, 1995 and 2005). Moreover, no onlooker can legitimately pass judgment on the severity of any particular impairment. This is what a biomedical perspective does; it offers an 'objective' assessment about someone's life. What needs to be recognized is that impairment can only be experienced from the inside, within the overall context of someone's life. These women rely upon their own bodily experiences to resist medicalization, and claim their own authoritative expertise.

From a biomedical perspective, each of us was for a time seriously ill, but has made a good or even excellent recovery. In this regard, many of us have exceeded our physicians' expectations.[14] Our residual impairments, however, are solely recognized as tragic, and are understood to mean that our lives have been transformed for the worse. According to the World Health Organization (2002: 3), we 'experience a decrement in health,' while, according to the DALY, our post-stroke lives have less worth than our pre-stroke lives, and we represent 'a net drain on society' (Groce, Chamie, & Me, 1997: 7). From this perspective, there is no border between illness, impairment, and disability; these are adverse conditions in need of elimination.

Biomedicine cannot possibly know how illness, impairment, and the experience of disability will transform a life. Few of the women I interviewed would agree that their lives have been transformed for the worse. On the contrary, most of us find much to celebrate about the changes we have been through. Grounded in our lived bodily experiences, we contest the assessment that our impairments represent nothing more than suffering, we reject the application of an illness label to our lives, and we claim that our lives cannot be understood through the lens of an illness paradigm. In so many ways, we contest the views of others, using our bodies as a source of authoritative expertise.

Acknowledgments

I would like to thank Pamela Moss for encouraging me to write this chapter and making suggestions along the way; Kathy Teghtsoonian for helpful comments in revising this chapter for publication; and Cindy Davis, Vicky Evans, and Ornella Marsico for sharing their stories with me.

NOTES

1 Conversely, illness is often perceived as a type of disability. Nevertheless, I am interested in the constitution of disability as illness, and not the reverse.
2 For example, persons who are too ill to seek or maintain employment may qualify for disability benefits in Canada (see Michael J. Prince, Chapter 2, this volume), but are not guaranteed to do so (see also Katherine Lippel, Chapter 3, this volume). Such practices work to sustain a view of disability as a health issue.
3 I define *suffering* as it is usually understood, as entailing pain and/or distress. Eric Cassell's (1991: 33) definition of suffering is also relevant: 'the state of severe distress associated with events that threaten the intactness of person.'
4 Susan Wendell (2001) argues for the need to recognize that chronic illness can be disabling and explores the ways in which illness and disability experiences are similar.
5 It has not always been the case that I have resisted medicalization of my arthritis, and it may not always be the case in the future. My point here is to give an example of what it means to resist an illness label.
6 To this extent, the concept of the DALY is at odds with the ICF which does not regard disability *solely* in terms of the individual, but says: 'Disability is

a complex phenomena [*sic*] that is both a problem at the level of a person's body, and a complex and primarily social phenomena' (WHO, 2002: 9).

7 This understanding of disability as an economic burden is repeated in the ICF document: 'We need information on the disability burden of various diseases and health conditions' (WHO, 2002: 7).

8 Susan Greenhalgh (2001) has written an autobiographical account of her attempts at getting appropriate medical treatment for her chronic illness. Her story includes a harrowing warning against placing too much trust in biomedical advice.

9 In this regard, I disagree with Patricia de Wolfe (2002: 263), who says, 'The notion of sick people arguing for "illness rights" akin to "disability rights" seems almost embarrassing, raising the spectre of a kind of whingers' charter.' On the contrary, there *is* a need for illness rights.

10 A research project funded by the Social Sciences and Humanities Research Council of Canada, grant no. 410-2002-0633.

11 I too am a survivor, and much of what my research participants say resonates with my own experience.

12 All research participant names are pseudonyms.

13 Marjorie DeVault (1999: 69) discusses these issues and the importance of paying attention to women's hesitant or inarticulate speech. My remark here is not meant to imply that Vicky was the only one who was thoughtful and felt strongly. Indeed, every woman I interviewed offered thoughtful, deeply felt commentary.

14 Another striking feature across many interviews was the frequency with which women would comment on how surprised their physicians were that they had recovered so well.

REFERENCES

Cassell, Eric J. (1991). *The nature of suffering: And the goals of medicine.* New York: Oxford University Press.

Charmaz, Kathy. (1991). *Good days, bad days: The self in chronic illness and time.* New Brunswick, NJ: Rutgers University Press.

Clare, Eli. (1999). *Exile and pride: Disability, queerness and liberation.* Cambridge, MA: South End Press.

Crow, Liz. (1996). Including all of our lives: Renewing the social model of disability. In Jenny Morris (Ed.), *Encounters with strangers: Feminism and disability* (pp. 206–226). London: Women's Press.

DeVault, Marjorie. (1999). Talking and listening from women's standpoint. In *Liberating method: Feminism and social research* (pp. 59–83). Philadelphia: Temple University Press.

de Wolfe, Patricia. (2002). Private tragedy in social context? Reflections on disability, illness and suffering. *Disability and Society, 17*(3), 255–267.

Freund, Peter E. S., McGuire, Meredith B., & Podhurst, Linda S. (2003). *Health, illness, and the social body: A critical sociology* (4th ed.). Upper Saddle River, NJ: Prentice-Hall.

Greenhalgh, Susan. (2001). *Under the medical gaze: Facts and fictions of chronic pain.* Berkeley and Los Angeles: University of California Press.

Groce, Nora Ellen, Chamie, Mary, & Me, Angela. (1999). Measuring the quality of life: Rethinking the World Bank's disability adjusted life year. *International Rehabilitation Review, 49*(1&2). Retrieved 11 Sept. 2005, from http://www.rehabinternational.org/publications/rivol49/measuringquality.html.

Herzlich, Claudine, & Pierret, Janine. (1987). *Illness and self in society.* Baltimore: Johns Hopkins University Press.

Hughes, Bill, & Paterson, Kevin. (1997). The social model of disability and the disappearing body: Towards a sociology of impairment. *Disability and Society, 12*(3), 325–340.

Hughner, Renée Shaw, & Kleine, Susan Schultz. (2004). Views of health in the lay sector: A compilation and review of how individuals think about health. *Health, 8*(4), 395–422.

Kleinman, Arthur. (1988). *The illness narratives: Suffering, healing, and the human condition.* New York: Basic Books.

Metts, Robert L. (2001). The fatal flaw in the disability adjusted life year. *Disability and Society, 16*(3), 449–452.

Morris, Jenny. (1991). *Pride against prejudice: Transforming attitudes to disability.* London: Women's Press.

Olsson, Craig A., Bond, L., Johnson, M.W., Forer, D.L., Boyce, M.F. & Sawyer, S.M. (2003). Adolescent chronic illness: A qualitative study of psychosocial adjustment. *Annals of the Academy of Medicine, Singapore, 32*(1), 43–50.

Rock, Melanie. (2000). Discounted lives? Weighing disability when measuring health and ruling on 'compassionate' murder. *Social Science and Medicine, 51*, 407–417.

Saltonstall, Robin. (1993). Healthy bodies, social bodies: Men's and women's concepts and practices of health in everyday life. *Social Science and Medicine, 36*(1), 7–14.

Stone, Sharon Dale. (1995). The myth of bodily perfection. *Disability and Society, 10*(4), 413–424.

Stone, Sharon Dale. (2005). Reactions to invisible disability: The experiences of young women survivors of hemorrhagic stroke. *Disability and Rehabilitation, 27,* 293–304.

Thomas, Carol. (1999). *Female forms: Experiencing and understanding disability.* Buckingham, UK: Open University Press.

Thorne, Sally, Paterson, Barbara, Acorn, Sonia, Canam, Connie, Joachim, Gloria, & Jillings, Carol. (2002). Chronic illness experience: Insights from a metastudy. *Qualitative Health Research, 12*(4), 437–452.

Tremain, Shelley. (2002). On the subject of impairment. In Marian Corker & Tom Shakespeare (Eds.), *Disability/postmodernity: Embodying disability theory* (pp. 32–47). London: Continuum.

Wakewich, Pamela. (2000). Contours of everyday life: Women's reflections on embodiment and health over time. In Baukje Miedema, Janet M. Stoppard, & Vivienne Anderson (Eds.), *Women's bodies, women's lives: Health, well-being and body image* (pp. 237–254). Toronto: Sumach Press.

Weitz, Rose. (2004). *Sociology of health, illness, and health care* (3rd ed.). Belmont, CA: Wadsworth.

Wendell, Susan. (1996). *The rejected body: Feminist philosophical reflections on disability.* New York and London: Routledge.

Wendell, Susan. (2001). Unhealthy disabled: Treating chronic illnesses as disabilities. *Hypatia, 16*(4), 17–33.

World Bank. (1993). *World Development Report 1993: Investing in health.* New York: Oxford University Press.

World Health Organization. (2002). *Towards a Common Language for Functioning, Disability and Health: ICF: The International Classification of Functioning, Disability and Health.* Geneva: World Health Organization.

12 The Race and Class Politics of Anorexia Nervosa: Unravelling White, Middle-Class Standards in Representations of Eating Problems

HELEN GREMILLION

Until quite late into the twentieth century, anorexia nervosa (hereafter referred to as anorexia) had been described almost exclusively as a white, middle-class phenomenon. Consider the following popular 1978 book titles, written at a time when the incidence of anorexia was increasing so dramatically that it was no longer considered an obscure illness (indeed, it was soon to obtain what some would call a 'quasi-epidemic' status): pioneer therapist Hilde Bruch (1978) wrote *The Golden Cage*; and prominent therapist Steven Levenkron (1978) penned *The Best Little Girl in the World*. These titles conjure up familiar stereotypes of young women and girls diagnosed with anorexia: they are bright, emotionally 'repressed,' and privileged perfectionists, presumed to be white and middle class. Although an increasing number of studies have challenged this generalized representation of 'anorexic'[1] patients, it remains highly influential in diagnosis and treatment. Indeed, most patient populations are overwhelmingly white and middle class, in part because of mental health professionals' assumptions about 'typical' patient profiles. During my fieldwork on the treatment of anorexia in a prestigious teaching and research hospital,[2] an intern in training remarked: 'I would get tired of working with anorexic patients all the time – nothing but blonde, repressed, middle-class girls.' In keeping with this comment, I noticed throughout my fieldwork that clinicians occasionally romanticized the more 'volatile' patients that were usually admitted for 'psychosomatic' problems other than anorexia; but at the same time, anorexic patients were often held up as 'model' patients and received better treatment than their (usually) underprivileged counterparts.

Since the mid-1980s, some scholars have cast doubt on the widespread assumption that anorexia is a white and middle-class phenomenon. As Ruth H. Striegel-Moore and Linda Smolak (2000: 228) note, 'Evidence has been accumulating ... that eating disorders cross ethnic and class boundaries. A growing number of case studies have provided clinical accounts of eating disorders in Black American, Native American, and Hispanic American girls or women' (for reviews, see Crago, Shisslak, & Estes, 1996; Root, 1990).[3] Note, however, that trends in literature on the prevalence of anorexia among ethnic minority groups are difficult to assess, in part because of methodological problems with studies that address this question and in part because of lack of comparability between such studies regarding categories of ethnic groups and of eating problems (Striegel-Moore & Smolak, 2000). In addition, there are divergent findings about anorexia's articulation with both race and class.

The varying designs of and divergent findings in this research literature muddy the analytic waters. However, taken together, these studies are instructive for a critical examination of anorexia's race and class politics – particularly the race and class politics of anorexia as a diagnostic category. This chapter asks: When authors stake out a particular position in this literature, how do they frame the implications of their work, either explicitly or implicitly, with regard to understanding anorexia as a clinical entity? When status quo understandings of anorexia are questioned in terms of the race and class 'composition' of sufferers, are dominant medical concepts of personhood and illness causality questioned as well, or are they preserved? I argue that debates in this literature, while apparently critically engaged with racialized and classed assumptions, often leave these assumptions intact because they are deeply embedded in diagnostic categories. Many researchers tend to reify race, ethnicity, and/or class in such a way that privileged – white and middle class – categories of personhood fail to receive adequate scrutiny. These categories of personhood, rendered invisible or unmarked in their articulation of desired sociocultural norms, have come to appear as neutral or naturalized features of anorexia. The privileging of diagnostic 'expertise' in defining anorexia here conceals from view, and therefore also perpetuates, the race and class particularities of the problem as we currently understand it.

In this chapter I assess research that explores the role of race and class in manifestations of eating disorders. Throughout, I critically analyse white, middle-class standards embedded in many scholars' and clinicians' representations of eating problems (anorexia in particular) in the United States. I am interested here in the question of how marginality and privilege are theorized in the literature on eating disorders. Ultimately, I suggest that an adequate accounting of marginality must include a thorough scrutiny of categories of privilege, which are, in this case, enshrined most clearly in medicalized definitions of 'true anorexic patients.' Extending the analysis of race and class discourses in therapies for anorexia that appeared in my book *Feeding Anorexia* (Gremillion, 2003), I hope to contribute to broader questions about theorizing subjectivity, marginality, power, and resistance in clinical contexts.

I frame my use of the concept of contestation in several different ways. First, I review the research literature that contests prevailing views of anorexia as a white and middle-class phenomenon and consider debates that surround these relatively new findings. I show in some detail how, ironically, these debates can have the effect of preserving white, middle-class norms at the heart of clinical assessments. Next, I consider research that unpacks categories of privilege more thoroughly by examining anorexia's location in multiple fields of power and cultural meaning. In particular, sociologist Becky Thompson shows that eating disorders may be more widespread than is currently believed, because assumptions about what counts as a 'true' eating disorder may obscure from view a wide range of significantly troubling, yet marginalized experiences with eating and food. I also discuss studies that richly contextualize clinical practice. I reconsider a section of my book *Feeding Anorexia* (Gremillion, 2003) that contests the racialized and classed power of clinical 'expertise,' and examines underprivileged patients' resistance against treatment practices that work to exclude them.

My overall argument is that effective forms of contestation must directly challenge the seeming neutrality of cultural and clinical norms. Contestation in the form of resistance against these norms – in either the research literature or clinical practice – will not by itself guarantee a shift in who is to count as 'eating disordered' or in how these disorders are treated. Treatment effectiveness is an abiding concern here, as anorexia has the highest mortality rate of any psychiatric illness (approximately 10 per cent), and most patients never fully recover (Gordon, 2000; Levenkron, 2000). As I discuss below, racialized and classed norms that are implicit in clinical assessments and treatment protocols arguably contribute to difficulties in therapy. This problem raises the question: How might research literature on the race and class politics of eating disorders contribute to helpful changes in clinical practice? We might also ask: How might contested forms of clinical practice shape agendas in the research literature? The conclusion of this chapter reflects on different sites for and modalities of contesting representations of anorexia as race and class neutral, and considers the potential here for productive traffic between research and practice.

White Standards in Research on Eating Problems

Most standard measures for eating disorders – such as the Appearance Orientation Scale, the Body Esteem Scale, and the Eating Disorder Examination–Questionnaire – focus on concerns about shape, weight, ideal bodies, and a perceived need for self-restraint. These measures reflect the preoccupations of white, middle-class women and girls who are faced with forms of social disadvantage that circulate primarily around gendered differentials of power. Although some argue that an often-cited 'tyranny of slenderness' (or 'culture of thinness') affects women and girls across racial/ethnic and economic groups (Bartky, 1988), this 'tyranny' is often expressed as an individualized effort to realize personal achievement through bodily control and through the exaggeration, or perfection, of contemporary Western female beauty ideals that clearly adhere to (heterosexual) middle-class and white standards (Gremillion, 2003). Note, however, that most medicalized questionnaires do not contain references to historically and culturally situated norms of female beauty; rather, they work from the assumption that generic, individual (and/or family) 'pathology' leads to eating disordered behaviour. In contrast, studies that focus on the racial and ethnic profiles of those who struggle with eating disorders do recognize, to some extent, that sufferers are not in fact simply 'generic individuals,' unmarked by categories of identity such as race, class, and gender.

However, the vast majority of studies that examine the role of race/ethnicity in eating disorder symptomatology 'simply compare ethnic groups to Caucasian groups on measures of eating pathology' (Striegel-Moore & Smolak, 2000: 229). In these studies, already established measures of eating problems – developed through research with white populations – are applied to research subjects across at least two different ethnic groups. Here, white standards in assessing eating problems are retained, and definitions of 'disorder' are left intact.

Results from such studies are widely divergent. These divergences are not surprising considering the fact that there is little or no effort to specify forms of diversity *within* ethnic groups that might explain a particular set of results. One indicative study 'tested for effects of race/ethnicity and gender on … body image measures while controlling for age, body size, social desirability, and socioeconomic status' (Miller et al., 2000: 310). By design, the Miller study reifies race/ethnicity as a 'risk factor.' The researchers' efforts to mitigate the white standards built into their assessment tools only highlight their reification of race/ethnicity: 'Body parts significant to race/ethnicity' were added to the Body Esteem Scale and were scored separately (ibid.: 312). The overall goal remained: identify non-whites' differences from, or similarities to, whites. The embedded assumption here is that eating disorders, including anorexia, are 'white problems' – and the implicit research question is: How 'white' (or not) are ethnic/racial 'Others'?

One consistent finding across many different (and differently designed) studies is that African-American girls and women are more satisfied with their bodies than are white women and girls. Some studies, noting a distinctive absence of African-Americans among patient populations, cite this finding as evidence that African-American 'culture' provides a buffer against the development of anorexia. However, others have pointed out that patient populations will not tell us very much about eating disorder symptoms among African-Americans, given clinicians' preconceived ideas about 'typical' patient profiles (Dolan, 1991; Thompson, 1994b),[4] and given social and regional differences in mental health service accessibility (Dolan, 1991). Some studies do document eating disorder symptoms, including symptoms of anorexia, among African-American women and girls (Cachelin, Veisel, Striegel-Moore, & Barzegarnazari, 2000; Striegel-Moore & Smolak, 2000; Thompson, 1994a). However, most scholars do not dispute the finding that, overall, African-American women and girls are relatively satisfied with their bodies.

In her book *Fat Talk*, Mimi Nichter (2000) attempts to parse out the particularities of African-American experiences and self-presentations that lead to a relatively high degree of bodily self-acceptance. In this regard, she works to move beyond vague representations of 'Black culture.' The project of Nichter's book as a whole is to distinguish between dieting *behaviours* and *verbal concern* about body size and food intake among white, Latina, and African-American teens in Tucson, Arizona. As such, her book is not about eating disorders per se, but

rather about the social functions of 'fat talk,' such as impression management. In fact, Nichter finds that relatively few girls engage in sustained dieting at all. However, because her book addresses key
measures such as satisfaction with one's body – often explored in analyses of anorexia – her representations of ethnicity are instructive for
the purposes of my analysis in this chapter.

Nichter (2000) found that while white and Latina girls diet less than
their verbal reports suggest, many of them 'watch what they eat' and
are dissatisfied with their bodies. In contrast, African-American girls
refuse to diet or watch what they eat (even though they too report dieting), and thus they reject dominant cultural messages about body size,
drawing instead on community and family traditions to create styles of
self-presentation that are flexible and that accommodate a range of
sizes (see also Parker et al., 1995). Nichter's discussion of 'alternative'
lived expressions of beauty and embodied selfhood offers many interesting insights, but she comes close to representing African-American
body and beauty ideals as Other to those of whites (Other in a positively valued sense). For example, she suggests that black girls are
more 'authentic' than white girls when they refuse dominant cultural
norms regarding appearance and the watchful monitoring of food
intake. Nichter's focus on (apparent) contrasts between black and
white girls is highlighted by the fact that she incorporates her data
from Latina girls into the category 'white' while developing a special
survey (and recruiting additional informants) to uncover 'difference'
in her black sample.

Nichter's somewhat romanticizing portrait of black girls is mitigated by her recognition of racism; she does point to ethnic strategies
of survival 'in a potentially hostile environment' (2000: 171). At the
same time – while she acknowledges the possibility of assimilation to
white ideals of beauty and body size[5] – Nichter's emphasis on core
meanings and practices in the black community that are arrayed
against otherwise pervasive cultural norms (themselves posited as
given) means that African-Americans are granted a solid Otherness in
her analysis.

Lisa R. Rubin, Mako L. Fitts, and Anne E. Becker (2003) take a different tack from Nichter, exploring the *simultaneity* of African-American –
and also Latina – women's engagement with and resistance against
dominant cultural norms surrounding eating difficulties. Working with
different findings from those that Nichter cites, Rubin, Fitts, and Becker
seek to explain why African-American and Latina women's relative

body satisfaction does not confer protection from eating problems. They develop a distinction between body aesthetics and an ethics of bodily acceptance, suggesting that while African-American and Latina women do not hold to specific bodily aesthetics that diverge from culturally powerful norms of slender femininity, they do espouse a multifaceted ethics of bodily acceptance, presentation, and care that can be called upon to resist dominant corporeal ideals.

Rubin, Fitts, and Becker (2003) illustrate the importance of debunking generic 'ethnic factors' when analysing eating problems. It may not even be wise to generalize about ethnicity and bodily satisfaction. Striegel-Moore and Smolak (2003: 228) note that 'when social pressure to be thin is experienced, it appears to be just as strongly related to body dissatisfaction … or to drive for thinness in Black as in White females.' They conclude that 'we must closely examine each ethnic group to identify differences [both between and within groups] and, more important, the *source* of these differences' (see also Phinney, 1996), such as 'ethnic identity, or minority status effects' (Striegel-Moore & Smolak, 2003: 244).

Reifications of Class

Clearly, some (if relatively few) authors have ceased to reify categories of race and ethnicity in studies of anorexia. The same cannot be said of analyses of anorexia and social class; in most of these analyses, 'class' appears as a stable entity in that it remains implicit and unquestioned in diagnoses of eating problems. This is true even when the rarely challenged association between anorexia and high socioeconomic status (SES) is taken to task.

The vast majority of studies on anorexia and social class link the problem with high SES. One influential 1996 review of the literature upsets this association. Maisie C.E. Gard and Chris P. Freeman (1996: 2) write that between 1983 and 1995, '13 studies have failed to find a relationship between high socioeconomic status and eating disorders,' including anorexia. They conclude that 'the relationship between anorexia nervosa and high socioeconomic status is not proven' (ibid.: 10) and is based primarily on a biased clinical impression and the faulty methodologies of earlier studies. Gard and Freeman suggest that anorexia goes undetected among the poor: 'The homeless are a good example of a population in which eating disorders are not expected, are not looked for, and are not treated' (ibid.).

Lisa McClelland and Arthur Crisp (2001) directly challenge Gard and Freeman's results. A retrospective analysis of 692 patients referred to a specialist centre for the assessment and treatment of anorexia between 1960 and 1993 revealed that nearly 70 per cent of the patients were of a high SES. McClelland and Crisp argue that referral bias was not at work here: 'The duration of illness at presentation did not differ significantly across the social classes. Therefore, it is unlikely that social class influenced access to our service' (2001: 153). The authors do note that, since 1975, an increasing number of patients have hailed from lower SES groups; they suggest that 'a particular set of attitudes, a middle class value system, has become more widespread in society' (ibid.: 155). They conclude that conflicts producing anorexia 'may remain social class bound but social class as such may be increasingly mobile from generation to generation' (ibid.: 155).

McClelland and Crisp's position is similar to 'assimilation' arguments used to explain the presence of eating disorder symptoms among ethnic minority groups. These arguments propose that populations not ordinarily predisposed towards eating disorders may develop such problems in an effort to approximate white, middle-class standards of living.[6] Assimilation arguments leave some important issues unexamined. While it seems clear that discourses of assimilation are indeed at work for some individuals in the development of eating disorders among non-white and low SES groups (Striegel-Moore & Smolak, 2000; Thompson, 1994a), 'we must explore as part of this picture the racialized and classed norms that define eating disorders in popular and clinical narratives. These norms may preclude the recognition of significant eating problems that are "nonstandard" and perhaps more widespread' (Gremillion, 2003: 158). To the extent that members of underprivileged groups are indeed 'assimilating' – applying white middle-class standards to their own lives – we must recognize that these standards themselves:

> are written through representations of [poor bodies and] female bodies of color as quintessentially fleshy and unproductive. In particular, the lingering image of the corpulent 'black mammy' haunts U.S. constructions of fit and beautiful female bodies in its position as other to these constructions ... This image, which has served historically to set white women apart from 'deviant' black femininities ... today informs representations of poor black welfare mothers as simultaneously lazy, fat, and insufficiently or improperly feminine. It may also contribute to

representations of African-American women's and girls' body ideals as healthier and less tightly controlled than those of middle- and upper-class white women and girls. (ibid.: 52)

In this light, we can see that Gard and Freeman (1996) – the authors discussed above who challenge assumptions linking eating disorders with high SES – also leave intact a definition of anorexia that is shaped by race and class discourses; they seek to identify anorexia 'as we know it' among the poor.

A similar difficulty arises with the 'ethnic risk factors' approach discussed above, and adopted by Striegel-Moore and Smolak, who write: 'Risk derives from multiple domains and, within each of these domains, theoretical models have to address the question of how these risk factors combine to raise risk ... Simply comparing ethnic groups along single-risk factors (e.g., body dissatisfaction) or along single-risk domains (e.g., personal vulnerability) is not an adequate approach to understanding ethnic differences in risk for developing an eating disorder. Moreover, research is needed to test the relative contribution of certain risk factors to overall risk' (2000: 244). While Striegel-Moore and Smolak work against the reification of race/ethnicity by refusing to treat these categories as generic wholes, the specification of multiple 'risk factors' scientizes ethnicity/race, failing to interrogate the racial/ ethnic *constitution* of anorexia as a diagnostic category.

A Constitutionalist Approach to Race and Class in Research on Eating Disorders

Becky Thompson offers what I call a constitutionalist perspective on the race and class politics of anorexia. A constitutionalist analysis forgoes any and all fixed categories of identity in favour of asking how these identities are forged in their social and cultural contexts, and at the intersection of multiple levels of power and meaning. Thompson (1994b: 373) points out that in addition to exploring the particulars of underprivileged identities, we should also 'clarify what constitutes "culture" in the culture-of-thinness model.' In other words, both 'marked' and 'unmarked,' privileged and underprivileged categories of personhood should be scrutinized. Examining the mutual constitution of these categories, as well as their hierarchized interrelationships, troubles any clear distinction between compliance with and resistance to normative beliefs and practices, and also avoids social Othering. In addition, it raises powerful and significant questions about anorexia as a diagnostic category.

Thompson's publication *A Hunger So Wide and So Deep* (1994a) is the only book-length study of eating problems concerning body size across a range of ethnicities, ages, classes, religious affiliations, and sexualities in the United States. Thompson's life-history interviews reveal that widespread pressures to be slim do articulate with narratives of assimilation – specifically, narratives of whitening, feminizing, and moving up the social ladder. These pressures also entail 'grooming girls to be heterosexual' (ibid.: 37). At the same time, Thompson argues that these discourses – while exerting powerful influences on people – do not by any means capture all the meanings of eating difficulties. She points out that 'dissatisfaction with appearance often serves as a stand-in for topics that are still invisible' (ibid.: 11) such as racism, poverty, ageism, and sexual abuse.

Unlike many of the authors cited above, who accept a pre-given (and race- and class- inflected) understanding of eating disorders and attempt to identify or measure ethnic or class 'factors' relative to this understanding, Thompson situates her data about eating problems in contextually specific fields of social power and cultural meaning that constitute people's experiences with food and their bodies. She writes:

> A thin girl may diet because her mother taught her to accept the strictures that await her in womanhood (Orbach, 1985), but a parent's actions may be motivated by other social forces as well. Jewish or African-American parents who cannot protect their daughters from anti-Semitism or racism may encourage thinness [often not consciously] to protect them from the further discrimination directed against fat people ... When a Puerto Rican mother feeds her 5-year old daughter a food supplement to gain weight, then ridicules her when she gains weight in adolescence, pressures of assimilation may account for the mother's change of heart. Doing justice to the social context in which difficulties with food arise requires an integrated analysis – one that accounts for the intersecting influence of gender, race, sexuality, nationality, and class. (ibid.: 359–60)

Thompson critically interrogates dominant cultural norms of thinness as part of her analysis. In her challenge to works on eating disorders that focus almost entirely on gender inequality, she argues that more than gender 'tyranny' is at work in institutional specifications for thin female bodies. She argues that a comprehensive analysis of beauty standards 'would also elucidate "tyranny" based on the glorification of white, young, heterosexual, and able-bodied people' (1994b: 360).

Thompson complicates standard representations of 'eating disordered' individuals (e.g., white and middle-class) by exploring not only the wider cultural politics of eating problems, but also the Othering of 'non-standard' individuals that is inscribed invisibly into narrow diagnostic profiles, which thereby exclude people by definition. Indeed, a number of cultural studies scholars and social scientists examine medical discourses about eating disorders as themselves cultural products that reflect particular norms of personhood (Austin, 1999; Eckermann, 1997; Gremillion, 1992, 2001, and 2003; Hepworth, 1999; Hepworth & Griffin, 1995; MacSween, 1993; Malson, 1991 and 1998; Swartz, 1985 and 1987; Vogler, 1993). Unlike Nichter (2000), these authors question any clear-cut distinction between eating problems as psychiatric conditions and the widespread, 'normal' management of diet and body shape among women and girls in particular. Much of this work focuses on anorexia, challenging its status as a 'pre-given medico-psychological entity' (Malson, 1991: 31). Several scholars analyse the culturally specific character of both illness and health in treatment, and some implicate science 'in a culture of disordered eating' (Austin, 1999: 245). All of these works refuse to exempt diagnostic labels and treatment practices from epistemological scrutiny, and many of them highlight the negotiated status of anorexia as a medicalized problem (Eckermann, 1997; Gremillion, 2003; Swartz, 1987).

In a chapter on the race and class politics of treatment in my book *Feeding Anorexia* (Gremillion, 2003), I argue that if medical discourses and practices related to eating problems such as anorexia are cultural products, and if dominant cultural representations of eating disorders are narrow and exclusionary (privileging readings of these problems that conform to expectations for a 'standard' white, middle-class profile), then one would expect hierarchies of race and class to permeate constructions of anorexia in the therapy process. Because of the potential to privilege some patients over others, the importance of critically examining powerful, unmarked categories of personhood is perhaps clearest in a clinical context. Drawing on 14 months of participant observation and interviewing in a prominent eating disorders treatment program in the western part of the United States, I track the ways in which non-white and working-class patients are excluded from full participation in treatment. My focus is on 'the rhetoric of exclusion that helps to produce the clinical norms against which certain "atypical" patients are measured' (Gremillion, 2003: 157).

'Good' patients behave in ways that fit a particular profile; these behaviours are expected of (and learned by) patients on this hospital unit. For instance, on the one hand, a 'typical' (good) patient will learn unit rules well regarding appropriate calorie intake at mealtimes and internalize these rules, even as she protests them quietly in a number of (expected) ways. On the other hand, 'atypical' patients – invariably non-white and/or working-class – are those who are considered 'externalizers' (as opposed to 'internalizers'); they refuse to incorporate unit rules into their identities. Sandra (a pseudonym) – a 16-year-old Chicana patient on welfare, and one of the few 'externalizers' diagnosed with anorexia during the time of my fieldwork – is a case in point:

> Sandra loudly tested, pushed, and challenged [unit] staff at every turn; in other words, she rarely internalized unit protocols. One evening at dinnertime, while most anorexic patients were quietly and nervously counting their calories, Sandra and Elsie, the nurse who was observing her, had the following dialogue:
>
> SANDRA: I'm not going to finish my calories, Elsie.
> ELSIE: Well, try.
> SANDRA: They never do anything to me when I don't.
> ELSIE: I'll have to call the doctors on call.
> SANDRA: You guys don't have to tell them everything!
> ELSIE: Yes, I do.
> SANDRA: I'm just going to eat one of these graham crackers.
> ELSIE: Good. You can eat that.
> SANDRA: I can't do it in just three minutes! [when mealtime ended]
> ELSIE: Yes, you can, eat fast. Chew, chew, chew! [pause] Try to eat two.
> SANDRA: Will you give me more time? [staff are not supposed to do this]
> ELSIE: If you eat really fast.
> SANDRA: No way.
> ELSIE: Well, just eat one, then.
> SANDRA: What did they say about me in [nursing] report?
> ELSIE: An order for unit restriction.
> SANDRA: Can I see it? [considered a 'cheeky' request] (Gremillion, 2003: 165–6)

This kind of overt 'testing' is considered a sign of a poor prognosis. What is more, clinicians actively took steps to shorten Sandra's hospital stay and to prevent future admissions to the unit (multiple admissions are quite common for 'typical' patients), claiming her anorexia was not her 'real' problem. Her real problem was deemed to be a (budding, and not formally diagnosed) 'borderline personality disorder.' This diagnostic category is notoriously vague and is applied in many clinical settings mostly to 'externalizing' (or 'acting out') female patients who are difficult to treat (Becker, 1997). Note that, while only three patients diagnosed with anorexia were excluded from full participation in the treatment program I studied during the time I was conducting fieldwork, all three were labelled 'borderline' (and externalizers), and all three were also both non-white and working class.

The race and class politics of determining which patients are 'treatable' are particularly clear when we compare medical professionals' approaches to 'anorexic' patients who are deemed borderline as they vary in their degree of sociocultural privilege. Although Sandra and another patient, Pam, were both considered borderline, no one ever floated the idea of shortening a hospital stay for Pam or refusing to admit her when she was not faring well as an outpatient. In fact, Pam had been allowed more than nine admissions over the course of three years by the time I met her, even though she was often suicidal and required a lot of individual attention. Either one of these situations was often cited as sufficient reason to refuse certain patients access to the treatment program. Pam is white and middle class, and her apparent willingness to work hard in the program and to try to internalize treatment protocols protected her status as a 'good enough' patient on the unit, even though she often failed to comply with the program. According to Pam herself, as well as the clinicians who worked with her, she was grateful for her treatment and felt a strong sense of responsibility for it. Most clinicians also considered Pam to be deeply thoughtful and articulate, both of which are features of internalizing identities.

Ironically, the exaggeration or perfection of internalizing identity features is itself considered a hallmark of anorexia. Here we can see how deeply implicated medical practice and ideology are in the support of racialized and classed norms that constitute anorexia (and help render it so difficult to 'cure') – the very processes of internalization encouraged in this treatment program mirror 'anorexic' ways of being. Some clinicians are reflective about this issue: 'most staff are white and middle class. So it's hard to be introspective: do I impose white, middle-class values on a white, middle-class [anorexic] population'? (Gremillion, 2003: 163–164). But for the most part, the race and class politics of treatment go unremarked; they are implicit in definitions of 'typical' (treatable, if usually intractable) patients and 'atypical' (untreatable) patients.

Like Becky Thompson (1994a and 1994b), I maintain that the very constitution of these categories of patient embed race and class ideologies.
These ideologies include notions that are not often taken into account in
'measures' of race/ethnic/class identifications – for example, particular
understandings of 'working hard' (or not), of what it means to play by
the rules (or openly challenge them), and of 'internalized' versus 'exter-
nalized' self-expression.

Considering that treatments can reinforce the problem, it is not
entirely a negative outcome for so-called borderline patients to be
excluded from full participation in the treatment program. But the
larger points here are that no one is receiving adequate treatment and
that race and class hierarchies are perpetuated in therapy. To fully
understand the extent of this latter problem, it is important to recognize that borderline patients are not simply excluded from treatment;
rather, 'typical' patient profiles are written through and against perceptions of seemingly untreatable (borderline) identities. Consider the
occasional romanticizing of 'borderline' emotional expression. Staff
sometimes complained that typical patients were difficult to work with
because they are so 'uptight' and 'rule-driven,' and in this context, the
seeming volatility of borderline patients (whether or not they were
diagnosed with anorexia)[7] was admired. In the end, however, 'borderline' emotional expressiveness was seen to go overboard. Clinicians
hoped that typical patients would borrow merely a fraction of atypical
passion and then craft more tempered, 'healthy,' and 'appropriate'
emotions than those expressed by patients who would 'never make it.'
In other words, privileged and marginalized identities are mutually
constituted in the treatment of anorexia.

Conclusion

In this chapter I have argued that an analysis of marginality must include
a scrutiny of privilege. When assessing the race and class 'composition' of
those who struggle with anorexia and other eating problems, or when
considering the possibility that anorexic 'symptoms' may not be uniform
across different social groups, it is imperative to examine critically the
various yardsticks that are taken to be normative. If we fail to acknowledge that categories of privilege and of marginality are always mutually
constructed, then we risk the Othering of underprivileged social groups.
We also miss an opportunity to explore the culturally contingent aspects
of mainstream treatments and diagnostic categories that may well be

problematic – for example, the recreation of 'anorexic' forms of internalization in the treatment process.

Subjectivity, including that of individual patients (or potential patients), is always crafted in relationship to interlocking or 'intersecting' fields of social power (Crenshaw, 1991). For this reason, we cannot account for eating disorders among ethnic minority groups strictly in terms of 'assimilation,' nor should we reflexively read a lack of eating disorder symptoms among a particular group of people as a sign of cultural resistance. Both stances presume a fixed and self-contained arena of cultural norms, which leads to a representation of non-normative 'Others' as existing in a space outside of these norms. But there is no stable or pure set of norms against which various groups can be measured. As rhetorician Judith Butler (1993: 8) argues, hegemonic instantiations of personhood always entail 'the constitutive force of exclusion, erasure … abjection and its disruptive return within the very terms of discursive legitimacy.'

These considerations lead to intriguing questions regarding deployments of power and contestation in clinical contexts. It is far from the case that we can single out atypical (underprivileged) 'anorexic' patients as those who resist treatment norms. *All* patients diagnosed with anorexia resist treatment; in fact, they are *expected* to. Resistance to treatment has become an (informal) diagnostic criterion and, in addition, a necessary 'phase' on the road to health. This latter idea is part of a psychiatric paradigm that measures health in part by the degree of self-control that one maintains over one's own body. In this way, medical 'cures' ironically reproduce 'symptoms' that are hallmarks of anorexia – and indeed anorexia remains one of the most difficult illnesses to cure. But the larger point here is that resistance itself cannot necessarily provide critical purchase on medical norms. The greater degree of resistance that underprivileged patients often seem to display on the hospital unit I studied is an exaggerated expression of resistances and subversions that are prevalent among 'typical' patients, who, for example, routinely hide food in their clothing, devise ways of feigning weight gain, and often reject medicalized assessments of eating problems.[8] I suggest that an adequate accounting of power and contestation in clinical contexts would examine the ways in which clinical norms are constituted through the production of a *range* of hierarchized Others: typical patients, Othered through medicalization, as well as atypical ones, Othered in more thoroughgoing ways (see Foucault, 1990). Only in this way can we begin to truly appreciate the race and class politics of medical categories. Furthermore, when we mark categories that have previously gone unmarked, they no longer appear to be 'natural' features of the problem at hand, and a greater range of choices – for treatment methods, for example – are, at least potentially, opened up to us.

I conclude here with a few reflections on the potential for productive traffic between the two types of literature I have discussed in this chapter: research literature on the prevalence of anorexia and other eating disorders within underprivileged groups, and critical literature on the race and class politics of clinical practice in the treatment of anorexia. As already noted, clinical contexts provide perhaps the clearest examples of the need to scrutinize categories of privilege in representations of eating problems. It is in the treatment of eating disorders that the extent and depth of exclusions based on race and class are most visible. Without a research agenda that is constitutionalist – that is, that seeks to contextualize fully racialized and classed identities in therapy – these exclusions can be easily justified through references to particular (usually underprivileged) patients' seeming intractability. In this process, and through exclusion itself, normative understandings of diagnostic categories are preserved.

As we have seen, status quo representations of diagnostic categories are also quite easily preserved in the research literature on the prevalence of anorexia within underprivileged groups. I suggest that this type of research ought to take its cue from constitutionalist approaches to eating problems, whether these approaches address clinical practice or, as is the case with Thompson's (1994a and 1994b) work, experiences with eating difficulties in the general population. Research that deeply contextualizes all aspects of eating problems stands the best chance of generating productive categories of analysis that query norms along with marginalized experiences and beliefs.

In turn, new 'constitutionalist' studies of the prevalence of eating disorders within various groups could help justify and support changes in treatment practices. These studies may well highlight variations in how these disorders become manifest, variations that might challenge diagnostic 'expertise' as we know it. On this note, I argue that the creation of clinical alternatives in the *absence* of careful critiques of the status quo risks the marginalization of new therapies, however effective they may be.[9] As I suggest in *Feeding Anorexia*, 'without a thoroughgoing examination of dominant medical and psychological models – one that contextualizes and questions the very terms of health and illness at work within these models – both the effectiveness and the institutional power of [treatment] alternatives may well be compromised' (Gremillion, 2003: xxii). In the end, of course, successful contestations of white, middle-class standards embedded in typical understandings of anorexia must include interventions in both theory and practice.

NOTES

1 I place quotes around the term 'anorexic' to signal my questioning of this pathologized and medicalized identity label.

2 Ethnographic research and interviews took place from July 1993 to September 1994 in a facility in the western part of the United States. See Gremillion (2003) for a full description of this research and its results.

3 Furthermore, several epidemiological studies have shown that increasing numbers of girls and women in non-Western societies also experience eating disorders (see, e.g., Lee, Hsu, & Wing, 1992). However, it is 'highly problematic that cross-cultural ... studies have proliferated in which case identification is based solely on survey questionnaires' that are developed in North America (Striegel-Moore & Smolak, 2000: 229). In this chapter I discuss problems with these questionnaires for cross-ethnic research in the United States. For discussions of methodological problems with the use of these questionnaires in cross-cultural research, see Katzman and Lee (1997) and Lee, Lee, and Leung (1998).

   Interestingly, several studies suggest that 'one of the core symptoms of eating disorders, body-image disturbances, may not be universal: for example, fear of fatness is not a prominent feature in patients with [anorexia] in Hong Kong ... Whether the absence of this feature means that these patients do not suffer from [anorexia] is a matter of considerable debate' (Lee, Lee, & Leung, 1998, cited in Striegel-Moore & Smolak, 2000: 229). For a discussion of the need for a broadened conceptualization of anorexia in China, see Lee, Lee, Ngai, Lee, and Wing (2001).

   These debates about cross-cultural manifestations of anorexia are interesting to consider in light of questions explored in this chapter about cross-ethnic research on eating problems in the United States.

4 Thompson (1994a: 374) explains that African-American (and Latina) women with eating problems are often misdiagnosed or receive a delayed diagnosis 'as a result of stereotypical thinking that these problems are restricted to white women.'

5 But see the discussion below of problems with too strong a reliance on notions of assimilation.

6 See Dawkins (1995) and Pate, Pumariega, Hester, and Garner (1992) for discussions of some of this literature.

7 Recall that the treatment program I studied admitted some patients with 'psychosomatic' problems other than anorexia.

8 See *Feeding Anorexia* (Gremillion, 2003) for a full description of 'typical' patients' resistances in treatment.

9 One alternative therapy for anorexia, 'narrative therapy' (Maisel, Epston, & Bordon, 2004; White & Epston, 1990), has emerged in important part precisely through such a careful critique of mainstream treatments. Narrative therapy fully contextualizes and politicizes anorexia, adopting a constitutionalist approach to both the problem and its resolution. Formal studies of the effectiveness of narrative work are lacking, but anecdotal evidence and pilot study results (Madigan & Goldner, 1999) suggest significant improvement in treatment outcomes.

REFERENCES

Austin, S. Bryn. (1999). Fat, loathing and public health: The complicity of science in a culture of disordered eating. *Culture, Medicine, and Psychiatry, 23,* 245–268.

Bartky, Sandra. (1988). Foucault, femininity and the modernization of patriarchal power. In Lee Quinby & Irene Diamond (Eds.), *Feminism and Foucault: Paths of resistance* (pp. 61–86). Boston: Northeastern University Press.

Becker, Dana. (1997). *Through the looking-glass: Women and Borderline Personality Disorder.* Boulder, CO: Westview Press.

Bruch, Hilde. (1978). *The golden cage: The enigma of anorexia nervosa.* Cambridge, MA: Harvard University Press.

Butler, Judith. (1993). *Bodies that matter: On the discursive limits of 'sex.'* New York and London: Routledge.

Cachelin, Fary M., Veisel, Catherine, Striegel-Moore, Ruth H., & Barzegarnazari, Emilia. (2000). Disordered eating, acculturation, and treatment-seeking in a community sample of Hispanic, Asian, Black, and white women. *Psychology of Women Quarterly, 24*(3), 244–253.

Crago, Marjorie, Shisslak, Catherine M., & Estes, Linda S. (1996). Eating disturbances among American minority groups. *International Journal of Eating Disorders, 19,* 239–248.

Crenshaw, Kimberle. (1991). Mapping the margins: Intersectionality, identity politics, and violence against women of color. *Stanford Law Review, 43*(6), 1241–1299.

Dawkins, Karon. (1995). The interaction of ethnicity, sociocultural factors, and gender in clinical psychopharmacology. *Psychopharmacology Bulletin, 32*(2), 283–289.

Dolan, Bridget. (1991). Cross-cultural aspects of anorexia nervosa and bulimia: A review. *International Journal of Eating Disorders, 10*(1), 67–78.

Eckermann, Liz. (1997). Foucault, embodiment and gendered subjectivities: The case of voluntary self-starvation. In Alan Petersen & Robin Bunton (Eds.), *Foucault, health and medicine* (pp. 151–169). New York and London: Routledge.

Foucault, Michel. (1990). *The history of sexuality, volume 1: An introduction*. (Robert Hurley, Trans.). New York: Vintage Books. (Original work published in 1978.)

Gard, Maisie C.E., & Freeman, Chris P. (1996). The dismantling of a myth: A review of eating disorders and socioeconomic status. *International Journal of Eating Disorders, 20*(1), 1–12.

Gordon, Richard A. (2000). *Eating disorders: Anatomy of a social epidemic* (2nd ed.). Malden, MA: Blackwell.

Gremillion, Helen. (1992). Psychiatry as social ordering: Anorexia nervosa, a paradigm. *Social Science and Medicine, 35*(1), 57–71.

Gremillion, Helen. (2001). In fitness and in health: Crafting bodies in the treatment of anorexia nervosa. *Signs, 27*(2), 381–414.

Gremillion, Helen. (2003). *Feeding anorexia: Gender and power at a treatment center*. Durham, NC: Duke University Press.

Hepworth, Julie. (1999). *The social construction of anorexia nervosa*. London: Sage.

Hepworth, Julie, & Griffin, Christine. (1995). Conflicting opinions? 'Anorexia nervosa,' medicine, and feminism. In Sue Wilkinson & Celia Kitzinger (Eds.), *Feminism and discourse: Psychological perspectives* (pp. 68–85). London: Sage.

Katzman, Melanie A. & Lee, Sing. (1997). Beyond body image: The integration of feminist and transcultural theories in the understanding of self-starvation. *International Journal of Eating Disorders, 22*, 385–394.

Lee, Sing, Hsu, L.K.G., & Wing, Y.K. (1992). Bulimia nervosa in Hong Kong Chinese patients. *British Journal of Psychiatry, 161*, 545–551.

Lee, Sing, Lee, Antoinette M., & Leung, Tony. (1998). Cross-cultural validity of the eating disorders inventory: A study of Chinese patients with eating disorders in Hong Kong. *International Journal of Eating Disorders, 23*, 177–188.

Lee, Sing, Lee, Antoinette M., Ngai, Emily, Lee, Dominic T.S., & Wing, Y.K. (2001). Rationales for food refusal in Chinese patients with anorexia nervosa. *International Journal of Eating Disorders, 29*, 224–229.

Levenkron, Steven. (1978). *The best little girl in the world*. Chicago: Contemporary Books.

Levenkron, Steven. (2000). *Anatomy of anorexia*. New York: W.W. Norton.

MacSween, Morag. (1993). *Anorexic bodies: A feminist and sociocultural perspective on anorexia nervosa*. New York and London: Routledge.

Madigan, Stephen P., & Goldner, Elliot M. (1999). Undermining anorexia through narrative therapy. In Raymond Lemberg with Leigh Cohn (Eds.), *Eating disorders: A reference sourcebook* (pp. 138–146). Phoenix, AZ: Oryx Press.

Maisel, Richard, Epston, David, & Borden, Ali. (2004). *Biting the hand that starves you: Inspiring resistance to anorexia/bulimia*. New York: W.W. Norton.

Malson, Helen. (1991, Winter). Hidden a-genders: The place of multiplicity and gender in theorizations of anorexia nervosa. *BPS Psychology of Women Section Newsletter*, 31–42.

Malson, Helen. (1998). *The thin woman: Feminism, post-structuralism and the social psychology of anorexia nervosa*. New York and London: Routledge.

McClelland, Lisa, & Crisp, Arthur. (2001). Anorexia nervosa and social class. *International Journal of Eating Disorders, 29*, 150–156.

Miller, Katherine J., Gleaves, David H., Hirsch, Tera G., Green, Bradley A., Snow, Alicia C., & Corbett, Chandra C. (2000). Comparisons of body image dimensions by race/ethnicity and gender in a university population. *International Journal of Eating Disorders, 27*, 310–316.

Nichter, Mimi. (2000). *Fat talk: What girls and their parents say about dieting*. Cambridge, MA: Harvard University Press.

Orbach, Susie. (1985). Accepting the symptom: A feminist psychoanalytic treatment of anorexia nervosa. In David M. Garner & Paul E. Garfinkel (Eds.), *Handbook of Psychotherapy for Anorexia Nervosa and Bulimia* (pp. 83–104). New York: Guilford.

Parker, Sheila, Nichter, Mimi, Nichter, Mark, Vuckovic, Nancy, Sims, Colette, & Ritenbaugh, Cheryl. (1995). Body image and weight concerns among African American and white adolescent females: Differences that make a difference. *Human Organization, 54*(2), 103–114.

Pate, Jennifer E., Pumariega, Andrés J., Hester, C., & Garner, David M. (1992). Cross-cultural patterns in eating disorders: A review. *Journal of the Academy of Child and Adolescent Psychiatry, 31*(5), 802–809.

Phinney, Jean S. (1996). When we talk about ethnic groups, what do we mean? *American Psychologist, 51*, 918–927.

Root, Maria P.P. (1990). Disordered eating in women of color. *Sex Roles, 22*, 525–536.

Rubin, Lisa R., Fitts, Mako L., & Becker, Anne E. (2003). 'Whatever feels good in my soul': Body ethics and aesthetics among African American and Latina women. *Culture, Medicine, and Psychiatry, 27*(1), 49–75.

Striegel-Moore, Ruth H., & Smolak, Linda. (2000). The influence of ethnicity on eating disorders in women. In Richard M. Eisler & Michael Hersen (Eds.), *Handbook of gender, culture, and health* (pp. 227–253). Mahwah, NJ: Lawrence Earlbaum Associates.

Swartz, Lesley. (1985). Anorexia nervosa as a culture-bound syndrome. *Social Science and Medicine, 20*(7), 725–730.

Swartz, Lesley. (1987). Illness negotiation: The case of eating disorders. *Social Science and Medicine, 24*(7), 613-618.

Thompson, Becky. (1994a). *A hunger so wide and so deep: American women speak out on eating problems.* Minneapolis: University of Minnesota Press.

Thompson, Becky. (1994b). Food, bodies, and growing up female: Childhood lessons about culture, race, and class. In Patricia Fallon, Melanie A. Katzman, & Susan C. Wooley (Eds.), *Feminist perspectives on eating disorders* (pp. 355–378). New York: Guilford.

Vogler, Robin Jane Marie. (1993). *The medicalization of eating: Social control in an eating disorders clinic.* Greenwich, CT: JAI Press.

White, Michael, & Epston, David. (1990). *Narrative means to therapeutic ends.* New York: W.W. Norton.

13 'More Labels Than a Jam Jar': The Gendered Dynamics of Diagnosis for Girls and Women with Autism[1]

JOYCE DAVIDSON

> Since I first heard of autism I have thought of it as 'my problem,' and this conviction only deepens as I learn more, and as I fail to change myself despite my best efforts. While professional diagnosis may be a comfort, professional denigration would be painful, which is why I have avoided exposing myself to anyone qualified to deny my self-diagnosis. The main reason for writing now is the hope of finding a support group of fellow adult recoverees. I would really like to find some company.
>
> Sharon, quoted in Szatmari, 2004: 59–60

Sharon wrote this excerpt in a letter to autism specialist, Peter Szatmari, who has since authored a popular text (2004) for those who care for and work with children with Autistic Spectrum Disorders (ASDs). Szatmari reproduces Sharon's letter in this text, wherein she articulates her reasons for writing in a way that is clear, insightful, and moving. The clinician includes a lengthy description of his subsequent meetings with Sharon, and his interpretations of her stories of a life lived on the autistic spectrum.

The unusually 'fuzzy' characteristics of autism (Hodge, 2005; Wing, 1997) are increasingly familiar to a lay population, informed through popular media of an explosion in diagnosed cases of the disorder, referred to variously as an increase of epidemic proportions (Nash, 2002) and an 'autism baby boom' (Baker, 2006: 16).[2] ASDs occupy more space in the popular cultural imagination than ever before; witness the phenomenal success of Mark Haddon's (2004) fictional account of an ASD child's detective story, predated by several cases of 'autism at the movies' (Waltz, 2005: 432). It has become common knowledge that ASD individuals experience and interact with people and places in a way that is very *different*. They are perceived to struggle with communication in all forms and to demonstrate interests and behave in ways that are noticeably unusual, highly focused, and perhaps fixated; they stand out from any crowd that they may find themselves part of. Most, however, strive to avoid the sensory overstimulation associated with unfamiliar or complex social and spatial situations, hence the common description of ASD individuals as occupying a 'world of their own' (Davidson, 2005).

Clinical guidelines have changed since Kanner and Asperger's independent descriptions in the 1940s (Frith, 1996), but most recent accounts, drawing on the *Diagnostic and Statistical Manual of Mental Disorders* (DSM-IV; American Psychiatric Association, 2000) and/or ICD-10 (World Health Organization, 1992), focus on the same triad of impairments initially identified – in social interaction, in communication, and in behaviour, which tends to be repetitive and restricted in nature (Tidmarsh & Volkmar, 2003: 517). As Szatmari makes plain, 'there is no blood test or brain scan that will tell us who has ASD and who does not' (2004: 77).

The diagnostic process tends to involve an extended period of observation accompanied by a slate of developmental tests (Bruey, 2004) and usually takes place with young children whose carers become aware of atypical development and seek professional help. Sharon's case appears to be unusual, given that clinical literature demonstrates an expectation for diagnosis at a young age – the DSM-IV criteria relate specifically to the disorder as it appears in early childhood. Adults present certain challenges for the diagnostic process, particularly in relation to the lack of so-called corroborating evidence and the need to rely on the individual's own account of her or his developmental history. Although hindsight may offer perspective and reflective clarity for Sharon, patient memory lacks the clinically preferable characteristics of being observable and objectively verifiable. Clinical presentation changes with age (Molloy & Vasil, 2002: 661; Seltzer et al., 2003), and difficulties may be compounded by the efforts that adult patients make to educate themselves about ASDs by the time they present to clinicians. This process can conceivably colour their memories and shift their accounts of childhood experience to fit the ASD profile.

Patient adulthood is a challenge, and, as with Sharon, gender complicates the picture further. Clinical estimates consistently demonstrate a male-to-female ratio of more than four to one. As Lee Tidmarsh and Fred Volkmar (2003: 522) state, 'The male predominance is striking, yet researchers have given it relatively little attention.' This may be changing, with Simon Baron-Cohen's (2003) investigations that suggest that autism is an expression of the 'extreme male brain'; this attention reinforces rather than challenges expectations that girls and women are far less likely to have an ASD diagnosis than boys and men. We cannot know to what extent or even *if* such considerations influenced Szatmari's final judgment of Sharon: 'In the end,' despite the fact that 'what she described to me was certainly analogous to the experiences of people with ASD,' he could not, in fact, 'give' her this diagnosis: Sharon's experience 'did not constitute a "true" disorder'; her 'insights into her own predicament were just too good' (Szatmari, 2004: 77).

Sharon's interests in this narrative are always mediated by her clinician, and they slip further from the centre of the therapeutic encounter as his account foregrounds other outcomes of the exchange. Szatmari uses the imagery of a gift to characterize their dialogue: 'I had given her a language for her predicament. But she had given me something more important: the language to understand the inner world of people with autism and AS (Asperger's Syndrome). I do not think it was a fair trade' (2004: 78). The extent to which Szatmari claims to have learned about ASDs from Sharon's experience is puzzling, given that he does not allow her to own the identification.

The vast majority of what we know about people with ASDs comes from accounts written by other kinds of experts, primarily professionals (in numerous monographs and dedicated journals) and, less prolifically, carers (e.g., Claiborne Park, 2001; Collins, 2004).[3] As Mitzi Waltz (2005: 432) discovered in her study of the social construction of ASDs, 'people with autism are denied primacy, and even agency, in all but the least-mediated personal texts.' Her analysis of clinical accounts details seemingly typical instances where the patient is portrayed as a mere 'object of study' and occasion for demonstration of professional omniscience. To discover the personalities, experiences, interests, and desires of women with autism, I turn to the least-mediated sources available, first-hand accounts of direct personal experience.[4]

A growing number of ASD women's autobiographical narratives have been published in recent years (see Table 13.1), and their accounts provide a rich source of insight into the gendered dynamics of experience and diagnosis.[5] Sharon's epistolary sentiments are fairly typical of women who self-identify as having an ASD and who crave the legitimacy and support that a professional diagnosis is perceived to bestow. Judy Singer (1999: 62), for example, states that diagnosis gave her 'an entry ticket to a new world of people whose struggle parallels mine.'

Sharon obviously did not receive such validation and, unfortunately, we cannot know how she has negotiated her way in the world in the aftermath of her therapeutic encounter; the story ends with her specialist saying goodbye to his 'subclinical' patient and going to collect his mail 'in hopeful anticipation of other gifts that might come my way' (Szatmari, 2004: 78).

Sharon's testimony brings to the fore a number of themes that I explore in this chapter. I use the term *testimony* in the politicized sense of self-advocacy intended by Mark Cresswell (2005) in his interpretation of writings by women who self-harm. With Cresswell, I endorse the accounts of authors who are self-described survivors of the psychiatric system and of 'societies which devalue our personal experience' (Campbell, 1992: 117, quoted in Creswell, 2005: 1674). By conceptually reframing autobiography as testimony I seek to emphasize the politics of knowledge and expertise, alongside questions of representation and power, of voices heard and voices marginalized. Furthermore, by highlighting the plurality and multiple meanings of autism in women's lives, I attempt to show what diagnosis might *mean* for those women like Sharon who actively pursue it. I seek to engage with those knowledges sidelined and subjugated by hegemonic clinical discourse, and take seriously the truth claims of those who would speak – in private letters and public accounts – their (autistic) minds.

Approaching Autism in Person: Notes on Methodology

Gunilla Gerland (2003: 53) writes in her autobiography that 'expressing words in writing was much easier for me than taking the long way round, as I experienced it, via speech.' Dawn Prince-Hughes, in the preface to an edited collection of personal stories by college students with autism, is similarly emphatic about the limitations of speech, and repeatedly states that writing is the best way for an autistic person to communicate: 'It allows time to form one's thoughts carefully, it has none of the overwhelming intensity of face-to-face conversation, and it affords the writer space to talk about one question or thesis without limit' (2002: xiii). Stressing a perceived need among ASD individuals for research on their experience, Prince-Hughes refers to writings in the anthology as self-produced 'ethnographic narratives' containing 'their truth. Our truth.' Such 'autistic autobiography is rare,' she states, 'and in my opinion valuable' (ibid.: xi). Furthermore, and most emphatically,

Table 13.1
First-Hand Accounts of Women with Autism

Cohen, Judith H. (2005). *Succeeding with autism: Hear my voice.* London and Philadelphia: Jessica Kingsley.

Cowhey, Sharon P. (2005). *Going through the motions: Coping with autism.* Baltimore, MD: PublishAmerica.

Gerland, Gunilla. (2003). *A real person: Life on the outside.* London: Souvenir Press.

Grandin, Temple. (1996). *Thinking in pictures: And other reports from my life with autism.* New York: Vintage Books.

Grandin, Temple, & Scariano, Margaret M. (1996). *Emergence labelled autistic.* New York: Warner Books.

Kearns Miller, Jean. (Ed.). (2003). *Women from another planet: Our lives in the universe of autism.* Bloomington: Dancing Minds.

Lawson, Wendy. (2005). *Life behind glass: A personal account of Autism Spectrum Disorder.* London and Philadelphia: Jessica Kingsley.

Prince-Hughes, Dawn. (Ed.). (2002). *Aquamarine blue 5: Personal stories of college students with autism.* Athens, OH: Swallow Press.

Prince-Hughes, Dawn. (2004). *Songs of the gorilla nation: My journey through autism.* New York: Harmony Books.

Singer, Judy. (1999). 'Why can't you be normal for once in your life?' From a 'problem with no name' to the emergence of a new category of difference. In Mairian Corker & Sally French (Eds.), *Disability discourse* (pp. 59–67). Buckingham, England: Open University Press.

Willey, Liane Holliday. (1999) *Pretending to be normal.* London and Philadelphia: Jessica Kingsley.

Willey, Liane Holliday. (2001). *Asperger Syndrome in the family: Redefining normal.* London and Philadelphia: Jessica Kingsley.

Williams, Donna. (1992). *Nobody nowhere: The extraordinary autobiography of an autistic.* New York: Random House.

Williams, Donna. (1994). *Somebody somewhere: Breaking free from the world of autism.* New York: Random House.

Williams, Donna. (2003). *Exposure anxiety, the invisible cage: An exploration of self-protection responses in the Autism Spectrum and beyond.* London and Philadelphia: Jessica Kingsley.

Williams, Donna. (2004). *Everyday heaven: Journeys beyond the stereotypes of autism.* London and Philadelphia: Jessica Kingsley.

'there is simply no way for nonautistic people to gather this kind of information through questionnaires or interviews, or through reading what nonautistic people have said about us' (ibid.: xiv).

The view that insufficient and even inappropriate research has taken place on ASD women's experience is relatively common, as is the sense that there are right and wrong ways to address this absence. In the introduction to her book entitled *Women From Another Planet: Our Lives in the Universe of Autism,* Jean Kearns Miller writes: 'Given the relative inattention of the research community to women with AS and our own dismay at the inadequacy of diagnostic description, especially as it pertains to women, we began the process of self-definition through interaction with each other ... We were, in effect, observer–participants in our own ethnography' (2003: xxiii). The women involved in the project explicitly challenge the reader to 'look beyond the clinical contours of their experience,' and I intend to take this invitation and recommendation to heart. As Prince-Hughes points out, 'many people with autism care little for the fine distinctions of category, preferring to focus on the common underpinnings of the phenomenon' (2002: xxii). Part of this project to re-centre the perspectives of ASD women involves taking seriously those diagnostic categories with which they themselves choose to identify, the labels that they elect to apply to themselves in preference to those many others they have often been stuck with.

Published accounts, despite their limitations,[6] present a still rare opportunity to gain insights into ASD experience, and so begin to address at least some of the exclusions and power imbalances found in existing clinical discourse. I have focused on writings that foreground experiential connections between gender and diagnosis.[7] I begin interpretative discussion of this theme by highlighting accounts of a subject of recurring and explicit significance for the majority of authors whose writing I am considering: what it feels like and means to have to *try* – deliberately, consciously, relentlessly – to be normal, and moreover, to be a passably normal woman.

Performing Gender and Passing as Normal

Some recent feminist and poststructuralist theorists have followed Judith Butler (1990 and 2004) in arguing that 'doing gender' involves significant elements of performance for all of us, neuro-typical or otherwise. The accounts of difficulties experienced by women with ASDs might lead us to think that they are merely rendering explicit what for all others is supposed to come more or less naturally. However, ASD women face additional and disabling barriers that further complicate their experience of difference and diagnosis. The body language of non-verbal behaviours such as hand gestures and eye contact communicate little if anything to the ASD individual, who often finds others' ability to understand and respond to such cues entirely mysterious.

Any supplementary input to conversation beyond the strictly verbal and straightforward (non-metaphorical and preferably factual) – only serves to confuse, to obfuscate rather than enrich or clarify the respondent's intentions. The inability to employ the usually intuitive language of hand and eye is often obvious to others. Authors' accounts suggest that few ever learn to intuit information from social cues independently, but rather learn to deduce information by entirely logical means. Autistic people do not usually comprehend small talk, and the inability to engage in gossip, constructed as central to the stereotypically feminine social identity (Coates, 1993: 135–6), can present particular difficulties for women. Although many can learn to make the right sounds, such that questions can be asked and apparently appropriate answers given, there are usually clear indications to the non-autistic person that information or understanding cannot be said to have been shared.

Donna Williams is fairly typical among ASD authors in her use of technological metaphors to convey something of ASD women's communicative coping techniques: 'Like files in a computer, people can mentally store copied performances of emotions, retrieve them and act them out. But that doesn't mean that performance is connected to a real feeling or that there is any understanding of a portrayed emotion beyond the pure mechanics of how and possibly when to emulate it' (2003: 214). Acting normal can thus be a purely imitative project, and authors refer to learning the art of mimicry in order to perform an(y) identity and survive the complexities of a necessarily social and unbearably demanding world: 'I was an empty jar that could be filled with anything. People's behaviour simply fell into the jar and I used it to try to feel myself someone, like a real person' (Gerland, 2003: 209). The acts of imitation are never managed entirely successfully, and at no point is the project completed. Although ASD individuals differ markedly from each other in their ability to accomplish and perform normality, none do so without enormous effort, and few fail to be marked out as different and labelled accordingly, always detrimentally: 'All the years of watching and studying what the normal people were about, I created my own piece of normality. In the eyes of my co-workers they thought of me as the crazy lady, bag lady or a drug user ... Trying to be normal made me act like a nut ... but at least [my co-workers] accepted me as some kind of person, even if some of them had me pegged as a big coke head' (Lawson, 2005: 29). Being *any*thing or any*one* is better than being nothing or nobody.

Enacting normalcy arguably presents challenges for women with ASDs more easily avoidable by men, given gendered stereotypes and expectations around communication styles. Women's speech and body language is culturally constructed around co-operation and connection, rather than competition and distinction, and doing gender appropriately for women often involves being more sociable, sympathetic, insightful, and polite (Holmes, 1995). Obviously, ASD men also have difficulties with social relations and spaces where mind-reading appears to take place. However, it is widely considered less permissible, and more deviant, for women to perform inadequate interaction in social (skills-based) spheres. As Kearns Miller explains: 'Consider how much of femininity is about taking a precise reading of all the social currents of a given moment and aligning (and if necessary, abnegating) oneself to serve the stability of the moment and the wellbeing of all those who inhabit it, whether this means sniffing out the exact social dress code ... the subculture, and occasion, or reading all the social clues in a group and occupying the niche most guaranteed to soothe, nurture, and harmonize all who are in it. This is not the role our wiring has created for us' (2003: xii).

The everyday telepathy that takes place between typical individuals of both sexes is an inexplicable mystery to those with ASDs. Jane Meyerding describes her own painful awareness of difference and disability at an early age – those around her simply knew 'how to be little girls together ... as if everyone else had studied a script and learned their parts beforehand' (2003:159). She was baffled by the 'natural ease with which they acquired their gender identity from the culture around them' (ibid.) and feels that our society makes it harder for girls and women than for boys and men to survive without such mysterious social skills. Judy Singer articulates her sense that those with ASDs are not 'real women,' at least 'not according to any of the known guidebooks,' and recounts examples of discrimination faced by autistic women: 'by employers on social grounds in jobs where social skills should not be part of the criteria; the pressure from families to act normal, to be more feminine, to have children. If this is hard enough for NT [neuro-typical] women, how much harder is it for us?' (2003: xi). Such potentially significant experiential and cultural considerations have been absent from clinical accounts, which almost invariably model the ASD individual in gender neutral (and so singularly male) terms.

Those at the higher-functioning end of the spectrum who can articulate such experience – at least in written form – are able to learn the rules of appropriate behaviour and social and spatial tactics to help them manage others' expectations. This ability to pass as appropriately gendered and neuro-typical at least some of the time presents particular difficulties when women eventually seek diagnostic confirmation.

Diagnosis: Engendering Autism Awareness

From Sharon's experiences, we know that diagnosis for adult women is complex and challenging, and ASD authors reveal that *mis*diagnoses are common. Many of the alternative explanations and labels that women collect are of a more stereotypically appropriate and common feminine form. Judy Singer reveals that, in email lists and meetings for ASD women, 'almost everyone has an anecdote about consulting their GP with suspicions of having some kind of developmental problem, to be told (in effect) "there's nothing wrong, stop being neurotic"' (1999: 65). There is a long and well-documented history of women's positioning as neurotic or hysterical by masculinist medical discourses that dismiss or delegitimize health complaints stereo/typically associated with women.[8] In relation to ASD and so many other cases, physicians apparently hear what they want (or expect) to hear, and see only what the lens of the powerful but misogynistic clinical gaze allows through, filtering out much of what matters from patient presentations (Goudsmit, 1994; Ussher, 1991).

Michelle (2002), for example, was cast as anorexic because of her troubled and apparently strange – but in fact typically autistic[9] – relationship with food. She had managed to pass as having relatively normal eating habits prior to leaving home to attend college. In this new environment, she was expected to eat with other students in the public cafeteria, a nerve-wracking place that failed to facilitate the development of a protective, comforting routine – few other students would request and indeed require the same foods everyday. Michelle's intolerance for disturbing colour and texture combinations severely restricted her options and she ate very little, with the following results: 'After a couple of weeks of telling me continuously that I wasn't fat (which struck me as odd, as I never thought I was), pressuring me to eat more, and monitoring every bite I took, they finally "turned me in" to the school counselor … It was a matter of shape up, or ship out' (2002: 46). Michelle was in fact threatened with admission to a psychiatric ward which, predictably, sent her anxiety 'through the roof. I took to rolling up into a little ball and rocking under tables again, something I hadn't done much since pre-school' (ibid.). Although Michelle was eventually able to negotiate a compromise satisfactory to the authorities, the consequences for her own health were dire. Forcing herself to eat in public, but literally unable to stomach available food combinations, she began regurgitating her meals, and felt forced to do so for some time until she was able to create a more mutually acceptable routine. The compromise required displaying two kinds of food on a plate at one time: less than two was unacceptable to others, more than two was unmanageable for her, but so long as 'they were the kinds of items that said, "We comprise a normal meal" to everyone who looked,' two items were satisfactory to all (ibid.: 48). As with other ASD women, Michelle had a great many unusual habits, but it was her disordered eating – more typical of women than men (Bordo, 1993) – that attracted the greatest attention and attempts at intervention and control.

Other misdiagnoses, including forms of mental ill-health, may be somewhat less stereotypically feminine in nature than anorexia or the chronic depression and anxiety so commonly encountered in diagnosis. However, the dismissal of ASD as a potential diagnostic outcome may in itself be significant for a gendered analysis. Misdiagnoses can be at least partially understood in terms of clinicians' presuppositions about male and female problems: when disordered women come to the attention of medical professionals, ASD may not be the first – or even the last – of those labels that enter their minds. The results can be immensely disruptive to the course of a woman's life.

Patricia Clark, for example, felt forced to adopt and adapt to the label bipolar, applied to her in her thirties. Clark took the prescribed medication for 13 years, 'terrified that I would end up institutionalized for insanity, having no idea what was going on, or that my behaviour was actually normal for a person in my circumstances' (2003: 82). Others have undergone a series of more typical and less disturbing diagnoses over many years before such disturbing labels were finally applied. At school, Wendy Lawson was 'considered lazy, slow and immature for my age … I remember one teacher saying that I was "educationally subnormal" … Other children called me "crazy" or "mad" and some didn't like to play with me' (2005: 30). Gunilla Gerland suffered similar misunderstandings as a school child, and was described in the following terms: 'Lazy. Doesn't listen. Doesn't help. Careless. Inattentive. Drags her feet. Hears only what she wants to hear. Sulks' (2003: 80). (She later adds 'silly, willful, stubborn, rude, spoilt, and defiant' to the growing list.)

Negative behavioural judgments and pseudo-diagnoses based particularly around perceived mental deficiencies are perhaps the most commonly applied to ASD children: 'I was a nut, a retard, a spastic. I threw "mentals" and couldn't act normal' (Williams, 2003: 11). The labelling process often becomes increasingly harsh and explicitly feminized with the growth of the girl towards womanhood: 'To some people my attitude either came off as being a bitch or mad' (Cowhey, 2005: 21); 'I was also thought of as being a witch' (ibid.: 127). As Jane Ussher argues, those positioned by experts as witches, bitches, wicked, or mad throughout the history of patriarchal society have almost invariably always been women. These labels are 'catch-all terms' of 'misogynistic annihilation,' and the women to whom they are applied are thus repeatedly assured of their 'guilty' and outsider status (Ussher, 1991: 43).

Lawson's experience of life and labels failed to improve following her troubling girlhood. On leaving school, she 'crashed' and suffered repeated admissions to institutions, but felt lucky to have avoided electroconvulsive therapy. She resolved: 'If they think I am mad, then I must prove them wrong' (2005: 77). She eventually did so, although it took 25 years to have the diagnosis of schizophrenia overturned. She was relieved by the ASD diagnosis, but states that it was 'also scary to realize I had some other ailment that had no cure' (ibid.). The new label provided her with an opportunity to arm herself with knowledge, and her 'hunger for information and understanding pursued me like a lost dog' (ibid.: 92). This determination to be informed about one's freshly labelled self is typical, although the search is often unsupported by professional involvement. Williams, for example, labouring under the same misdiagnosis as Lawson, describes searching for insight in the medical section of her local library: 'I buried my head in books on schizophrenia and searched desperately to find a sense of belonging within those pages that would give me a word to put to all of this. Suddenly it jumped out at me from the page … "Autism," it read, "not to be confused with schizophrenia."' (1992: 187). Following further research, Williams felt 'both angered and found … I hadn't realized that my "quirks" and "difficulties" were anything other than my mad, bad, or sad personality' (ibid.).

The perceived accuracy of the new label can provide legitimacy and an opportunity to seek out support: 'At the time that we as autistic people finally get a diagnosis – especially if that diagnosis occurs in adulthood – we are relieved just to know there are others like us out there' (Prince-Hughes, 2002: xxii). There may not be a program of treatment to pursue – it is too late for the social skills training they might have accessed in childhood – but knowledge is itself a form of power, at least partially enabling women to make sense of and take control over their unusual lives. For Prince-Hughes (2004: 175), changes in diet and medication to help with compulsive symptoms improved her quality of life immediately, and enabled her to communicate to her partner her determination that she did not intend to live life as a 'diagnostic description.'

Despite the sense that such changes could have been made much earlier with an appropriate diagnosis, Prince-Hughes (2002 and 2004) and others are largely sympathetic to the challenges that clinicians face when presented with their symptoms, already complex, and further complicated when presented through the prism of wildly differing quirks and eccentric personalities. Kearns Miller, for example, recognizes that 'the diagnostic difficulty is rooted in the diversity of autism itself, which is neither unitary, nor binary, but plural' (2003: xix). Women's survival strategies also undermine their efforts to obtain an accurate diagnosis: many 'develop a lifetime pattern of using their intelligence to find ways to appear normal' (ibid.: xxii), meaning that ASD 'is hard to diagnose in adulthood because we can learn to compensate and cover' (Angie, 2002: 77). There are many ways in which ASD traits might be concealed, and not all are deliberate. Although ASD women seem relatively unskilled at doing gender appropriately, they are not immune from cultural pressures to conform to type. Exposure to everyday processes of socialization may in fact mean that ASDs are bound to manifest differently in girls and women, who might, for example, 'have the same passion for facts but less drive to exhibit that knowledge' (Kearns Miller, 2003: xxi). In many circumstances, whether institutional, social, or familial, it may be more acceptable and *normal* for girls to be seen and not heard – and so hide neurological difference – than it is for boys, typically expected and so culturally encouraged to act out. Somewhat paradoxically, the intersections between feminine and ASD traits can present particular challenges, but they might also offer a degree of protection from unwanted attention.

Many ASD women choose to lead very private lives, based around home and family. In societies where it is still not unusual for women to be full-time carers, they have cultural permission to 'live in the kind of seclusion vital to her functioning' (Kearns Miller, 2003: xxii), at the same time as fulfilling a highly valued social role that deflects institutional interference. Testimonies reveal that entering into a heterosexual partnership can be a survival decision, providing the appearance of normality as well as a source of support in the form of someone to help navigate the world. Having a model to demonstrate the correct responses to continual tests of normality – such as when and what it is appropriate to eat – can be experienced as a positive outcome of gender role stereotypes. For others, such as Williams (2003), the attempt to find a comfortable woman's place was less normatively successful. For many years she served as a 'domestic prostitute' to a series of men, trading her body for the stability of a home life that she knew no other way to obtain. Gerland too used sex in attempts to be normal: 'Normality included relationships, and I discovered that sex worked. I could have sex with anyone, for it required no special closeness. It became a way of having relations without having them, a way of making my life look normal. If it was also destructive, this was the price I was prepared to pay in order to feel real' (2003: 167). Although some of the acceptable roles for women provide a cover for ASD traits, this survival strategy further contributes to diagnostic marginalization. Clinicians unaware of such tactics continue to operate with and perpetuate an inaccurate picture of ASDs from which women remain conspicuously absent. The efficacy of theories and treatments – and those who might otherwise benefit – suffer as a result.

Women seeking diagnosis might be thought to clash with an increasingly prevalent view, in some activist and academic circles at least, that pathologizing (particularly psychiatric) labels are best avoided wherever possible (Burstow & Weitz, 1988; Shimrat, 1997). There is, however, a powerful difference, emphasized by ASD authors, between the involuntary receipt of (mis)diagnoses at the hand of a clinician and the positively experienced, voluntary identification with and indeed *claiming* of a diagnosis: 'Whereas the traditional image of "diagnosis" is of something reluctantly sought, dreaded, resisted and imposed from outside, people with "marginal" neurological differences, clamour at the gates, self-diagnosed and demanding to be let in' (Singer, 1999: 65).

The desire for access to this world of difference and acceptance ought to be taken seriously, but we should not assume that the decision to identify with a diagnostic label is uncritical of or complicit with definitions and exclusions as they currently function. As we have seen, ASD women's published accounts often contest the medical(izing) definition of autism and the ways in which the label tends to be applied. The search for diagnosis, and the project of writing about this search, can then be viewed as performance of political activism, an attempt at self-advocacy through testimony that publicly challenges predominant conceptions of ASDs.

Accepting Diagnosis/Contesting Medical Power

First-hand accounts emphasize that there are multiple meanings of autism and that definitions and discourses can be reworked for emancipatory purposes. For Lawson, 'Dr Asperger may have defined the syndrome I was born with, but I have decided his descriptions of my limitations will be the means to remove the bars from my cage – not reinforce them' (2005: ii-iii). Instead of focusing on the pathology and symptoms, deficits and weaknesses, most first-hand accounts of ASDs in fact highlight traits such as unique personality and perspective, alternative knowledge, and individual strengths, traits that arguably amount to neurological *difference* rather than disability. I have focused specifically on the gendered dynamics of diagnosis, but cannot ignore the extent to which authors also communicate a powerful sense of genuine self-worth, a sense that they have worked hard to find and to nurture, despite (or perhaps because of?) their ASD identity. There are many instances where ASD traits are presented positively in the broader context of individuals' lives: 'My world was a rich one, full of colour and music that seemed to splash over and around me wherever I walked' (Lawson, 2005: 40). There are few – if any – where authors accept that textbook criteria have *author*ity over their lives. These women write their own stories, advocating for acceptance of their own difference, and challenging the societal barriers and widespread prejudice that disables their participation in neuro-typical culture.[10]

The desire to create an alternative culture is not uncommon among members of a marginalized group struggling to be heard. To want to find oneself in a community of Others who have claimed a similar positioning and identity – as with political, consciousness-raising, and rights-claiming projects – often involves creating a means of expression, claiming a *voice*. It need not involve passive acceptance of marginalization from 'normal' culture, conceptualized as, for example, 'malestream,' heterosexist, able-bodied, or neuro-typical, depending on the form of exclusion being contested. Commenting on the painful absence of such a positive space for herself and the mother and daughter with whom she shares a place on the autistic spectrum, Singer writes: 'By now [the 1980s], groups of women, queers, crips, had all found their voices, their communities. It seemed that only my family was left without a group to belong to, who could speak for us and with us' (1999: 61).

ASD women authors have through their writing begun to address this absence; an alternative space for the neurologically divergent group to which they choose to belong is coming into existence, and a culture of and for that group is emerging. Interestingly, for those who describe their communicative style in technological terms, and who struggle with face-to-face meetings, it is the Internet that enables access to a shared space of comfortable conversational exchange and the emergence of positive and politicized identities: 'With their own communication medium autistics are beginning to see themselves not as blighted individuals, but as a different ethnicity' (Singer, 1999: 67). In the words of Prince-Hughes: 'Autistic culture is new and dynamic, it is in an initial phase of growth, and it comprises people who do not easily form relationships. Unlike "deaf culture" or "blind culture," autistic culture has only become possible in the age of the internet' (2002: xi).

The connection made here with a group who has used the cultural mechanism of sign language to negotiate the 'natural' impairment of deafness is telling. Deaf culture is empowering and increasingly power-ful in its ability to challenge medical models of disability (Valentine & Skelton, 2003). Cultural commentators on neurological difference stress the similarities between ASD activism and other such (counter)cultural projects, drawing attention to the empowering potential of taking pride in being 'differently brained' (Gevers, 2000). We might then see a com-parison between ASD accounts and the contestational yet celebratory nature of queer coming-out narratives. Both can be seen as simulta-neously expressing and contributing to the creation of a cultural differ-ence. Autistic culture also strives to demonstrate that there are other ways to participate meaningfully in society.

Acknowledgments

Thanks to all workshop participants for a genuinely enriching experi-ence, and especially to Pamela Moss and Kathy Teghtsoonian for orga-nizing the event and following through with such dedicated care – fantastic editors both. Thanks also to Liz Bardi, Victoria Henderson, Leah form the basis for this work.

NOTES

1   The title is taken from a biographical note on the back cover of Donna Williams' 2004 book, *Everyday Heaven: Journeys Beyond the Stereotypes of Autism:* 'She grew up with more labels than a jam jar and like many people

with autism born in the 60s and earlier, she was not formally diagnosed with autism until adulthood.'

2 The clinical jury is still out on whether the 10-fold increase in recorded cases over the past two decades is representative of increased prevalence or reflects, instead, changes in diagnostic criteria, along with increased awareness and referral (Baker, 2006: 16). Recent epidemiological studies suggest figures as high as 60 per 10,000 (Fombonne, 2003a: 504, and 2003b).

3 See Gray (2001, 2002, and 2003) for examples of qualitative research *with* carers.

4 Such research is still rare, but see Jones, Quigney, & Huws (2003) and Jones, Zahl, & Huws (2001) for notable exceptions.

5 The Internet also constitutes a user-friendly communications medium for a group who struggle with face-to-face interaction. Email lists and chat rooms are apparently popular with ASD Internet users, and will no doubt become an increasingly prominent site of future research (see Jones, Quigney, & Huws, 2003, and Jones, Zahl, & Huws, 2001, for existing examples). Internet-based research does, however, have its own methodological risks and limitations (Brownlow & O'Dell, 2002; Mann & Stewart, 2000).

6 Clearly, there are a number of limitations to the methodology employed by this project. Many of those with ASDs lack the skills or resources – whether cognitive, social, or financial – to present their accounts in a publishable form. My focus on book-based autobiography therefore screens out the vast majority of – and probably more typical – ASD experiences.

7 Among those autobiographical sources identified for this study (a sample no doubt far from exhaustive), there are numerous themes that could be highlighted as deserving significant attention. The book titles themselves are suggestive; consider, e.g., the environmental and affective alienation suggested by *Life on the Outside* (Gerland, 2003), *Life behind Glass* (Lawson, 2005), and *Exposure Anxiety, the Invisible Cage* (Williams, 2003).

8 Reviewed by Lorber (1997); see also Davidson (2002) for discussion in specific relation to agoraphobia.

9 Susan, e.g., 'made the same thing for dinner for two years (club sandwiches with French fries and a pickle pear)' (in Prince-Hughes, 2002: 104). Atypical eating habits are recognized as characteristic of ASDs in the clinical literature (Tidmarsh & Volkmar, 2003: 520).

10 The authors represented in this chapter would not deny the material reality of their disorder or suggest that their neurological difference could somehow be socially reconstructed out of existence. Most describe their impairments as causing extraordinary challenges, and although few have lived less than very difficult lives, it seems they would not leave ASD traits behind if they

were able (see the arguments in Stone, Chapter 10, this volume). In *Pretending to be Normal*, Liane Willey, for example, explains that she would never want a 'cure' for an ASD, experienced as thoroughly enmeshed with her personality and sense of self: 'What I wish for, is a cure for the common ill that pervades too many lives; the ill that makes people compare themselves to a normal that is measured in terms of perfect and absolute standards, most of which are impossible for anyone to reach' (1999: 121).

REFERENCES

American Psychiatric Association. (2000). *Diagnostic and statistical manual of mental disorders* (4th ed. – Text Revision). Washington: Author.

Angie. (2002). Angie. In Dawn Prince-Hughes (Ed.), *Aquamarine blue 5: Personal stories of college students with autism* (pp. 76–78). Athens, OH: Swallow Press.

Baker, Dana Lee. (2006). Neurodiversity, neurological disability and the public sector: Notes on the autism spectrum. *Disability and Society, 21*(1), 15–29.

Baron-Cohen, Simon. (2003). *The essential difference: Male and female brains and the truth about autism*. New York: Basic Books.

Bordo, Susan. (1993). *Unbearable weight: Feminism, western culture and the body*. Berkeley: University of California Press.

Brownlow, Charlotte, & O'Dell, Lindsay. (2002). Ethical issues for qualitative research in on-line communities. *Disability and Society, 17*(6), 685–694.

Bruey, Carolyn Thorwarth. (2004). *Demystifying Autism Spectrum Disorders: A guide to diagnosis for parents and professionals*. Bethesda, MD: Woodbine House.

Burstow, Bonnie, & Weitz, Don. (Eds.). (1988). *Shrink resistant: The struggle against psychiatry in Canada*. Vancouver: New Star Books.

Butler, Judith. (1990). *Gender trouble: Feminism and the subversion of identity*. New York and London: Routledge.

Butler, Judith. (2004). *Undoing gender*. New York and London: Routledge.

Campbell, Peter. (1992). The service user/survivor movement. In Craig Newnes, Guy Holmes, & Cailzie Dunn (Eds.), *This is madness: A critical look at psychiatry and the future of mental health services* (pp. 357–363). Ross on Wye, England: PCCS Books.

Claiborne Park, Clara. (2001). *Exiting nirvana: A daughter's life with autism*. Boston, New York, and London: Little, Brown.

Clark, Patricia. (2003). The perils of diagnosis (Or how I became bipolar?). In Jean Kearns Miller (Ed.), *Women from another planet? Our lives in the universe of autism* (pp. 81–82). Bloomington: Dancing Minds.

Coates, Jennifer. (1993). *Women, men and language*. London and New York: Longman.

Collins, Paul. (2004). *Not even wrong: Adventures in autism*. New York and London: Bloomsbury.

Cowhey, Sharon P. (2005). *Going through the motions: Coping with autism*. Baltimore: PublishAmerica.

Cresswell, Mark. (2005). Psychiatric 'survivors' and testimonies of self-harm. *Social Science and Medicine, 61*, 1668–1677.

Davidson, Joyce. (2002). 'All in the mind?' Women, agoraphobia and the subject of self-help. In Liz Bondi, Hannah Avis, Ruth Bankey, Amanda Bingley, Joyce Davidson, Rosaleen Duffy, Victoria Ingrid Einagel, Anje-Maaike Green, Lynda Johnston, Susan Lilley, Carina Listerborn, Shonah McEwan, Mona Marshy, Niamh O'Connor, Gillian Rose, Bella Vivat, & Nichola Wood, *Subjectivities, Knowledges, and Feminist Geographies* (pp. 44–56). Lanham, MD: Rowman and Littlefield.

Davidson, Joyce. (2005, April). *'In a world of her own … ': An emotional geography of autism*. Paper presented at the Annual Meeting of the Association of American Geographers, Denver, Colorado.

Fombonne, Eric. (2003a). Modern views of autism. *Canadian Journal of Psychiatry, 48*(8), 503–505.

Fombonne, Eric. (2003b). Epidemiological surveys of autism and other pervasive developmental disorders: An update. *Journal of Autism and Developmental Disorders, 33*(4), 365–382.

Frith, Uta. (1996). Asperger and his syndrome. In Uta Frith (Ed.), *Autism and Asperger Syndrome* (pp. 1–36). Cambridge: Cambridge University Press.

Gerland, Gunilla. (2003). *A real person: Life on the outside*. London: Souvenir Press.

Gevers, Ine. (2000). Subversive tactics of neurologically diverse cultures. *Journal of Cognitive Liberties, 2*(1), 43–60.

Goudsmit, Ellen M. (1994). All in her mind! Stereotypic views and the psychologisation of women's illness. In Sue Wilkinson & Celia Kitzinger (Eds.), *Women and health: Feminist perspectives* (pp. 7–12). Bristol, England: Taylor and Francis.

Gray, David E. (2001). Accommodation, resistance and transcendence: Three narratives of autism. *Social Science and Medicine, 53*, 1247–1257.

Gray, David E. (2002). 'Everybody just freezes. Everybody is just so embarrassed': Felt and enacted stigma among parents of children with high-functioning autism. *Sociology of Health and Illness, 24*(6), 734–749.

Gray, David E. (2003). Gender and coping: The parents of children with high functioning autism. *Social Science and Medicine, 56*, 631–642.

Haddon, Mark. (2004). *The curious incident of the dog in the night-time*. Toronto: Anchor Canada.

Hodge, Nick. (2005). Reflections on diagnosing autism spectrum disorders. *Disability and Society, 20*(3), 345–349.

Holmes, Janet. (1995). *Women, men and politeness*. Harlow, England: Longman.

Jones, Robert S.P., Quigney, Ciara, & Huws, Jaci C. (2003). First-hand accounts of sensory perceptual experiences in autism: A qualitative analysis. *Journal of Intellectual and Developmental Disability, 28*(2), 112–121.

Jones, Robert S.P., Zahl, Andrew, & Huws, Jaci C. (2001). First-hand accounts of emotional experiences in autism: A qualitative analysis. *Disability and Society, 16*(3), 393–401.

Kearns Miller, Jean. (Ed.). (2003). *Women from another planet: Our lives in the universe of autism*. Bloomington: Dancing Minds.

Lawson, Wendy. (2005). *Life behind glass: A personal account of autism spectrum disorder*. London and Philadelphia: Jessica Kingsley.

Lorber, Judith. (1997). *Gender and the social construction of illness*. London and Thousand Oaks: Sage.

Mann, Chris, & Stewart, Fiona. (2000). *Internet communication and qualitative research: A handbook for researching online*. Thousand Oaks: Sage.

Meyerding, Jane. (2003). Growing up genderless. In Jean Kearns Miller (Ed.), *Women from another planet? Our lives in the universe of autism* (pp. 157–169). Bloomington: Dancing Minds.

Michelle. (2002). Michelle. In Dawn Prince-Hughes (Ed.), *Aquamarine blue 5: Personal stories of college students with autism* (pp. 43–49). Athens, OH: Swallow Press.

Molloy, Harvey, & Vasil, Latika (2002). The social construction of Asperger Syndrome: The pathologising of difference? *Disability and Society, 17*(6), 659–669.

Nash, J. Madeleine. (2002, 6 May). The secrets of autism: The number of children diagnosed with autism and Asperger's in the US is exploding. Why? *Time, 159*, 47–56.

Prince-Hughes, Dawn. (Ed.). (2002). *Aquamarine blue 5: Personal stories of college students with autism*. Athens, OH: Swallow Press.

Prince-Hughes, Dawn. (2004). *Songs of the gorilla nation: My journey through autism*. New York: Harmony Books.

Seltzer, M.M., Krauss, M.W., Shattuck, P.T., Orsmond, G., Swe, A., & Lord, C. (2003). The symptoms of autism spectrum disorders in adolescence and adulthood. *Journal of Autism and Developmental Disorders, 33*(6), 565–581.

Shimrat, Irit. (1997). *Call me crazy: Stories from the mad movement*. Vancouver: Press Gang.

Singer, Judy. (1999). 'Why can't you be normal for once in your life?' From a 'problem with no name' to the emergence of a new category of difference.

In Mairian Corker & Sally French (Eds.), *Disability discourse* (pp. 59–67). Buckingham, England: Open University Press.

Singer, Judy. (2003). Foreword: Travels in parallel space: An invitation. In Jean Kearns Miller (Ed.), *Women from another planet? Our lives in the universe of autism* (xi–xiii). Bloomington: Dancing Minds.

Szatmari, Peter. (2004). *A mind apart: Understanding children with autism and Asperger Syndrome.* New York and London: Guilford.

Tidmarsh, Lee, & Volkmar, Fred R. (2003). Diagnosis and epidemiology of autism spectrum disorders. *Canadian Journal of Psychiatry, 48*(8), 517–525.

Ussher, Jane. (1991). *Women's madness: Misogyny or mental illness?* New York: Harvester Wheatsheaf.

Valentine, Gill, & Skelton, Tracey. (2003). Living on the edge: The marginalization and 'resistance' of D/deaf youth. *Environment and Planning A, 35,* 301–321.

Waltz, Mitzi. (2005). Reading case studies of people with autistic spectrum disorders: A cultural studies approach to disability representation. *Disability and Society, 20*(4), 421–435.

Williams, Donna. (1992). *Nobody nowhere: The extraordinary autobiography of an autistic.* New York: Random House.

Williams, Donna. (2003). *Exposure anxiety, the invisible cage: An exploration of self-protection responses in the Autism Spectrum and beyond.* London and Philadelphia: Jessica Kingsley.

Willey, Liane Holliday. (1999). *Pretending to be normal: Living with Asperger's syndrome.* London and Philadelphia: Jessica Kingsley.

Wing, Lorna. (1997). Syndromes of autism and atypical development. In Donald J. Cohen & Fred R. Volkmar (Eds.), *Handbook of Autism and Pervasive Developmental Disorders* (pp. 148–170). New York: Wiley.

World Health Organization. (1992). *The ICD-10 classification of mental and behavioural disorders: Clinical descriptions and diagnostic guidelines.* Geneva: Author.

14 The Female Sexual Dysfunction Debate: Different 'Problems,' New Drugs – More Pressures?

ANNIE POTTS

Women's sexuality in Western culture has historically been constructed as problematic (Tuana, 1993), and women's bodies continue to be 'a site of struggle for definition and control' (Braun & Wilkinson, 2001: 17). The contemporary debate around women's sexual problems – their causes and remedies – centres on the increasing influence of the biomedical model of sexuality and provides the latest example of such a struggle for meaning and control. In this chapter, I examine the key contributors to and perspectives in the Female Sexual Dysfunction (FSD) debate: those who endorse biophysiological explanations for sexual difficulties and promote the use of new sexuopharmaceuticals for treatment versus those who oppose the expanding influence of bio-medicine in everyday life, arguing that sexuality is a complex phenom-enon irreducible to mere physical processes and responses.

To place the debate in context, I provide a brief overview of the medical model of sexuality, including a critical analysis of the central-ity of the human sexual response cycle to this paradigm's conceptions of functionality and dysfunctionality. Next, I explore the recent push by the medical establishment to redefine women's sexual difficulties in terms of recognized biophysical disorders, particularly in light of the advent of sexuopharmaceuticals such as Viagra for the treatment of erectile dysfunction (ED) in men and the ensuing impetus to locate similarly effective – and highly profitable – drugs targeting women. I also outline the key arguments advanced by those associated with the political campaign for a new view of women's sexual problems who have contested the authoritative medical model of FSD. Members of the New View Working Group actively oppose the biomedicalized commercialization of women's sexuality associated with the pharma-ceutical industry's growing influence on conceptualizations of health and illness. Following my examination of the two main sides of this debate (the proponents and opponents of FSD), I engage with the perspectives and experiences of women themselves in relation to the medical model of sexual dysfunction and the development of so-called pink Viagra.[1] I conclude with a discussion of the possibilities for new norms, expectations, pressures, and demands to be produced as a result of the biomedicalization of women's sexual concerns.

The Medical Model of Functional/Dysfunctional Sex

The medical model of sexuality, which gained authority post-1960s, subscribes to a mechanistic view of the body, in which sexual response is broken down into a series of consecutive stages as part of a supposedly universal human sexual response cycle (HSRC). This cycle, considered to be a biological given, is assumed to operate within individuals regardless of cultural or historical factors (Tiefer, 2001), although it is more or less acknowledged that its usual trajectory may be compromised by such influences. William Masters and Virginia Johnson (1966 and 1970), the pioneers of the HSRC, posit that men and women respond sexually in a similar manner, which they reduce to physiological changes associated with vasocongestion and muscular tension. For example, in the excitement phase of the HSRC, penile erection is considered neurophysiologically parallel to vaginal lubrication (Segal, 1994).

Deviation from the 'normal' sexual response cycle constitutes a 'sexual dysfunction' in medical discourse and is understood to manifest itself through various symptoms. For instance, the American Psychiatric Association's 4th edition of the *Diagnostic and Statistical Manual of Mental Disorders* (DSM-IV) describes sexual dysfunction as 'a disturbance in the processes that characterize the sexual response cycle or by pain associated with sexual intercourse' (APA, 1994: 493). The original form of this cycle consisted of excitement, plateau, orgasm, and resolution phases (Masters & Johnson, 1966); however, a triphasic version is currently employed by the DSM-IV, comprising desire, arousal, and orgasmic phases. These phases correspond with disorders of desire, disorders of arousal (and orgasm), and pain disorders (Nicholi, 1999).

Masters and Johnson's (1966) model of the HSRC has attracted strong criticism. Feminist scholars have disputed its androcentric bias (female sexuality is assumed to follow the observed 'normal' trajectory of male sexuality), universalist claims (one cycle fits all), and reductionism (it diminishes sexual pleasure to physiological responses,

women's and men's bodies to genitalia, normal sexual practice to heterosexual intercourse, and healthy sexual response to orgasm) (Potts,
2002; Tiefer, 1995). The various sexual dysfunctions constructed
according to the stages of the HSRC are similarly censured. Moreover,
the HSRC assumes that some sort of sexuality is necessary and healthy
for everyone; there is no space for someone who is not sexual, who
does not care for genital contact, or who is not interested in sex per se
to be viewed as healthy or normal (Potts, 2002).

Twenty-First Century Biomedicalization and Sexuopharmacology

Ideas about normal sexual response – and functional/dysfunctional sex
– filtered into popular culture and everyday talk in the latter half of the
twentieth century, forged by their association with the authoritative
medical model. Medical constructions of normal and abnormal sexuality
now affect women's own understandings and experiences of sexual
pleasure in profound ways (Potts, 2002). The term *medicalization* refers to
the process whereby 'diverse areas of human behaviour are brought
within a medical frame of discourse both conceptually and institution-
ally' (Tiefer, 2001: 65). One consequence of the medicalization of sexuality involves the framing of women's sexual concerns as primarily
physiologically based and, hence, able to be treated by physical means.

Since the advent of Viagra – following its approval by the U.S. Food
and Drug Administration for the treatment of erectile difficulties in 1998
– attention has turned to the new phenomenon of *biomedicalization*.
Adele Clarke and her colleagues (Clarke, Shim, Mamo, Fosken, & Fishman, 2003: 161) argue that the process of biomedicalization marks a new
transformation in medicine, whereby medicalization is 'extended and
reconstituted through the new social forms of highly technoscientific
biomedicine.' Significantly, the process of biomedicalization is inti-
mately linked to the world of late capitalism and especially to the pharmaceutical industry – referred to by critics as Big Pharma (Elliot, 2003;
Healy, 2004; Loe, 2004; Metzl, 2003; Moynihan & Cassels, 2005; Tiefer,
2004). Clarke and her colleagues go on to contend there has been a shift
from *normalization* of bodies – achieved through the process of medicalization – to *customization* (tailor-made drugs, niche marketing, and 'bou-
tique medicine'), associated with biomedicalization and with the
pharmaceutical industry's concentration on so-called lifestyle drugs.
These are medications that improve or enhance one's life but that may not
address any actual disease process: 'Viagra exemplifies this movement

towards enhancement and the concern with "treating" the signs of aging' (Clarke et al., 2003: 181).

The expanding influence of the biomedical model is demonstrated in the shift over the past 5 to 10 years to viewing women's sexual problems as more likely to be physically derived (rooted in the body, rather than psychologically-, emotionally-, or relationally-based) and, therefore, more readily addressed through organic solutions such as medications. For example, in his examination of the content of four key academic sexuality journals published between 1967 and 2000, Mark Winton (2001) identified a marked transfer from psychological to biophysiological explanations for women's sexual difficulties – particularly arousal and orgasmic disorders – occurring between 1999 and 2000.[2]

The contemporary dispute around definitions, classifications, and treatments related to 'Female Sexual Dysfunction' foregrounds the relationship between the medical establishment and Big Pharma: on one side are urologists, psychiatrists, and sexologists, supported financially by drug companies, who endorse the biophysiological nature of FSD, and the use of pharmacological remedies; on the other side are critics of the biomedical model who protest this reductionist framing of sexuality and expose the insidious influence of Big Pharma in our everyday lives. Critics of biomedicalization argue that the 'cure,' in the form of freshly developed (and potentially highly profitable) drugs, tends to precede and determine the illness or condition (i.e., the nature of new diagnostic categories). Drug companies manufacture their own markets through defining everyday ailments as pathological and then supplying remedies for these newly recognized diseases (Healy, 2004; Marshall, 2002; Metzl, 2003).

The FSD Debate

Proponents of Biomedicalization: The Consensus Committee

The biomedicalization of women's sexual difficulties at the turn of the twenty-first century can be traced through several important events and publications sponsored, in the main, by drug companies and taking place in the period 1997 to date (Loe, 2004; Moynihan, 2003; Tiefer, 2004; Treacher, 2003). Shortly after the advent of Viagra for men, there was a flurry of activity to identify similarly effective and profitable drugs that might work for women. First, however, there were some hurdles to clear in the race to manufacture a 'pink Viagra.' For example, since identification and classification are the cornerstones of the medical model (Hartley & Tiefer, 2003), exactly what problem(s) or condition(s) would this drug treat? And, given the long history of constructing women's sexuality as mysterious, complex, and contentious, how might a drug like Viagra be expected to work for women as effectively, and in the same straightforward manner, as it appeared to be working for men (Fishman, 2002)? How would any drug's impact on women be *measured* in easily quantifiable terms befitting the medical model – i.e., in the way a 'restored' erection had counted for successful treatment of erectile difficulties in men (Tiefer, 2003)?

In answer to these questions, a party of 19 leading international sexuality researchers and clinicians, 18 of whom had financial links to pharmaceutical companies (Moynihan, 2003), came together under the rubric of 'The Consensus Committee on FSD,' to revise the DSM-IV's existing nomenclature on sexual difficulties affecting women, a task accomplished by providing revamped norms of female sexual response and clearer definitions of dysfunction. Alongside the establishment of this committee, annual meetings foregrounding biomedical perspectives on FSD (known as the Boston Forums) have been hosted by Boston University School of Medicine's Department of Urology. Following the first Boston Forum in 1999, a new organization was established, called the Female Sexual Function Forum (FSFF).

The perceived need for such a forum on FSD was based on a study published in February 1999 in the *Journal of the American Medical Association* – authored by consultants to Pfizer, the company manufacturing Viagra (Hartley & Tiefer, 2003), which claimed that sexual dysfunction affected 43 per cent of women in America (Laumann, Paik, & Rosen, 1999). This statistic is apparently routinely employed in drug company advertising, despite the fact that the authors of this study have since argued that their figures did not equate with clinical diagnosis and that they were not suggesting that 43 per cent of women actually experienced FSD (Moynihan & Cassels, 2005).

The biomedical faction is represented by several prominent urologists, psychiatrists, gynaecologists, and sexologists (see Basson et al., 2003). Foremost is Irwin Goldstein, a urologist and specialist in ED, who has produced numerous articles asserting the significance of organic etiology in sexual difficulties (and who is notable for his perspective that sex is basically a mechanical event, albeit one that is more complicated for women). Goldstein's position is supported by 'the Berman sisters' (as they are commonly known), urologist Jennifer and sex therapist

Laura, a duo who have achieved celebrity status as the front-people promoting FSD through their appearances on prime time television and via their popular co-authored books (see, e.g., Berman & Berman, 2001). The Berman sisters contend that in the majority of cases, an organic disorder precedes an emotional one, and they are outspoken advocates of allocating drugs such as Viagra to women off-label.

The key changes to the medical categorization of women's sexual difficulties resulting from the Boston meetings included expanding existing nomenclature, adding a clause to each category regarding 'personal distress,' and amending diagnostic criteria in ways that made physical treatments more acceptable for the treatment of FSD of unknown or psychological etiology (Treacher, 2003). In the 1994 version of the DSM, female sexual disorders are classified under the following headings: Hypoactive Sexual Desire Disorder (HSDD), Female Sexual Arousal Disorder (FSAD), Female Orgasmic Disorder (FOD), and the pain disorders (such as dyspareunia) (APA, 1994). The proposed revised classifications of FSD consist of expanded versions of FSAD to include four different types (Combined Sexual Arousal Disorder, Subjective Sexual Arousal Disorder, Genital Arousal Disorder, and Persistent Arousal Disorder), and the addition of two new disorders (Persistent Arousal Disorder and Non-Coital Sexual Pain Disorder).

In the bevy of publications related to the so-called consensus-based categorizations of FSD, the authors claim to have paid attention to the concerns of feminists and other critics regarding earlier classification systems that failed to take into account contextual, relational, and gender factors (Basson, 2000, 2001, 2004a, 2004b, and 2005; Basson et al., 2003; Sugrue & Whipple, 2001). To address criticism of the masculinist assumptions of previous models of the HSRC, several versions of the female sexual response cycle have been proposed. For example, Rosemary Basson (2001) suggests that women's sexual response follows different trajectories: one version that she describes shows arousal occurring prior to desire, a sequence she claims is usual for many women but which, according to Masters and Johnson's depiction of the HSRC, would be diagnosed as dysfunctional.

BASIC TENETS OF THE BIOMEDICAL MODEL

The biomedical model of women's sexuality subscribes to two key positions. First, the body is treated as the problem (or at least any problem can be treated *through* the body). Thus, the experts in FSD focus primarily on the biophysiology of sexuality, for example, poor circulation and/or deficient or overly abundant amounts of certain hormones are blamed for insufficient or excessive stimulation or arousal (Loe, 2004). Because the body is positioned as problematic in this framing, management of these new conditions also increasingly favours the use of medications. The growing importance placed on biophysiological aspects of sexuality is demonstrated in changing patterns of research and treatment regimes in the years from 1998 to 2004, the period of the Boston meetings. The report on the first consensus meeting regarding FSD recommended clinical trials of drugs alongside efficacy studies of psychotherapy for sexual difficulties; 3 years later, the terrain shifted to a focus only on pharmacological interventions (usually off-label) with drugs such as androgens, estrogens, and dopamine agonists for the sexual desire disorders; prostaglandins for Genital Arousal Disorder; Selective Serotonin Reuptake Inhibitors (SSRIs) for Persistent Sexual Arousal Disorder; and tricyclic antidepressants for dyspareunia (see Basson, 2004b and 2005).

Second, the biomedical model assumes that women's sexuality is more complex and difficult than men's. FSD meetings over the past 5 years have consistently employed the model of a complex-looking mechanical contraption, bearing numerous buttons and switches, to represent women's sexuality, while at the same time men's supposedly straightforward sexual response is portrayed using a similar machine sporting just one on/off switch (Fishman, 2002). Of course, this representation continues the tradition of viewing women's sexualized bodies as mysterious, aberrant, and unpredictable, and requiring more control or management (Tiefer, 2003).

DISSENT FROM WITHIN THE MEDICAL MODEL

Although the new classifications of FSD devised by the Consensus Committee received backing from many experts in the fields of sexual science and medicine, dissenters also emerged from within the medical establishment. These people do not necessarily reject the idea of organic influences on sexual problems, but they do argue that the causes of women's sexual concerns extend beyond the body, and are as much – if not more – located in lifestyle, relationships, and other sociocultural factors. For example, John Bancroft, former director of the Kinsey Institute, disputes the use of the term Female Sexual Dysfunction, claiming that it paints a false picture of a disordered organic process, where in fact, it may be the case that a woman's lack of desire for sex, or difficulty feeling aroused, stems from everyday stress and tiredness (Bancroft, 2002).

Sandra Leiblum, psychiatrist and instigator of the additional diagnostic category Persistent Sexual Arousal Disorder (see Leiblum & Nathan, 2001), has also voiced doubts about the new classification system of FSD. Leiblum is one of the few medical experts (along with Bancroft) who acknowledges the historical pathologization of women's sexuality within masculinist frameworks (Loe, 2004). At the 2001 Boston Forum, she also stressed the importance of another non-organic factor that affects women's sexual well-being, something she termed the 'Steve Problem,' which emphasized the part (heterosexual) women's sexual partners play in dissatisfying sexual experiences (reported in Loe, 2004: 154).

Psychiatrist Rosemary Basson, a member of the Female Sexual Function Forum, is the lead author of many publications advocating changes to the previous classification system of women's sexual problems. As mentioned, Basson has also provided alternative (although medically influenced) models of women's sexual response to the standard HSRC proposed by Masters and Johnson and employed in DSM-IV (APA, 1994). Basson's (2000, 2001, 2004a, 2004b, and 2005) versions recognize contextual factors, such as the impact of long-term sexual relationships, on women's sexual experiences.

The New View Approach to Women's Sexual Problems:
'A Historically Situated Attempt to Contest Medicalization'[3]

> Ever since Viagra proved to the pharmaceutical industry that contemporary sexual confusions and dissatisfactions could be medicalized and marketed (to the sweet cash register ring of billions of dollars and Euros), companies have been searching for some way to make women into sex problem consumer-patients.
>
> Tiefer, 2003: 2

During the last decades of the twentieth century, feminist scholars mounted a concerted challenge to medicine's reductionist, androcentric constructions of normative sexuality: Leonore Tiefer (1995) critiqued the HSRC and definitions of sexual dysfunction derived from this model. Nellie Oudshoorn (1994) and Jennifer Harding (1998) interrogated the ways in which hormones came to be reified as determinants of male and female sexualities. Lana Thompson (1999) and Carol Groneman (2001) traced the history of cultural fallacies such as 'the wandering womb' and 'nymphomania' respectively. Rachel Maines (1999) analysed the medical treatment of 'hysteria' at the turn of the twentieth century (which involved doctors inducing orgasms in women via the use of early vibrators). Paula Nicolson (1993) identified three key discourses prevailing in medical and popular cultural definitions of 'normal' sexuality (the coital, orgasmic, and biological imperatives).

These feminist critiques of – and counter-perspectives to – the medical model continue in relation to the contemporary biomedicalization of women's sexuality. In response to the early meetings arranged by Goldstein, New York–based clinical psychologist and sexologist Leonore Tiefer brought together a group of social scientists, clinicians, and feminist activists to form a group called 'The New View Working Group,' which has provided effective and highly publicized opposition to this latest bid to define and control women's sexuality. Tiefer exposed the closed-door invitation-only nature of the original meeting in 1998, as well as the drug company affiliations of almost all of the contributors at this gathering, and questioned its timing – 6 months after FDA approval and launch of Viagra. She is also largely responsible for critiquing the so-called objectivity of the consensus report and the revised framings of FSD (Tiefer, 2001).[4]

New View campaigners argue that the recently developed classification system for FSD centres on the continued medicalization of women's bodies and sexualities in more intensely technologized and commercialized modes. While acknowledging that medical problems do exist, the group is concerned about the primacy of biophysiological explanations and solutions for women's sexual problems endorsed by a medical establishment now heavily influenced by the corporate world of the pharmaceutical industry. Advocates of the New View argue that commercial interests are central to moves in the field of FSD: 'Because there are no magic bullets for the socio-cultural, political, psychological, social or relational bases of women's sexual problems, pharmaceutical companies are supporting research and public relations programs, focused on fixing the body, especially the genitals. The infusion of industry funding into sex research and the incessant media publicity about "breakthrough" treatments have put physical problems in the spotlight and isolated them from broader contexts' (New View Working Group, 2001: 4). This is a process that Geraldine Treacher, in her examination of the FSD controversy, eloquently describes as 'FSD as pharmaceutical project' (2003: 30).

BASIC TENETS OF THE NEW VIEW APPROACH

To challenge the predominance of the medical model of FSD, the New View group has devised their own counter-document to the Consensus

Committee's report, which critiques current trends in the diagnosis and treatment of women's sexual concerns and offers a more expansive, holistic classification system. This manifesto, called *A New View of Women's Sexual Problems*, co-authored by 12 clinicians and social scientists in 2001, targets the medical model for its universalist underpinnings, arguing that this approach promotes a 'false notion of sexual equivalency between men and women,' leads to the 'erasure of the relational context of sexuality,' and fails to address diversity among women (New View Working Group, 2001: 3).

The categorization system devised by the New View group focuses on several key dimensions: *'sexual problems due to socio-cultural, political, or economic factors'* (including inadequate access to information about such matters as sexual biology, contraception and abortion, sexual trauma, and STD prevention, and issues such as shame about one's body and confusion about sexual identity); *'sexual problems relating to partner and relationship'* (including sexual concerns due to relationship conflicts or communication problems); *'sexual problems due to psychological factors'* (including depression and anxiety, negative past experiences, fear of consequences of pregnancy and pain, etc.); and *'sexual problems due to medical factors'* (e.g., neurological, neurovascular, and endocrine conditions; side effects of drugs; iatrogenic conditions; pregnancy; STIs; etc.) (New View Working Group, 2001: 4, emphases added).

Members of the New View campaign contend that its strength lies in its re-situation of women's sexuality in the political, rather than medical, domain (Hartley & Tiefer, 2003). By highlighting the insights of women's studies and critical sex research, and focusing on preventative strategies that offset the sociopolitical and economic causes of sexual problems, the New View approach disrupts simplistic biomedical frameworks of FSD.

The New View campaign has received significant publicity through numerous publications (including an edited volume and a teaching manual), via its Website (www.fsd-alert.org), and through two conferences, the first in San Francisco in 1999 and the second (and closing conference of the campaign) in Montreal in 2005.

Women's Own Perspectives on 'Pink Viagra'

While the expert voices of the proponents and opponents of FSD have been heard through the media and various medical and academic forums, the opinions of women themselves have received less attention.

To date, few studies exist specifically focusing on women's perspectives on the construction of sexual problems within medicalized frameworks and/or the development and advent of sexuopharmaceuticals targeting women (although, see Treacher, 2003). However, women participating in research on the impact of men's use of Viagra (for the treatment of erectile difficulties) have provided some insights (Askew & Davey, 2004; Loe, 2004; Potts, 2005; Potts, Gavey, Grace, & Vares, 2003; Potts, Grace, Gavey, & Vares, 2004). This section concentrates on the accounts of women in one such study, a qualitative project undertaken between 2001 and 2004, which was funded by the Health Research Council of New Zealand (Grace, Potts, Gavey, & Vares, 2006; Potts, Grace, Vares, & Gavey, 2006; Potts et al., 2003 and 2004).[5] The chief purpose of the interviews with the 27 women taking part in this study was to explore their experiences of erectile difficulties and Viagra use in the context of their relationships with men; however, women also took the opportunity to talk about the development of drugs to treat women's sexual difficulties. Because few, if any, of the women in this study were aware of the FSD controversy, which was occurring at the time of their interviews, the women's responses pertain more to speculations on the anticipated advent of a Viagra-type drug for women than to any informed engagement with this particular debate. Nevertheless, and perhaps not surprisingly, the responses of women in the New Zealand study resonate with both the pro- and anti-biomedicalization perspectives on FSD.

Perceived Benefits

KEEPING SEXUALLY ACTIVE
Several women in the New Zealand study expressed enthusiasm for the advent of a 'pink Viagra.' One woman (aged 52) commented:

> The faster they can get them on the market the better … Once you hit 60 I think, well, that's it. But what do you do? I mean you could have a raging sex life in your old age, if you organized it properly, and if you get your health straight … You've got to be fit, and I think the fitness factor for older people is going to be absolutely crucial.

This woman frames the new impetus to keep fit and active (including sexually) as essential to health in mid- to later life. Critical gerontologists Barbara Marshall and Stephen Katz (2002) have read this contemporary drive to maintain 'busy bodies' in older age as a new form of social pressure associated with late capitalism and biomedicalization. They argue that sexuality is one field receiving the hardest push, especially by pharmaceutical companies urging potential consumers to purchase the latest sex drug that will enable them to remain 'forever functional' (i.e., sexually active for life).

EQUAL RIGHTS TO SEXUOPHARMACEUTICALS

Another woman (aged 53), who had tried Viagra (without any noticeable effect), argued that sexuopharmaceuticals should be readily accessible for women as a matter of gender equity. She contended that men's sexual needs had historically been prioritized and that it was a matter of equality – women were entitled to the same (potential) benefits as men:

> What I do have difficulty with is drugs aren't available for women. I feel annoyed about that … It seems like men's sexuality is catered for on many different levels, and I don't think ours is … For example, there hasn't been the interest in women's sexuality to the same degree … I would like women to have the freedom to take something – as long as it was comparatively safe. I think women should have that option.

In their London-based study of women's experiences of Viagra use within heterosexual relationships, Julie Askew and Maureen Davey (2004) noted similar responses from three of the four women they interviewed. These women were particularly interested in drugs that might enhance arousal. Similarly, several women in Meika Loe's (2004) U.S. study reported that some form of pink Viagra would be welcomed by them. However, Loe (2004: 105) argues that women's desire for Viagra-type drugs may be motivated by different factors than those driving men's desire for Viagra: 'While men may need the drug to help them continue their sexual pleasure, women may want the drug to discover theirs for the first time.'

Interestingly, one woman in the New Zealand study (aged 50) speculated that, while women should have the same access to sexuopharmaceuticals as men, men would not want them to. She based this assumption on the idea that men need to be the experts on women's sexuality and to feel they have produced pleasure (through orgasm) for their partners; a pill consumed by women would take this sense of sexual authority and know-how away from men.

Women's Concerns

NEW PRESSURES

Women participating in the New Zealand research communicated various concerns about the use of Viagra by men within sexual relationships. These included pressure to have sex following a partner's consumption of Viagra, an increased focus on intercourse to the detriment of other forms of sexual activities, and difficulties negotiating sex following use of the drug (Potts et al., 2003). For example, several interviewees reported it felt more difficult to decline sex once they knew their partners had used Viagra; once a pill was taken, it 'committed' them to sex; and some spoke about 'putting up with sex' when they really didn't feel like it (ibid.). The difficulty declining sex was in some cases associated with a concern to please one's partner – 'not to let him down.' In her U.S. investigation of senior women's attitudes to Viagra use by men, Loe (2004) also noted this kind of response, with participants conveying that they felt pressure to please their partners following use of the drug, as part of a 'wifely obligation.'

When asked about the implications of pink Viagra, some women in the New Zealand study speculated that this could place *even more* pressure on women. For instance, new demands might come from men wanting women to take drugs too, in order to match the new-found youthful virility associated with their own use of Viagra or other sexuopharmaceuticals. This concern is exemplified in the following excerpt, in which a 60-year-old woman expresses doubts about the less intimate experience of sexual relations that this might produce:

> [My husband] was also wanting *me* to take Viagra … because apparently it's supposed to work on women too, and I said what I would have liked … was a little bit of *romance back in the relationship*, but it wasn't like that at all. It was Viagra, right, you make an appointment for sex, and now I have to know *x* number of hours before and so there's no use me taking this pill and then you not being receptive and so on, and I'm thinking to myself … *oh*, I don't know if I want to bloody feel like that today, you know?

REJECTING A 'QUICK FIX'

Women also challenged the notion of drugs as a quick fix for sexual problems. For some, the use of sexuopharmaceuticals by partners had, in effect, *caused* new problems (tension and conflict) within relationships, rather than resolved issues (Potts et al., 2004). Several women commented that medication was an inadequate solution for sexual difficulties that were as much about relational problems as organic ones. One woman (aged 51) disputed the perceived artificiality of any drug, which she considered posed a problem for women's 'natural' sexuality:

> I think a woman should be left natural, it should be a natural instinct to a woman, and if she doesn't feel like having sex, or is having problems, there's usually an underlying reason why. And I don't think that can be overcome or fixed by just poking drugs into her. A lot of women, they're just tired, they're stressed out and so forth ... I'm not in agreement with women taking artificial things to boost them.

Interestingly, a few women reported that when Viagra or other medical interventions had not been able to rectify erectile difficulties, they had actually noticed an improvement in sexual relations with male partners. They tended to explain this phenomenon in terms of an expansion of sexual repertoires since certain habitual modes of relating sexually (such as penetrative sex) were no longer an option. One 50-year-old woman explained:

> It's actually probably made it better ... You try other things as well, because it's not that easy, so you do more of other foreplay and all sorts of things ... so it actually probably has improved things, rather than not ... I guess we are doing different and more things than we were doing before.

Thus, the very problems that the medical model of sexuality identifies and targets for rectification (i.e., non-erections in men, inability to complete coital sex) were actually experienced as non-problematic in the context of this relationship, and medical definitions of dysfunctionality did not necessarily apply.

RESISTING THE PHARMACEUTICAL INDUSTRY

The involvement of the pharmaceutical industry in the increasing hype around women's sexual difficulties did not escape scrutiny in the New Zealand study. One woman (aged 27) argued that drug companies were putting pressure on women and men to fixate on physical aspects of sexuality and worry about whether or not their sexual relations were adequate (in the context of medicalized assumptions about normality):

> I actually feel a bit sick when I see these drug companies coming out …
> and saying that women have to take this and this. It's like a flipping pill to
> fix this, and a pill to fix that … without actually addressing perhaps some
> of the deeper issues that a woman is facing like extra pressures of being a
> mother and subsuming her own sexual desires for the male, you know,
> living in a patriarchal society and all those kind of things which are prob-
> ably *more* likely to inhibit her sexual arousal than anything that's kind of
> physiological. Yet the drug companies jump on the bandwagon and say
> take this cream and it'll fix you … It's quite sickening really.

This criticism of the pharmaceutical industry's creation of the need
for sexuopharmaceuticals (a position that is upheld by the New View
group) has also been expressed by men and women in a focus group
study about representations of Viagra in direct-to-consumer advertising.[6] Participants in this study blamed drug companies for producing
assumptions about the benefit of drugs like Viagra through 'peddling
fear' – creating 'performance anxieties' – in 'normally functioning'
people (Vares, Potts, Gavey, & Grace, 2003: 101). This concern was also
raised by a 60-year-old woman who contended that the 'hard sell' surrounding Viagra had caused people to believe they were defective:

> Up until Viagra … nature took care of it and men's ability went down
> equally with women getting older, losing the same desire that they had
> when they were young women … I think Viagra has made a lot of people
> feel inadequate … Everybody's on the defence about how often they have
> sex and so on, in the older age group.

This participant viewed the changes in sexuality associated with aging, for
example, as part of a natural rather than pathological (or disease) process.

Dysfunctional Women or Dysfunctional Medicine?

Although the construction of women's sexuality as irregular or deviant
has a long history in Western culture, in the twenty-first century we are
witnessing the growing impact of biomedicalization on categorizations
of normal and pathological sexuality, forms of diagnosis, and modes of
treatment. In line with the biomedical perspective's propensity to view
sexual difficulties as either having organic foundations, or at least the
capacity to be treated by physical means, pharmacological preparations
are increasingly considered first-choice quick-fix interventions on the

road to recovery from sexual problems. Accordingly, sexual experiences are likely to be more and more understood within a framework emphasizing anatomical and biophysiological 'facts' about the sexual body and the importance of blood flow and hormones on 'genital wellness.' FSD has emerged as a new term that more or less reframes previous 'problems' such as frigidity (Askew, 2004), nymphomania, and hysteria as desire, arousal, and orgasmic disorders. However, FSD remains a contested illness, the debate between pro-biomedicalization and anti-medicalization factions persists, and the treatment of women's sexual difficulties with sexuopharmaceuticals continues to be controversial.[7]

Although they do not express an overt awareness of the contemporary FSD debate, women's perspectives on the advent of pink Viagra are influenced by the same kinds of arguments that prevail on each side of this dispute. This indicates that medicalized constructions of women's sexuality (and sexual difficulties) are being contested at institutional levels (e.g., in the language and debate of the experts) *and* at discursive and experiential levels (in women's everyday lives and talk). Some women endorse the development of a pink version of Viagra, citing reasons such as the need for gender equity in access to such drugs and the perceived benefits of these drugs in maintaining sexual fitness and function across the lifespan. Other women are less convinced about the advantages of sexuopharmaceuticals, expressing reservations about the increasing influence of the medical model and Big Pharma on sexuality, relationships, and other aspects of everyday life. Once *both* partners are medicated for sex, women may well be left with little room to determine (and insist on) their own preferred forms of sexual pleasure, including those that do not involve penetration.

The biomedical perspective, in its advocacy of a universal body and a universal sexual response, has tended to rely on generalizations about sexuality, producing a concept of sexual normality (heterosexual, coital, orgasmic, with masculine sexuality understood as more active and penetrative and feminine as receptive or passive) against which other forms of sexuality, sexual practice, sexual response, and sexual experience are measured and rendered abnormal, disordered, diseased, or dysfunctional. Within this reductionist model, the complexities of *both* women's *and* men's sexualities and relationships are by-passed or rendered problematic, and there is limited scope for alternative sexualities or experiences. Those not conforming to the conventional notion of normality are marginalized and pathologized.

With new sexual biotechnologies on hand, the sexual landscape may change in ways that limit the negotiation of differences in desire and sexual pleasure in a relationship: arguably, women's desires will be expected to accommodate men's. This is perhaps more so the case for older women whose relationships are based on traditional notions of heterosexuality and wifely obligations within marriage. In the wake of increasing biomedicalization and the race to develop and market pink Viagra, it therefore seems crucial to ensure that alternative sexual practices and pleasures (such as heterosex without erections, and non-penetrative sex) are not marginalized or trivialized, but instead visibly promoted as viable, sexy alternatives.

Acknowledgments

I am grateful to Pamela Moss and Kathy Teghtsoonian for the invitation to report on the FSD debate, as well as to the Institute of Gender and Health of the Canadian Institutes for Health Research and to the Social Sciences and Humanities Research Council of Canada (grant no. 646-2004-1531) for funding my participation at the *Illness and the Contours of Contestation* workshop, in Victoria, British Columbia. Thanks also to the participants – and to my colleagues – on the Health Research Council of New Zealand funded project 'Sex for life?' (grant no. HRC 00/287), and especially Geraldine Treacher for her pioneering work in this area in the New Zealand context.

NOTES

1   The term 'pink Viagra' entered popular vernacular through journalistic reports and popular media.
2   Another trend connected to the increasing biomedicalization of women's sexual problems is the promotion of FSD by urologists; this is a relatively new phenomenon, and one which Heather Hartley and Leonore Tiefer (2003) connect with a desire on the part of urologists to move the classification system for sexual problems from the arena of mental health into the field of physical medicine (a change that would also assist the promotion of drugs for sexual complaints).
3   From Tiefer (2001: 89).
4   Tiefer's work is complemented by the arguments of those involved in anti-psychiatry activism, including several prominent authors with medical backgrounds (Elliot, 2003; Healy, 2004; Metzl, 2003), and by journalists and others critical of the increasing influence of Big Pharma (Moynihan, 2003; Moynihan & Cassels, 2005).

5 'Sex for life? The socio-cultural implications of prosexual pharmaceuticals for men and women' (Principal Investigator: Annie Potts; Co-investigators: Victoria Grace, Nicola Gavey, and Tiina Vares). Twenty seven women volunteered to take part in the study; ages ranged from 33 to 68 years, with the average age being 53. Participants came from a variety of socioeconomic backgrounds; the majority were Pakeha (i.e., non-Maori New Zealanders, of European descent) and heterosexual. Interviews (conducted in 2001) lasted between 1 and 2 hours, and followed a semi-structured format, focusing on women's perspectives and experiences of Viagra use by male partners. Interviews generally began with women being asked to relay their own 'story' of Viagra use in their relationship, and then moved on to unpack specific issues and topics including: the impact of sexual changes or difficulties on relationships, self-esteem, and quality of life; the effects of Viagra use on the relationship (including sexual relations); their views on the implications of greater attention to sexual difficulties (and the various treatment options) for our understandings about sexuality and older people, and for our ideas about and experiences of female sexuality and male sexuality; and their opinions about the development of sexuopharmaceuticals for women. All interviews were audio-taped and transcribed in full. The research team conducted close readings of all transcripts to identify key themes and issues.

6 Direct-to-consumer advertising (DTC) permits the direct promotion of drugs (including lifestyle drugs like Viagra) to potential consumers (via television, radio, and magazine advertisements). DTC is legal in the United States and New Zealand.

7 An important victory of sorts was achieved by advocates of the New View group in December 2004 when the FDA declined to approve a hormonal preparation (Intrinsa) manufactured by Proctor and Gamble for the treatment of Female Sexual Arousal Disorder. Although those connected with the anti-medicalization group who were present at the FDA hearing drew attention to numerous potential problems for women associated with use of this drug, it was the medical risk factors that held the most weight: Intrinsa was rejected on the grounds that it may increase the likelihood of breast cancer, heart attack, or stroke (Spark, 2005).

REFERENCES

American Psychiatric Association (APA). (1994). *Diagnostic and statistical manual of mental disorders* (4th ed.). Washington: Author.

Askew, Julie. (2004). Reproductive success and the social construction of 'frigidity': Do women 'go off' sexual intercourse because they are 'ill'? *Sexualities, Evolution and Gender, 6*(1), 55–57.

Askew, Julie, & Davey, Maureen. (2004). Women living with men who use Viagra: An exploratory study. *Journal of Couple and Relationship Therapy, 3*(4), 23–42.

Bancroft, John. (2002). The medicalization of female sexual dysfunction: The need for caution. *Archives of Sexual Behavior, 31*(5), 451–456.

Basson, Rosemary. (2000). The female sexual response: A different model. *Journal of Sex and Marital Therapy, 26*, 51–65.

Basson, Rosemary. (2001). Are the complexities of women's sexual function reflected in the new consensus definitions of dysfunction? *Journal of Sex and Marital Therapy, 27*, 105–112.

Basson, Rosemary. (2004a). Recent advances in women's sexual function and dysfunction. *Menopause: The Journal of the North American Menopause Society. 11*(6), 714–725.

Basson, Rosemary. (2004b). Pharmacotherapy for sexual dysfunction in women. *Expert Opinion on Pharmacotherapy, 5*, 1045–1059.

Basson, Rosemary. (2005). Women's sexual dysfunction: Revised and expanded definitions. *Canadian Medical Association Journal, 10*, 1327–1333.

Basson, Rosemary, Leiblum, Sandra, Brotto, Lori, Derogatis, Leonard, Fourcroy, Jean, Fugl-Meyer, Kerstin, et al., (2003). Revised definitions of women's sexual dysfunction. *Journal of Sexual Medicine, 1*(1), 40–48.

Berman, Jennifer, & Berman, Laura. (2001). *For women only: A revolutionary guide to reclaiming your sex life*. London: Virago.

Braun, Virginia, & Wilkinson, Sue. (2001). Socio-cultural representations of the vagina. *Journal of Reproductive and Infant Psychology, 19*(1), 17–32.

Clarke, Adele E., Shim, Janet K., Mamo, Laura, Fosket, Jennifer Ruth, & Fishman, Jennifer R. (2003). Biomedicalization: Technoscientific transformations of health, illness, and US biomedicine. *American Sociological Review, 68*(2), 161–194.

Elliot, Carl. (2003). *Better than well: American medicine meets the American dream*. New York: W.W. Norton.

Fishman, Jennifer. (2002). Sex, drugs, and clinical research, *Molecular Interventions, 2*(1), 12–16.

Grace, Victoria, Potts, Annie, Gavey, Nicola, & Vares, Tiina. (2006). The discursive condition of Viagra. *Sexualities, 9*(3), 295–315.

Groneman, Carol. (2001). *Nymphomania: A history*. New York: W.W. Norton.

Harding, Jennifer. (1998). *Sex acts: Practices of femininity and masculinity*. London: Sage.

Hartley, Heather, & Tiefer, Leonore. (2003). Taking a biological turn: The push for a 'female Viagra' and the medicalization of women's sexual problems. *Women's Studies Quarterly, 31*(1/2), 42–46.

Healy, David. (2004). *Let them eat Prozac: The unhealthy relationship between the pharmaceutical industry and depression.* New York: New York University Press.

Laumann, Edward, Paik, Anthony, & Rosen, Raymond. (1999). Sexual dysfunction in the United States: Prevalence and predictors. *Journal of the American Medical Association, 281,* 537–544.

Leiblum, Sandra, & Nathan, Sharon. (2001). Persistent sexual arousal disorder: A newly discovered pattern of female sexuality. *Journal of Sex and Marital Therapy, 27,* 365–380.

Loe, Meika. (2004). *The rise of Viagra: How the little blue pill changed sex in America.* New York: New York University Press.

Maines, Rachel. (1999). *The technology of orgasm: 'Hysteria,' the vibrator, and women's sexual satisfaction.* Baltimore: Johns Hopkins University Press.

Marshall, Barbara. (2002). 'Hard science': Gendered constructions of sexual dysfunction in the 'Viagra age.' *Sexualities, 5*(2), 131–158.

Marshall, Barbara, & Katz, Stephen. (2002). Forever functional: Sexual fitness and the aging male body. *Body and Society, 8*(4), 43–70.

Masters, William H., & Johnston, Virginia E. (1966). *Human sexual response.* Boston: Little, Brown.

Masters, William H., & Johnston, Virginia E. (1970). *Human sexual inadequacy.* Boston: Little, Brown.

Metzl, Jonathan. (2003). *Prozac on the couch: Prescribing gender in the era of wonder drugs.* Durham, NC: Duke University Press.

Moynihan, Ray. (2003). The making of a disease: Female sexual dysfunction. *British Medical Journal, 326,* 45–47.

Moynihan, Ray, & Cassels, Alan. (2005). *Selling sickness: How drug companies are turning us all into patients.* Crows Nest, Australia: Allen and Unwin.

New View Working Group. (2001). A new view of women's sexual problems. In Ellyn Kaschak & Leonore Tiefer (Eds.), *A New View of Women's Sexual Problems* (pp. 1–8). New York: Haworth Press.

Nicholi, Armand. (Ed.). (1999). *The Harvard Guide to Psychiatry* (3rd ed.). Cambridge, MA: Belknap Press of Harvard University Press.

Nicolson, Paula. (1993). Public values and private beliefs: Why do women refer themselves for sex therapy? In Jane M. Ussher & Christine D. Baker (Eds.), *Psychological perspectives on sexual problems* (pp. 56–78). New York and London: Routledge.

Oudshoorn, Nellie. (1994). *Beyond the natural body: An archeology of sex hormones.* New York and London: Routledge.

Potts, Annie. (2002). *The science/fiction of sex: Feminist deconstruction and the vocabularies of heterosex.* New York and London: Routledge.

Potts, Annie. (2005). Cyborg masculinity in the Viagra era. *Sexualities, Evolution and Gender, 7*(1), 3–16.

Potts, Annie, Gavey, Nicola, Grace, Victoria, & Vares, Tiina. (2003). The downside of Viagra: Women's experiences and concerns about Viagra use by men. *Sociology of Health and Illness, 25*(7), 697–719.

Potts, Annie, Grace, Victoria, Gavey, Nicola, & Vares, Tiina. (2004). 'Viagra stories': Challenging 'erectile dysfunction.' *Social Science and Medicine, 59*, 489–499.

Potts, Annie, Grace, Victoria, Vares, Tiina, & Gavey, Nicola (2006). 'Sex for life?' Men's counter-stories on 'erectile dysfunction,' male sexuality and ageing. *Sociology of Health and Illness, 28*(3), 306–329.

Segal, Lynne. (1994). *Straight sex: The politics of pleasure.* London: Virago.

Spark, R.F. (2005). Intrinsa fails to impress FDA advisory panel. *International Journal of Impotence Research, 17*, 283–284.

Sugrue, Dennis, & Whipple, Beverly. (2001). The consensus-based classification of female sexual dysfunction: Barriers to universal acceptance. *Journal of Sex and Marital Therapy, 27*, 221–226.

Tiefer, Leonore. (1995). *Sex is not a natural act and other essays.* Boulder, CO: Westview Press.

Tiefer, Leonore. (2001). Arriving at a 'new view' of women's sexual problems: Background, theory, and activism. In Ellyn Kaschak & Leonore Tiefer (Eds.), *A new view of women's sexual problems* (pp. 63–98). New York: Haworth Press.

Tiefer, Leonore. (2003). The pink Viagra story. We have the drug, but what's the disease? *Radical Philosophy, 21*, 2–5.

Tiefer, Leonore. (2004). *Sex is not a natural act* (2nd Ed.). Boulder, CO: Westview Press.

Thompson, Lana. (1999). *The wandering womb: A cultural history of outrageous beliefs about women.* New York: Prometheus Books.

Treacher, Geraldine. (2003). *Sex drugs and women: Exploring the construction of technologies and sexualities in the development and use of sexuopharmaceuticals for women.* Unpublished Master's Thesis, University of Canterbury, Christchurch, New Zealand.

Tuana, Nancy. (1993). *The less noble sex: Scientific, religious, and philosophical conceptions of woman's nature.* Bloomington and Indianapolis: Indiana University Press.

Vares, Tiina, Potts, Annie, Gavey, Nicola, & Grace, Victoria. (2003). Hard sell, soft sell: Men read Viagra ads. *Media International Australia, 108,* 101–114.

Winton, Mark Alan. (2001). Paradigm change and female sexual dysfunctions: An analysis of sexology journals. *Canadian Journal of Human Sexuality, 10*(1–2), 19–24.

15 Moving from Settled to Contested: Transformations in the Anatomo-Politics of Breast Cancer, 1970–1990

MAREN KLAWITER

In the late 1980s and early 1990s, new forms of cancer organizing and activism mushroomed across the United States. Over the course of the next few years, a politically powerful, patient-led social movement emerged that challenged and changed many of the practices through which breast cancer had been discursively represented, scientifically investigated, medically managed, and publicly administered. Breast cancer thus joined a growing number of health conditions politicized by those who directly suffer from them. Unlike many contested illnesses, however, whose sufferers struggle for medical legitimacy and recognition, breast cancer was a 'routinely diagnosed condition' (Brown, 1995) long before it became the linchpin of a new social movement. How, then, we might ask, did this routinely diagnosed condition move from settled to contested?

Activists' accounts of the U.S. breast cancer movement have made it abundantly clear that the movement was tightly tethered to the construction of a new collective identity, a new sense of 'we-ness' and solidarity among women diagnosed with breast cancer (see, e.g., Altman, 1996; Batt, 1994; Brenner, 2000; Love & Lindsey, 1995; Stocker, 1991 and 1993). The salience of collective identity – especially in movements of socially stigmatized people – is not, of course, unexpected; and collective identity has, in fact, been an important area of research in social movements scholarship for more than 20 years (for reviews, see Bernstein, 2005; Polletta & Jasper, 2001). What we do not fully understand in the case of breast cancer, however, is why a deep and abiding sense of collective identity among women with breast cancer took root in the 1990s when it failed to do so earlier. Or, to put the question a bit differently: Why, in the 1990s, did the experience of being a breast cancer patient become a springboard to collective action when, until then, it had served as a segue to silence, isolation, and invisibility?

In addition to the activists' accounts cited above, scholarly studies of the breast cancer movement have taught us a great deal about individual pathways to politicization and the construction of collective identities (Anglin, 1997; Blackstone, 2004; Boehmer, 2000; Kaufert, 1998; Taylor & Van Willigen, 1996). They have likewise taught us a great deal about the process of mobilization and the movement's success in the domain of federal policy-making (Casamayou, 2001; Dickersin & Schnaper, 1996; Kolker, 2004; Myhre, 2001; Weisman, 2000). Finally, they have taught us a great deal about the diverse goals, targets, strategies, identities, and cultures of action that proliferated within the larger social movement (Klawiter, 1999a, 2000, and 2003; McCormick, Brown, & Zavestoski, 2003; Zavestoski, Brown, & McCormick, 2004; Zavestoski et al., 2004). With rare exception, however, accounts of the breast cancer movement have ignored the cancer clinic as a source of insight into these new identity formations.

My sense, after studying the breast cancer movement for more than 10 years, is that there are three main reasons why the threshold of the cancer clinic has not been crossed. The first reason is that one of the main rallying cries of the breast cancer movement was activists' contention that nothing had changed for decades in the clinical treatment of breast cancer. Typically, this claim was linked to the closely related contention that breast cancer had been ignored by male politicians and marginalized by the cancer research establishment because it was considered to be a women's disease.

The second reason that the cancer clinic has been ignored by social movement scholars is that sociologists and political scientists who study the structural influences and sources of social movements, by and large, work with theoretical models that focus attention on the terrain of the state and the organizations of civil society. These models, and this is no exaggeration, simply ignore the role of medicine (which, in the United States, cannot be equated with the state), science, and technology in the development of social movements.

The third reason that scholars have not looked inside the cancer clinic for insight into the breast cancer movement is that medical sociologists and anthropologists (the groups most likely to feel comfortable poking around inside the clinic) have tended to conceptualize medicine as an institution of social control that individualizes and depoliticizes the experience of illness. Why, following this logic, should we examine this individualizing, depoliticizing institution for insights into collective, political action? Given these three mutually reinforcing orientations, it is no surprise that activists and academics have ignored what, on the surface, might strike the uninitiated as one of the more obvious places to look for insight into the breast cancer movement.

In this chapter I shift the focus of attention to the cancer clinic. The purpose of this shift is threefold. First, I want to show that the clinical management of breast cancer *did* change in a number of important ways during the 1970s and 1980s. Second, I want to show how these changes reconfigured breast cancer patients (subjects), their bodies, and the social relations of disease. Third, I want to persuade other scholars, activists, and interested parties that we cannot afford to ignore the space of the cancer clinic if we want to understand the emergence of new forms of identity and solidarity among women with breast cancer.

In this chapter I introduce the concept of *disease regime* and use it to 'reread' the history of breast cancer in the United States as a history of two regimes. My analysis focuses on the medical diagnosis, treatment, and 'rehabilitation' of women with breast cancer, emphasizing changes that occurred in these practices during the 1970s and 1980s. I argue that, although these changes did not improve breast cancer mortality rates during this period, they *did* transform the human subjects and social relations of the disease regime. They did so in ways that enlarged the role of breast cancer patients, complicated and lengthened their experiences of treatment, and created new forms of 'biosociality' (Rabinow, 1992) that diminished their isolation and invisibility. Ultimately, these changes transformed women diagnosed with breast cancer into permanent subjects of the disease regime.

The Concept of Disease Regime[1]

The concept of *disease regime* draws heavily on Michel Foucault's theorization of biopower and his approach to studying how it operates. According to Foucault, the technologies of biopower that arose in the West at the end of the eighteenth century fed the development, rationalization, and proliferation of modern institutions, which shaped the bodies and psyches of modern subjects. The 'bio' part of this term indexes the growing involvement of modern institutions in the management of the lives, and even the biological processes, of individual subjects and subject populations. Biopower, in this sense, is 'life power,' or power over life. Unlike the centralized sovereign power that it gradually colonized from below, however, biopower is exercised through technologies of discipline, surveillance, and knowledge production. Unlike the heavy-handed domination and repression that characterized the exercise of sovereign power, Foucault argued, biopower is constructive, dynamic, optimizing, and enabling.

In an essay on methods, Foucault argued (1987: 102) that the 'target' of analysis should not be 'institutions,' 'theories,' or 'ideology,' but rather 'regimes of practices.' He used this term to refer to the apparatus of practices organized around a shared problematic that 'possess[es] up to a point [its] own specific regularities, logic, strategy, self-evidence, and "reason"' (ibid.: 102–3). In analysing historically specific regimes of practices, Foucault also argued that the analysis of power should begin 'with the question of the body and the effects of power on it' (1980c: 59). The human body, as Foucault's genealogies of public health, medicine, madness, sexuality, deviance, and discipline so provocatively revealed, is not a transhistorical object but a culturally and politically invested product of specific regimes of practices (Foucault, 1965, 1973, 1978, 1979, and 1980a).

The body, however, is more than the *object* of specific regimes of practices, it is also the material means by which human beings become historical *subjects*. 'The individual,' Foucault argued (1980b: 73–74), 'with his [or her] identity and characteristics, is the product of a relation of power exercised over bodies [and] multiplicities.' Different regimes of practices, as Foucault's genealogies demonstrate, produce different human bodies and different human subjects.

Analytically, Foucault mapped biopower and its regimes of practices along two axes. The first, the *anatomo-politics of the human body*, is exercised through biopractices that target individual bodies, optimize their capabilities, and enhance their functioning (Foucault, 1990). The second, the *biopolitics of populations*, consists of biopractices that operate at the level of populations – the species body – making possible their social control and regulation while enhancing their biological and social functioning and productivity (ibid.). The genealogy of anatomo-politics can be traced to scientific medicine, what Foucault termed the 'clinical' or 'medical gaze' (1973). Public health, or what we might call the 'epidemiological gaze,' is linked more directly to the biopolitics of populations. Thus, health, for Foucault, is a particularly dense point of transfer within the modern circuitry of power. Although these two dimensions are analytically distinct, in practice they often intertwine.

Diseases, like other dimensions of human experience, are managed, produced, represented, and administered through specific regimes of practices. Different regimes of practices, in turn, constitute different bodies, subjects, and social relations of disease. In my conceptualization, a disease regime consists of the interlinked practices through which a disease is medically managed in individual bodies and publicly administered across populations. In addition to the screening, diagnostic, treatment, and rehabilitative technologies of public health and biomedicine, the medical management and public administration of disease includes the practices of scientific investigation and discursive representation that are part and parcel of these health institutions.

Neither the subjects of a disease regime, however, nor the regime's practices, are fixed or automatic. Scientific discourses of disease can change over time, screening practices can rise and fall, diagnostic categories can expand and contract, new technologies can be invented, old technologies can be abandoned, the use of existing technologies can change, and patient scripts can be tightened, relaxed, and rewritten. Significant changes in the practices of a disease regime can, and often do, alter the subjects and social relations of disease, as well as its temporal, visual, and spatial dimensions. Finally, changes in the practices of a disease regime can both enable and inhibit the formation of disease-based identities, social networks, solidarities, and sensibilities. These forms of 'biosociality' (Rabinow, 1992), in turn, are key ingredients in the mobilization and success of social movements.

In studying disease regimes, we can map them along the two axes of biopower that Foucault specified. The first, the anatomo-politics of individual bodies, includes the discourses and practices of clinical medicine: diagnosis, treatment, and the clinical sciences (e.g., clinical trials). I refer to this dimension as the medical management of disease. The second, the biopolitics of populations, includes the discourses and practices of public health education, screening, population surveillance, and the sciences of public health (e.g., epidemiology). I refer to this dimension as the public administration of disease. Some practices operate along both axes. Screening, for example, is a biopolitical technology of populations, but because the technology targets individuals, it is also an anatomo-technology of bodies.

Disease regimes do not, of course, wholly determine their subjects' experiences of disease. They do, however, deeply shape those experiences, they set limits, and they make various outcomes and possibilities – such as the development of social relationships, solidarities, and identities – more and less likely. This sounds abstract, but it is actually quite concrete and specific, as I show in the remainder of this chapter. In the analysis that follows, I trace changes over time in the anatomo-politics of breast cancer, highlighting the period from 1970 to 1990, when the regime of medicalization that arose during the first few decades of the twentieth century gradually gave way to a new regime of practices, the regime of biomedicalization.[2]

The Regime of Medicalization

Diseases of the breast have been claimed by various medical traditions for thousands of years. It was not until the first few decades of the twentieth century, however, that scientific medicine achieved a virtual monopoly in the United States over the treatment of women with breast cancer. Prior to that time 'regular' (allopathic) and 'irregular' physicians (homeopaths, hydrotherapists, herbalists, Eclectics, Thomsonians, etc.), midwives, folk healers, and sellers of patent medicines competed for patients in a teeming medical marketplace that was largely unregulated (Patterson, 1987; Starr, 1982). In fact, prior to the twentieth century, 'regular' physicians who practised 'heroic' medicine were avoided by a significant portion of the population, including people with cancer, in favour of therapeutic approaches that were equally ineffective but much less painful (Patterson, 1987).

During the first few decades of the twentieth century, however, breast cancer was successfully claimed by a new breed of physicians who, in the provocative words of historian Barron Lerner (2000: 25), 'invented' breast cancer as 'a curable disease.' The transition from an era of therapeutic pluralism to the regime of medicalization was tied to a broader transition in the practice of medicine that included the rising status and professionalization of 'regular' physicians, the growing power of the American Medical Association (AMA), the standardization of medical education, the establishment of state-based medical licensing systems, the movement of medical treatment from the home to the hospital, and the transformation of hospitals from poor houses to citadels of scientific medicine (Starr, 1982).

In the domain of breast cancer, however, the regime of medicalization did not flow simply or straightforwardly from these transformations in American medicine. The regime of medicalization was the outcome of two simultaneous campaigns. The first campaign was designed to convince ordinary physicians that cancer diagnosed early could be cured by a competent surgeon. The second campaign was designed to teach ordinary women to recognize the 'danger signals' of cancer and respond, without delay, by consulting a physician. These 'cancer is curable' and 'do not delay' campaigns were the brainchild of the American Society for the Control of Cancer (ASCC), a surgeon-dominated, 'lay' organization that was later renamed the American Cancer Society (Aronowitz, 2001; Breslow & Wilner, 1979; Gardner, 1999; Patterson, 1987; Reagan, 1997; Ross, 1987).

During the regime of medicalization the Halsted radical mastectomy was installed as the one-size-fits-all surgical treatment for women diagnosed with breast cancer. The Halsted was a deforming, often debilitating procedure that entailed the surgical removal of the chest muscles and surrounding lymph nodes, along with all of the breast tissue. Whenever possible, the radical mastectomy was performed during the same operation as the diagnostic biopsy. The advantage of this one-step procedure, from the perspective of surgeons, was that it saved both the patient and the surgeon from undergoing (and performing) an additional operation (Austoker, 1985; Fisher, 1999; Lerner, 2000 and 2001; Montini & Ruzek, 1989).

The one-step procedure required that patients sign in advance a consent form authorizing their surgeons to perform an immediate mastectomy if they decided, after conducting a biopsy of the tumour, that a mastectomy was necessary. Practically speaking, this meant that patients who entered the hospital expecting nothing more than a surgical biopsy often discovered, upon awakening, that their breast had been amputated and their chest muscles and lymph nodes had been surgically removed. In these circumstances, however, they were also often informed that the surgery had been a success and they were 'cured.' A surgical cure meant, in essence, that no local evidence of breast cancer remained. As Barron Lerner and other medical historians have shown, however, the meaning of 'cure' varied tremendously and by no means implied that other parts of the body were cancer-free or that the cancer would not reappear, metastasize, and kill the 'cured' patient (Austoker, 1985; Fisher, 1999; Lerner, 2000 and 2001; Montini & Ruzek, 1989).

Accompanying the rise of the regime of medicalization, a new social script, later dubbed the 'sick role' by Talcott Parsons (1951), was institutionalized. The sick role was a set of institutionalized mechanisms that, in the words of Parsons (ibid.: 477), 'channel[ed] deviance so that the two most dangerous potentialities, namely, *group formation* and *successful establishment of the claim to legitimacy* are avoided' (emphasis added). The sick role was a *temporary* role that required patients to comply with the doctor's orders, endeavour to exit the sick role as quickly as possible, and return to 'normal' and assume their normal roles and duties. The sick role, by definition, entailed the segregation of 'the sick' from 'the non-sick' and required the isolation of patients from each other. 'The sick are tied up,' Parsons wrote, 'not with other deviants to form a "subculture" of the sick, but each with a group of non-sick … above all, physicians' (ibid.). Thus, one of the most important functions of the sick role, according to Parsons, was that it 'deprived' patients 'of the possibility of forming a solidary collectivity' (ibid.).

In the context of breast cancer, the sick role co-constituted the imperial authority of surgeons, along with the isolation and obedience of breast cancer patients. Because the sick role was a temporary role, it required new 'mastectomees' – women who had undergone a breast amputation – to hide the evidence of their surgery and return, following a short convalescence, to their normal lives and duties. The architecture of the closet that greeted mastectomees when they exited the hospital thus complemented and reinforced the practices of normalization that accompanied the sick role script.

In addition, the norms of non-disclosure adhered to by surgeons and physicians further mitigated against the development of illness identities among 'mastectomees.' These norms of non-disclosure, which held sway well into the 1960s, strongly encouraged surgeons and family physicians to deliberately mislead their patients regarding the truth – even the existence – of their cancer diagnoses (Leopold, 1999; Lund, 1946; Oken, 1961; Patterson, 1987). Although these norms of non-disclosure were paternalistic, there is no evidence that the sex of the cancer patient affected the disclosure practices of physicians. Male cancer patients, in other words, were just as misled as women.

Whether their patients were women or men, 'physicians,' in the melodramatic words of James Patterson, 'conspired with frightened relatives to hide the "awful truth" of cancer' (1987: 69). In practice, 'hiding the awful truth' involved a number of different strategies, including the use of euphemistic language, dexterous dissembling, and when all else failed, old-fashioned, bald-faced lying (Leopold, 1999; Lund, 1946; Oken, 1961; Patterson, 1987). Even Rachel Carson, a professional scientist, was lied to by her surgeon in 1960 after he performed a radical mastectomy. When Carson asked her surgeon, point blank, if the tumour in her amputated breast was malignant, he told her only that she had a 'condition bordering on malignancy' (Leopold, 1999: 111). Carson died from the 'condition bordering on malignancy' in 1964, shortly after publishing *Silent Spring* (1962). By then, Carson had learned of her condition from a maverick surgeon who believed that patients had a right to know their diagnoses. Carson carefully guarded this information, however, fearing that her work on the environment would be discredited if other scientists believed that the author had an axe to grind.

Whether or not these practices of non-disclosure, which were clearly part of the physician's role, were detrimental or beneficial to patients is entirely beside the point. What matters, for the purposes of this discussion, is that breast cancer patients were not told that they were breast cancer patients. Developing an identity as a breast cancer patient was therefore, quite literally, unthinkable. At most, a woman could develop an identity as a mastectomee. Even this, however, as we shall shortly see, was deliberately and explicitly discouraged.

In sum, during the regime of medicalization, women with breast cancer were misled about their cancer diagnoses, isolated from each other, temporarily segregated from the rest of society, and channelled back into their 'normal' roles, identities, and responsibilities following their recuperation from surgery. The medicalization of breast cancer during the first seven or so decades of the twentieth century thus created a subject population of temporarily sick patients and invisible, post-surgical mastectomees. Practices of non-disclosure, the temporary nature of the sick role, the isolation of cancer patients from each other, and the architecture of the closet made the construction of a public, collectively shared breast cancer identity virtually impossible.

The Regime of Biomedicalization

During the 1970s and 1980s new practices arose within the cancer clinic that, cumulatively, transformed the regime of medicalization into a new regime of practices with its own 'specific regularities, logic, strategy, self-evidence, and "reason"' (Foucault, 1987: 102). In the emergent regime, the regime of biomedicalization, norms of non-disclosure were replaced by legal standards of informed consent, the space of patient decision-making expanded, and the sick role was gradually replaced by a more active and informed patient role and script. At the same time, the Halsted radical mastectomy was eliminated, diagnostic and treatment options proliferated, the complexity and longevity of treatment increased dramatically, and adjuvant therapies expanded further into patients' lives and bodies. Finally, new forms of patient support and rehabilitation were institutionalized. These new forms of patient support and rehabilitation diminished the isolation of breast cancer patients, created new forms of 'biosociality' (Rabinow, 1992), and challenged the absolute authority of physicians.

Within this new regime of practices there was greater transparency and communication among the involuntary subjects of the regime, yet at the same time, there was a heightened sense of uncertainty, a greater awareness of the limitations of medicine, and a growing recognition of permanent risk. Taken together, these changes transformed the experience of breast cancer and created new openings and opportunities. These shifts in the anatomo-politics of breast cancer are traced in greater detail in the sections that follow.

Informed Consent and Surgery

During the 1960s and 1970s, the norms of non-disclosure among surgeons and other physicians underwent a dramatic shift. Results of a study published in 1960, for example, indicated that 90 per cent of the physicians surveyed believed it was often best *not* to tell cancer patients the truth about their diagnoses, and a clear majority claimed that they *never* or *seldom* told their patients the truth (Good, Good, Shaffer, & Lind, 1990; Oken, 1961). By 1977 a full 98 per cent of the physicians surveyed reported that disclosure was their usual policy and that they believed cancer patients had the right to know their diagnoses (Novack et al., 1979).

Although by the late 1970s it was common practice for physicians to disclose their diagnoses to cancer patients, breast cancer patients were still being informed of their diagnoses *post-operatively*, after they had already received a radical mastectomy. Thus, beyond the logic of disclosure, lay the question of informed consent and the issue of patient participation in decision-making. Unlike professional norms of (non)-disclosure, however, informed consent emerged as a legal concept that was encoded in case law and legislation (Berg, Applebaum, Parker, & Lidz, 2001; Daugherty, 1999). In the case of breast cancer, battles over informed consent first emerged around the issue of surgery and surgical alternatives to the Halsted radical mastectomy. In the case of breast cancer, however, the practical utility of informed consent was dependent upon the fulfilment of two tightly linked preconditions: the abandonment of the one-step procedure and the willingness of American surgeons to offer an alternative to the radical mastectomy. In other words, informed consent was meaningless in the absence of alternatives.

In 1979, prompted by several years of public controversies over the one-step procedure and the continuing hegemony of the Halsted radical mastectomy, the National Institutes of Health (NIH) convened a consensus development conference entitled 'The Treatment of Primary Breast Cancer: Management of Local Disease.' A consensus statement issued by the NIH panel of experts explicitly encouraged physicians to abandon the one-step procedure so that breast cancer patients could consider their options before proceeding with treatment (NIH, 1979: n.p.). Although the consensus statement did not have the force of law behind it, it constituted a symbolically loaded nod towards the growing rights of breast cancer patients.

That same year Massachusetts became the first state to pass breast cancer informed consent legislation, and a year later California became the second. By the end of the decade, breast cancer informed consent legislation had been proposed in 22 states and adopted in 14 (Montini, 1991, 1996, and 1997; Montini & Ruzek, 1989). Breast cancer informed consent campaigns were typically launched by a handful of current and former patients (Montini, 1996). In most cases, these patient–activists were not organizationally linked to the women's health or patients' rights movements, nor did they create enduring organizations that advocated for the interests of breast cancer patients (Montini, 1996). The implementation of informed consent and the two-step procedure did not happen overnight, and it varied tremendously from patient to patient, surgeon to surgeon, state to state, and even region to region. During the 1980s, however, breast cancer patients finally gained the right to 'gaze back' at their physicians and participate in their treatment as conscious, speaking, agentic subjects (see Purkis & van Mossel, Chapter 8, this volume).

The 1979 NIH consensus conference that encouraged physicians to abandon the one-step procedure also sounded the death-knell for the Halsted radical mastectomy. The panel of assembled experts concluded that 'total mastectomy with axillary lymph node dissection with or without radiotherapy' provided 'an equivalent benefit' and 'should be recognized as the current treatment standard' (NIH, 1979: n.p.). The demands of women's health activists, the preferences of breast cancer patients, the results of European clinical trials of less radical surgeries, and the NIH consensus statement increased the pressure on U.S. surgeons to offer less radical surgeries (Kushner, 1986; Lerner, 2000 and 2001; Montini & Ruzek, 1989). By 1983 the number of Halsteds performed by U.S. surgeons had declined from a high of 54,000 to a new low of 5,000 (Montini & Ruzek, 1989).

The retraction of the Halsted radical mastectomy occurred hand in hand with the expansion of breast-conserving surgeries. These surgeries included total mastectomies that left the chest muscles intact, partial mastectomies that left some breast tissue, and lumpectomies that removed the tumour and a 'safe margin' of surrounding breast tissue but left the nipple and breast largely intact. The performance of less radical mastectomies opened the door to breast reconstruction, which rapidly expanded during the 1980s, along with the development of new breast implant technologies (Kushner, 1986; Trabulsy, Anthony, & Mathes, 1994).

Adjuvant Therapy

The transformation of the Halsted radical mastectomy into a relic of an earlier regime was only one of several important changes that took place in breast cancer therapeutics. During the 1980s adjuvant therapy became part of the standard treatment regimen for a growing number of breast cancer patients. Radiation therapy, a local treatment, was incorporated into the post-surgical treatment regimens of a growing number of women. Unlike the one-step procedure, radiation therapy was intensive and often required breast cancer patients to return to the hospital on a daily basis for a period of several weeks. Radiation therapy introduced new side effects into the treatment experience of a growing number of women. Short-term side effects included nausea, skin burns, and extreme fatigue. Long-term side effects included an elevated risk of other cancers since radiation is, after all, a carcinogen. The growing use of radiation therapy thus meant that women undergoing treatment for breast cancer could no longer quickly return to normal after surgery.

At the same time, cytotoxic chemotherapy, a systemic treatment, was also incorporated into the standard treatment regimens of a growing number of breast cancer patients. In 1976, for example, the vast majority of breast cancer patients were treated by surgery alone and only 7 per cent of breast cancer patients received chemotherapy (Kushner, 1986). In 1985, however, the NIH held a second consensus development conference on chemotherapy for women with breast cancer (the first was held in 1980) to review the results of recent clinical trials. The panel of experts issued a consensus statement recommending multi-agent cytotoxic chemotherapy as the standard treatment for women with lymph node positive, estrogen receptor negative breast cancer (NIH, 1985), a recommendation that extended the use of chemotherapy into new patient populations. The most dramatic expansion of chemotherapy took place in 1988 when the National Cancer Institute issued a Clinical Alert to all physicians urging them to administer chemotherapy to *all* breast cancer patients, regardless of their tumour biology or cancer stage (see especially Hillner & Smith, 1991; Johnson et al., 1994; Mariotto et al., 2002).

Cytotoxic chemotherapy, in the words of Rose Kushner (1984), 'literally made healthy people sick' – and not just a little bit. Common side effects of chemotherapy, often experienced as the *main* effects of chemotherapy, included crushing fatigue, severe nausea, hair loss all over the body, dry skin, disintegrating nails, loss of vaginal lubrication, painful intercourse, diminished fertility, premature menopause, thrush, and other opportunistic infections affecting those with weakened immune systems. In addition, chemotherapy regimens – which were conducted sequentially, not simultaneously, with radiation therapy – lasted for many months, sometimes for more than a year.

The expansion of adjuvant therapies, often performed on an outpatient basis, meant that women with breast cancer were no longer confined to the private space of the hospital; rather, they entered and exited the physical and temporal space of treatment repeatedly over the course of a year (or more). Because its side effects were so visible, because it was administered over an extended period, and because it was typically administered to patients who were not confined to the hospital, cytotoxic chemotherapy further challenged the architecture of the closet, the segregation of the sick from the healthy, and the temporary nature of the sick role. As a result, the spatial and temporal boundaries of the regime of biomedicalization expanded and, simultaneously, became more fluid, fuzzy, and transparent.

A third type of adjuvant therapy, tamoxifen (brand name Nolvadex), a hormone therapy, was approved by the U.S. Food and Drug Administration for the treatment of women with metastatic breast cancer in 1978. Over the course of the next 10 years, tamoxifen was gradually incorporated into the treatment regimens of women with metastatic breast cancer, as well as women diagnosed with earlier stage disease.[3] Unlike cytotoxic chemotherapies, which were administered intravenously, tamoxifen was self-administered in pill form by breast cancer patients in the privacy of their home. Tamoxifen therapy typically begins after surgery and other adjuvant therapies have been completed and lasts for 5 or more years (5 years is currently the recommended length of treatment). Tamoxifen reminds women on a daily basis of their membership in the 'remission society' – the society of people who, in the words of Arthur Frank (1995: 8), 'were effectively well but could never be considered cured.' Like all drugs, tamoxifen introduced new risks (including uterine cancer, blood clots, and stroke) and side effects. Compared with cytotoxic chemotherapy, however, it was relatively well-tolerated.

Thus, during the 1980s local and systemic adjuvant therapy in the form of radiation, cytotoxic chemotherapy, and hormone therapy embraced a wider band of breast cancer patients. Adjuvant chemotherapy prolonged the treatment experience over time and expanded treatment into parts of women's bodies left untouched by the previous regime.[4] Unlike women diagnosed with breast cancer in the previous regime, who were subjected to a physically and emotionally brutal surgery but were then cast out of the sick role, women in the second regime re-enacted their patient status over and over and over again. Unlike women in the first regime, they did so with the knowledge that they were cancer patients. Finally, during the regime of biomedicalization the discourse of curative surgery gradually gave way to the less absolutist, less reassuring discourse of risk reduction. Surgery and adjuvant therapies were increasingly conceptualized not as curative technologies, but as technologies for reducing the risk of recurrence.

Rehabilitation

During the 1970s and 1980s new opportunities for social interactions increasingly challenged the isolation of breast cancer patients. This shift was fed by two key developments. First, a program known as 'Reach to Recovery' was adopted and institutionalized by the American Cancer Society (ACS). Second, cancer support groups began to proliferate.

A former breast cancer patient, Terese Lasser, founded Reach to Recovery in 1952 and ran it as a private citizen until 1969, when it was finally adopted as a national program by the ACS (Lasser & Clarke, 1972). Lasser designed Reach to Recovery as a peer-based, one-on-one, self-help, hospital-based visitation program for new mastectomees that was modelled after Alcoholics Anonymous. Reach to

Recovery trained former breast cancer patients (mastectomees) to visit post-operative breast cancer patients in the hospital, provide practical advice, and model for them a successful exit from the sick role. Reach to Recovery volunteers provided new mastectomees with temporary breast prostheses (for use in the hospital), information about obtaining a permanent prosthesis, and practical instruction in rehabilitative exercises (physical therapy) to aid in their physical recovery. Reach to Recovery quickly became one of the largest and most successful programs of the American Cancer Society (Breslow & Wilner, 1979; Kushner, 1975; Lasser & Clarke, 1972; Ross, 1987).

To discourage mastectomees from thinking of breast cancer as an ongoing problem or a disability, however, Reach to Recovery volunteers were discouraged from maintaining contact with the women they visited.[5] The experience of breast cancer – and this was clearly consistent with the sick role script – was viewed as a temporary setback, not a permanent disability. Ongoing relationships with former breast cancer patients, the ACS believed, would make it more difficult for new mastectomees to exit the sick role, resume their former roles and responsibilities, and put the experience behind them. A statement from a Reach to Recovery representative, quoted by Kushner, illustrates this philosophy: 'We didn't want Reach to Recovery to become a crutch … After all, the whole point of Reach to Recovery is to convince women they do not have a disabling handicap. We talked about having a mastectomy club … But that would have defeated our whole purpose. Having a mastectomy is *not* a permanent handicap, and even the worst of scars can be hidden by a well-fitting prosthesis and the right clothing. So we decided we would help the patient for just a few weeks, and then leave her to her own psychological recovery' (1975: 211).

Ironically, although the principles and programmatic design of Reach to Recovery were consistent with the sick role script, in practice, Reach to Recovery challenged one of its central features: the isolation of patients from each other. At the same time, however, the programmatic structure of Reach to Recovery limited the social contacts between new and experienced mastectomees to one-on-one peer support delivered over a very brief period of time – typically, just one meeting. The option of becoming a Reach to Recovery volunteer opened the door for a small number of women to maintain an ongoing relationship to the mastectomy underground, but the degree to which the disease could become a collectively shared experience, and thus the foundation of a collective identity, was limited by the anti-identity philosophy of Reach to Recovery.

Reach to Recovery laid the groundwork for the development of a disease-based identity, but it was the development of support groups – groups of women with breast cancer meeting together – that directly facilitated the construction of this collective identity. In the San Francisco Bay Area, the focus of my fieldwork, support groups were first developed outside of, and at the margins of, medicine. During the 1990s, however, support groups were gradually institutionalized within the Bay Area health care system. Initially resisted by physicians, support groups were eventually reconceptualized as just another, albeit optional, form of adjuvant therapy.

Regardless of the model they adopted, support groups expanded and deepened the space available for the formation of new social networks, solidarities, and collective identities. Regardless of their therapeutic philosophy, they challenged the structural barriers that separated women with breast cancer from one another. Support groups facilitated the development of new relationships, friendships, and support systems, all of which provided patients with access to a much wider body of knowledge and experience. Before the widespread use of the Internet, support groups provided access to medical information that was still closely guarded by scientists and physicians.

Support groups reconfigured the social relations of disease in ways that undermined the norms of patient segregation, isolation, individualization, silence, and invisibility. Support groups also, however, deepened patients' awareness of the limitations of medicine, the uncertainty of treatment outcomes, and the permanent risk of recurrence. Support groups facilitated the construction of collective identities out of patients' shared experiences as subjects of the regime of biomedicalization.

Unsettling Anatomo-Politics

Taken individually, many of these changes in the anatomo-politics of the cancer clinic were minor and incremental. Cumulatively, however, they created a new regime of practices with its own 'specific regularities, logic, strategy, self-evidence, and "reason"' (Foucault, 1987: 102). Women diagnosed with breast cancer during the 1970s and 1980s faced a qualitatively and quantitatively different disease regime than had the generations that preceded them.

Although these changes in the cancer clinic did not improve breast cancer mortality rates during this period, they *did* transform the bodies and subjectivities of breast cancer patients and the social relations of disease. They did so in ways that enlarged the role of patients, complicated and lengthened their experiences of treatment, diminished their social isolation and invisibility, softened the spatial boundaries that segregated them from the rest of society, and expanded the temporal boundaries of the regime. It was these 'unsettling' changes in the cancer clinic, I contend, that helped create a new breed of subjects who succeeded during the 1990s in moving breast cancer from settled to contested.

NOTES

1 The concept of disease regimes that I develop in this chapter emerged from 4 years of ethnographic research on women's cancer support groups that I conducted in the San Francisco Bay Area as part of a larger ethnographic study of breast cancer activism (Klawiter, 1999b). Between 1994 and 1998 I observed four cancer support groups in different institutional settings for periods ranging from 2 months to more than 2 years: a private hospital (2 months), a public hospital (more than 2 years), an independent feminist cancer centre (more than 2 years), and an independent cancer support community (more than 2 months). The discussions that took place in the cancer support groups revolved around the physical and emotional demands of treatment, and the spiritual and psychological challenges of living with permanent risk and uncertainty. In addition to my observation of support groups, I conducted 24 interviews with support group participants, probing more deeply into their experiences of screening, diagnosis, surgery, radiation, chemotherapy, support groups, and permanent risk. The specific regime of practices that they experienced, as I discovered through historical research, was a relatively recent phenomenon. Despite the absence of new treatment modalities, these women were incorporated into a very different regime of practices than earlier generations of women had been and, as a result, experienced breast cancer very differently. These differences, it seemed to me, were consequential for the formation of a collective identity capable of launching a breast cancer movement. Thus, although they do not directly appear in the historical narrative of this chapter, it was the stories shared by support group participants that led me to rethink the relationships between bodies, identities, and the medical management of disease. These ideas and the historical and observational research on which they are based are elaborated in greater detail in Klawiter (forthcoming).

2 An examination of the biopolitics of populations, the second dimension of the regime of breast cancer, lies beyond the scope of this chapter (but see Klawiter, forthcoming). The term *biomedicalization* is borrowed from Clarke, Shim, Mamo, Fosket, and Fishman (2003).

3 In 1998 tamoxifen became the first (and is still the only) drug approved by the FDA for the reduction of cancer risk among healthy, 'high risk' women. Shortly thereafter, tamoxifen was approved by the FDA for the treatment of women with ductal carcinoma in situ of the breast, a 'non-' or 'pre-' invasive form of breast cancer. For an analysis of tamoxifen's role in the construction of the breast cancer continuum, see Klawiter (2002).

4 Chemotherapy and radiation therapy were used as well to treat cancer patients in the first disease regime, but they were most often used to treat patients with advanced cancer, often for the purposes of palliation. What changed in the second regime was that these therapies became a standard part of the treatment regimen for women with earlier stage, non-metastatic breast cancer.

5 Kushner's experiences with Reach to Recovery are revealing. When she began doing research on the experiences of women who had been treated for breast cancer, Kushner contacted the ACS and its Reach to Recovery program to ask for assistance in identifying women who were not immediately 'post-op.' They were unable to assist her, however, because Reach to Recovery did not maintain contact with women who had been served by their program (Kushner, 1975). For additional patient perspectives on Reach to Recovery, see Lorde (1980), Batt (1994), and Klawiter (2004).

REFERENCES

Altman, Roberta. (1996). *Waking up, fighting back: The politics of breast cancer.* Boston: Little, Brown.

Anglin, Mary K. (1997). Working from the inside out: Implications of breast cancer activism for biomedical policies and practices. *Social Science and Medicine, 44*(9), 1403–1415.

Aronowitz, Robert. (2001). Do not delay: Breast cancer and time, 1900–1970. *Milbank Quarterly, 79*(3), 355–386.

Austoker, Joan. (1985). The 'treatment of choice': Breast cancer surgery 1860–1985. *Society for the History of Medicine Bulletin, 38*, 100–107.

Batt, Sharon. (1994). *Patient no more: The politics of breast cancer.* Charlottetown, PEI: gynergy books.

Berg, Jessica W., Applebaum, Paul S., Parker, Lisa S., & Lidz, Charles W. (2001). *Informed consent: Legal theory and clinical practice* (2nd ed.). New York: Oxford University Press.

Bernstein, Mary. (2005). Identity politics. *Annual Review of Sociology, 31*, 47–74.

Blackstone, Amy. (2004). 'It's just about being fair': Activism and the politics of volunteering in the breast cancer movement. *Gender and Society, 18*(3), 350–368.

Boehmer, Ulrike. (2000). *The personal is political: Women's activism in response to the breast cancer and AIDS epidemics*. Albany: State University of New York Press.

Brenner, Barbara. (2000). Sister support: Women create a breast cancer movement. In Anne S. Kasper & Susan J. Ferguson (Eds.), *Breast cancer: Society shapes an epidemic* (pp. 325–354). New York: St Martin's Press.

Breslow, Lester, & Wilner, Danile. (1979). *A history of cancer control in the United States with emphasis on the period 1946–1971*. Prepared for the History of Cancer Control Project, Division of Cancer Control and Rehabilitation, National Cancer Institute. Department of Health, Education, and Welfare, Publication No. 79–1516. Washington: Government Printing Office.

Brown, Phil. (1995). Naming and framing: The social construction of diagnosis and illness. *Journal of Health and Social Behavior, Extra Issue*, 34–52.

Carson, Rachel. (1962). *Silent spring*. New York: Houghton Mifflin.

Casamayou, Maureen H. (2001). *The politics of breast cancer*. Washington: Georgetown University Press.

Clarke, Adele, Shim, Janet K., Mamo, Laura, Fosket, Jennifer Ruth, & Fishman, Jennifer. (2003). Biomedicalization: Technoscientific transformations of health, illness, and U.S. biomedicine. *American Sociological Review, 68*(2), 161–194.

Daugherty, Christopher K. (1999). Impact of therapeutic research on informed consent and the ethics of clinical trials: A medical oncology perspective. *Journal of Clinical Oncology, 17*(5), 1601–1617.

Dickersin, Kay, & Schnaper, Lauren. (1996). Reinventing medical research. In Kary L. Moss (Ed.), *Man-made medicine: Women's health, public policy, and reform* (pp. 57–76). Durham, NC: Duke University Press.

Fisher, Bernard. (1999). From Halsted to prevention and beyond: Advances in the management of breast cancer during the twentieth century. *European Journal of Cancer, 35*(14), 1963–1973.

Foucault, Michel. (1965). *Madness and civilization*. London: Tavistock.

Foucault, Michel. (1973). *The birth of the clinic: An archaeology of medical perception*. New York: Vintage Books.

Foucault, Michel. (1979). *Discipline and punish: The birth of the prison*. New York: Vintage Books.

Foucault, Michel. (1980a). The politics of health in the eighteenth century. In Colin Gordon (Ed.), *Power/knowledge: Selected interviews and other writings 1972–1977* (pp. 166–182). New York: Pantheon Books.

Foucault, Michel. (1980b). Questions on geography. In Colin Gordon (Ed.), *Power/knowledge: Selected interviews and other writings 1972–1977* (pp. 63-77). New York: Pantheon Books.

Foucault, Michel. (1980c). Body/power. In Colin Gordon (Ed.), *Power/knowledge: selected interviews and other writings 1972–1977* (pp. 55–62). New York: Pantheon Books.

Foucault, Michel. (1987). Questions of method: An interview with Michel Foucault. In Kenneth Baynes, James Bohman, & Thomas A. McCarty (Eds.), *After philosophy: End or transformation?* (pp. 100–117). Boston: MIT Press.

Foucault, Michel. (1990). *The history of sexuality, volume 1: An introduction.* (Robert Hurley, Trans.). New York: Pantheon. (Original work published in 1978.)

Frank, Arthur W. (1995). *The wounded storyteller: Body, illness, and ethics.* Chicago and London: University of Chicago Press.

Gardner, Kirsten E. (1999). *'By women, for women, with women': A history of female cancer awareness efforts in the United States, 1913–1970s.* Cincinnati: University of Cincinnati.

Good, Mary-Jo Del Vecchio, Good, Byron J., Shaffer, Cynthia, & Lind, Stuart. (1990). American oncology and the discourse on hope. *Culture, Medicine and Psychiatry, 14,* 59–79.

Hillner, B.E., & Smith, T.J. (1991). Efficacy and cost effectiveness of adjuvant chemotherapy in women with node-negative breast cancer: A decision-analysis model. *New England Journal of Medicine, 324*(3), 160–168.

Johnson, T.P., Ford, L., Warnecke, R.B., Nayfield, S.G., Kaluzny, A., Cutter, G., Gillings, D., Sondik, E., & Ozer, H. (1994). Effect of a National Cancer Institute clinical alert on breast cancer practice patterns. *Journal of Clinical Oncology, 12,* 1783–1788.

Kaufert, Patricia A. (1998). Women, resistance, and the breast cancer movement. In Margaret M. Lock & Patricia A. Kaufert (Eds.), *Pragmatic women and body politics* (pp. 287–309). New York: Cambridge University Press.

Klawiter, Maren. (1999a). Racing for the cure, walking women, and toxic touring: Mapping cultures of action within the Bay Area terrain of breast cancer. *Social Problems, 46*(1), 104–126.

Klawiter, Maren. (1999b). *Reshaping the contours of breast cancer: From private stigma to public actions.* Unpublished doctoral dissertation, University of California, Berkeley.

Klawiter, Maren. (2000). From private stigma to global assembly: Transforming the terrain of breast cancer. In Michael Burawoy, Joe Blum, Sheba George,

Zsuzsa Gille, Theresa Gowan, Lynne Haney, Maren Klawiter, Steve Lopez, Seán Ó Riain, & Millie Thayer (Eds.), *Global ethnography: Forces, connections, and imaginations in a postmodern world* (pp. 299–334). Berkeley: University of California Press.

Klawiter, Maren. (2002). Risk, prevention and the breast cancer continuum: The NCI, the FDA, health activism and the pharmaceutical industry. *History and Technology, 18*(4), 309–353.

Klawiter, Maren. (2003). Chemicals, cancer, and prevention: The synergy of synthetic social movements. In Monica J. Casper (Ed.), *Synthetic planet: Chemical politics and the hazards of modern life* (pp. 155–176). New York and London: Routledge.

Klawiter, Maren. (2004). Breast cancer in two regimes: The impact of social movements on illness experience. *Sociology of Health and Illness, 26*(6), 845–874.

Klawiter, Maren. (forthcoming). *The biopolitics of breast cancer: Changing cultures of disease and activism*. Minneapolis: University of Minnesota Press.

Kolker, Emily S. (2004). Framing as a cultural resource in health social movements: Funding activism and the breast cancer movement in the U.S. 1990–1993. *Sociology of Health and Illness, 26*(6), 820–844.

Kushner, Rose. (1975). *Breast cancer: A personal history and an investigative report.* New York: Harcourt Brace Jovanovich.

Kushner, Rose. (1984). Is aggressive adjuvant chemotherapy the Halsted radical of the '80s? *CA – A Journal for Clinicians, 34*, 345–351.

Kushner, Rose. (1986). *Alternatives: New developments in the war on breast cancer.* New York: Warner Books.

Lasser, Terese, & Clarke, William Kendall. (1972). *Reach to recovery.* New York: Simon and Schuster.

Leopold, Ellen (1999). *A darker ribbon: Breast cancer, women, and their doctors in the twentieth century.* Boston: Beacon Press.

Lerner, Barron H. (2000). Inventing a curable disease: Historical perspectives on breast cancer. In Anne S. Kasper & Susan J. Ferguson (Eds.), *Breast cancer: Society shapes an epidemic* (pp. 25–49). New York: St Martin's Press.

Lerner, Barron H. (2001). *The breast cancer wars: Hope, fear, and the pursuit of a cure in twentieth-century America.* Oxford: Oxford University Press.

Lorde, Audre. (1980). *The cancer journals.* San Francisco: aunt lute books.

Love, Susan M., & Lindsey, Karen. (1995). *Dr. Susan Love's breast book* (2nd ed.). New York: Addison-Wesley.

Lund, Charles C. (1946). The doctor, the patient, and the truth. *Annals of Internal Medicine, 24*(6), 955–959.

Mariotto, Angela, Feuer, Eric J., Harlan, Linda C., Wun, Lap-Ming, Johnson, Karen A., & Abrams, Jeffrey. (2002). Trends in use of adjuvant multi-agent chemotherapy and tamoxifen for breast cancer in the United States: 1975–1999. *Journal of the National Cancer Institute, 94*(21), 1626–1634.

McCormick, Sabrina, Brown, Phil, & Zavestoski, Stephen. (2003). The personal is scientific, the scientific is political: The environmental breast cancer movement. *Sociological Forum, 18*(4), 545–576.

Montini, Theresa. (1991). *Women's activism for breast cancer informed consent laws.* Unpublished doctoral dissertation, University of California, San Francisco.

Montini, Theresa. (1996). Gender and emotion in the advocacy of breast cancer informed consent legislation. *Gender and Society, 10*(1), 9–23.

Montini, Theresa. (1997). Resist and redirect: Physicians respond to breast cancer informed consent legislation. *Women and Health, 26*(1), 85–105.

Montini, Theresa, & Ruzek, Sheryl. (1989). Overturning orthodoxy: The emergence of breast cancer treatment policy. *Research in the Sociology of Health Care, 8*, 3-32.

Myhre, Jennifer. (2001). *Medical mavens: Gender, science, and the consensus politics of breast cancer.* Unpublished doctoral dissertation. University of California, Davis.

National Institutes of Health (NIH). (1979). The treatment of primary breast cancer and management of local disease. NIH Consensus Statement Online, 2(5), 29–30. Retrieved 5 May 2004, from http://consensus.nih.gov.

National Institutes of Health (NIH). (1985). Adjuvant chemotherapy for breast cancer. NIH Consensus Statement Online, 5(2), 1–19. Retrieved 14 October 2004, from http://consensus.nih.gov.

Novack, Denis H., Plumer, Robin, Smith, Raymond, L., Ochitill, Herbert, Morrow, Gary R., & Bennett, John M. (1979). Changes in physicians' attitudes toward telling the cancer patient. *Journal of the American Medical Association, 241*(9), 897–900.

Oken, Donald. (1961). What to tell cancer patients: A study of medical attitudes. *Journal of the American Medical Association, 175*, 1120–1128.

Parsons, Talcott. (1951). Social structure and dynamic process: The case of modern medical practice. In *The Social System* (pp. 428–479). New York: Free Press.

Patterson, James T. (1987). *The dread disease: Cancer and modern American culture.* Cambridge: Harvard University Press.

Polletta, Francesca, & Jasper, James M. (2001). Collective identity and social movements. *Annual Review of Sociology, 27*, 283-305.

Rabinow, Paul. (1992). Artificiality and enlightenment: From sociobiology to biosociality. In Jonathan Crary & Sanford Kwinter (Eds.), *Incorporations* (pp. 234–252). New York: Urzone.

Reagan, Leslie J. (1997). Engendering the dread disease: Women, men, and cancer. *American Journal of Public Health, 87*(11), 1779–1787.

Ross, Walter S. (1987). *Crusade: The official history of the American Cancer Society.* New York: Arbor House.

Starr, Paul. (1982). *The social transformation of American medicine.* New York: Basic Books.

Stocker, Midge. (Ed). (1991). *Cancer as a women's issue: Scratching the surface.* Chicago: Third Side Press.

Stocker, Midge. (Ed). (1993). *Confronting cancer, constructing change: New perspectives on women and cancer.* Chicago: Third Side Press.

Taylor, Verta, & Van Willigen, Marieke. (1996). Women's self-help and the reconstruction of gender: The postpartum support and breast cancer movements. *Mobilization: An International Journal, 1*(2), 123–143.

Trabulsy, Philip P., Anthony, James P., & Mathes, Stephen J. (1994). Changing trends in postmastectomy breast reconstruction: A 13 year experience. *Plastic and Reconstructive Surgery, 93*(7), 1418–1427.

Weisman, Carol S. (2000). Breast cancer policymaking. In Anne S. Kasper & Susan J. Ferguson (Eds.), *Breast cancer: Society shapes an epidemic* (pp. 213–243). New York: St Martin's Press.

Zavestoski, Stephen, Brown, Phil, & McCormick, Sabrina. (2004). Gendered bodies and disease: Environmental breast cancer activists' challenges to science, the biomedical model, and policy. *Science as Culture, 13*(4), 563-586.

Zavestoski, Stephen, Morello-Frosch, Rachel, Brown, Phil, Mayer, Brian, McCormick, Sabrina, & Gasior Altman, Rebecca. (2004). Embodied health movements and challenges to the dominant epidemiological paradigm. *Research in Social Movements, Conflict and Change, 25*, 255–280.

16 Environments, Bodies, and the Cultural Imaginary: Imagining Ecological Impairment

STEVE KROLL-SMITH AND JOSHUA KELLEY

This chapter is written as a gloss, an all-too-brief tour of several complex and nuanced topics held together by a thin thread that we are calling the *cultural imaginary*. Imagining, to paraphrase Wittgenstein, is an act of human creation (1967: 7 and 23). It is a mindful form of life rooted in language and, more deeply, in a cultural fabric of the actual and the possible. The cultural imaginary expresses itself in characterizations, figures, perceptions, and reflections; in mental images of ourselves, others, and the social and biophysical worlds that we inhabit. Our interest is in how, over time, popular and biomedical cultures imagine the intersections of environments and bodies.[1]

Consider a contemporary example. A magazine advertisement for a popular antihistamine states boldly, 'Your body and ragweed don't always get along' (*Ladies' Home Journal*, May 1999: 14). Biologist Sandra Steingraber would appear to agree with the *Journal*. In her book, *Living Downstream: An Ecologist Looks at Cancer and the Environment*, Steingraber writes, 'In one important sense, our bodies are internal environments that are ecologically linked to broader environments' (1997: 12). This advertisement in a popular magazine and this complementary conclusion by a respected scientist are not likely to arouse much opposition among contemporary readers. Both share a certain intuitive appeal. Few would find problems with either statement; together they represent part of the way that we imagine and talk about ourselves and the places we inhabit. The constellation of bodies, ragweed, and sinus misery constitutes one among dozens of modern figures that convey a nexus between humans and environments. Yoked together by their unavoidable contiguity – as Steingraber imagines – it makes sense to see the two as if in a dance, moving and changing in a roughly complementary fashion.

Tinker with a place – change its ambient air, its flora, its fauna, or the quality of its water, for example – and the body responds by making physiological, organic, and perhaps, at times, psychical changes. The retina contracts smartly when exposed to bright light; a sinus detects cat dander and as a defence releases millions of histamines; far more troubling, reduce the ozone in the atmosphere and ultraviolet radiation creates metastasizing skin cells. And the dance goes on.

There is nothing divine and timeless, however, about this imaginative characterization of bodies and environments. Like all texts, these are fragments of a broader social, cultural, and political cloth. Imagining the interplay of bodies, ragweed, and sinus misery becomes possible in a historical era marked by a volume of scientific research on immune systems, direct-to-consumer advertising of sinus medications, and an increasingly reflexive public poised to read any untoward change in the behaviour of the body as a reason for concern. Sinus misery is, in other words, historical, subject to alteration, and rooted in mass advertising, medical practices, and the cultural politics of the modern body.

This chapter explores the nexus between body and environment as a historical relationship, a mental and emotional image that shifts and changes with time. The first part of the chapter is a brief account of the various ways in which we have imagined our somatic connections with environments. Juxtaposing the historical present with its predecessors in the historical past, we can discern at least three figurative relationships: *bodies in environments*, *bodies and industrial environments*, and *industrial environments in bodies*. This last imaginative figure, *industrial environments in bodies*, is proving to be a vexing problem for both medical practice and an increasing number of ordinary people whose bodies appear to be rebelling against the invasive nature of contemporary places. In the second part of the chapter, we offer a modest suggestion for altering the conventional imagery of the person impaired by modern environments but unable to secure a legitimate medical diagnosis. The increasingly complex intersections between human bodies and modern molecular environments, we argue, begs an imaginative leap, one that joins the idea of impairment to *both* bodies *and* places.

Bodies in Environments

Writing in the 1880s on the salubrious effects of American resorts on the bodies of the middle and upper classes, Bushrod James (1889: 9–10) expounds on Montesquieu's eighteenth-century idea of climate: '"The empire of climate is the most powerful of all empires," capable, as it is, of making and molding its subjects physically and mentally, of bestowing life and death upon them.' The good physician, James opines, should 'be able to locate his patients both geographically and therapeutically' (ibid.: 17).

Imagining bodies in environments was tied in complex ways to migratory, pre-industrial America. The migration of people on the eastern seaboard to the west created a heightened sense of the relationship between bodies, health, and environments (Deacon, 2005; Valencius, 2002). A medical treatise written in 1929 emphasized 'in whatever latitude man locates himself, he assumes certain characteristic modifications' (Valencius, 2002: 22). These changes forged a 'relationship' with 'that particular atmosphere, and the various objects which surround him' (ibid.).

During much of the nineteenth century, as this passage illustrates, environment was often imagined as climate. For one writer, climate was the 'sum total of the extrinsic physical influences amid which we breathe.' For another it was 'the sum of the influences exerted upon atmosphere by temperature, pressure, soil proximity to the sea, lakes, rivers, plains, forests, light' and so on (James, 1889: 10). Bodies were enveloped in environments; the two were inextricably joined. Changing environments was thought to alter or change the body. In the nineteenth century there were, it was said, three reasons for travel: infirmity of the body, imbecility of the mind, or inevitable necessity (Deacon, 2005: 279).

With the invention of the thermometer, barometer, and devices for measuring wind velocity and rainfall, physicians developed skills in what came to be called 'medical meteorology' (Hannaway, 1993: 297): 'The editor of the leading California medical journal urged that "Every physician should train himself as an observer of meteorological phenomena. The thermometer, the hygrometer, the currents of wind and cloud, should be as familiar to him as the stethoscope, the microscope, and the speculum"' (Nash, 2003: par. 14).

Throughout the nineteenth century, physicians, farmers, businessmen, and others subscribed to a persuasive image of bodies existing *in* environments. Within this image were the close and unavoidable associations of types of environments and human health. Indeed, in this period, medicine, environment, and disease were closely allied in public consciousness through the images of 'landscape' and 'topography.'

Common sense directed people's attention to the types of physical and biological places that they inhabited or were likely to visit. Both popular and medical reasoning portrayed environments as surrounding and encompassing bodies. By the middle of the nineteenth century, the idea of medical tourism and the 'medical tourist' called attention to the efforts of the propertied classes to seek health in salubrious climates (Valencius, 2004).

The imaginative authority of bodies in environments was, eventually, eclipsed by another variation on the inventive continuum of body–environment relationships. Although it would lose its distinguished place in popular and professional imagination, *bodies in environments* would continue as a motif with a considerable claim on truth. In 1981, for example, 92 years after James heralded 'the empire of climate' on human well-being, Alan Nursall and David Phillips began to scientifically study the effects of weather on migraine in Canada. In their study, Nursall and Phillips (1980) concluded that Phase 4 weather had an adverse impact on migraine, and high pressure, sunny and dry weather had ameliorating effects on migraine.[2]

Bodies and Industrial Environments

From 1900 to the early 1960s, the ideas, notions, and images of bodies and their relationships with environments get mixed and recombined into a quite different cultural imaginary. In this second, industrialized period, medicine achieves an unprecedented degree of professionalization and the seminal idea of the germ and the germ theory of disease eclipses, but does not replace, the once prominent role of landscapes and topographies in explaining sick and healthy bodies. Moreover, industrial capitalism, as predicted, triumphs over industrial communalism, and manufacturing is now exclusively profit-driven. Social health is increasingly linked to the health of the economy, which in turn is a barometer of the health of industry. To an unprecedented degree, environments, once natural, fast became industrial (Mitman, Murphy, & Sellers, 2004; Nash, 2003).

The common-sense idea of bodies *in* environments is not simply erased by a new cultural imaginary; it is still visible if one chooses to see it, but it no longer dictates popular and professional thinking on the matter. Instead a quite different configuration exists, one that seems particularly suited for the times: bodies are now paramount in understanding and treating disease. Importantly, for our purposes, bodies are severed from the increasing expansion of industrial environments and imagined to coexist alongside them. A simple shift in prepositions signals this complex transformation from bodies *in* environments to bodies *and* industrial environments.

The cultural figure 'bodies *and* industrial environments' favoured the unfettered development of an industrial landscape replete with the flotsam and jetsam of wood, coal, chemical, and synthetic particulate wastes. Perhaps separating bodies from environments and re-imagining them as discrete spheres was necessary in order to pursue aggressively a heavy machine-based and high-waste mode of production. If disease is now principally a germ problem – a microbe seeking to enter the body – then environmental disease etiologies are likely to fade in importance, obscured by a medical, political, and public emphasis on personal hygiene and public health.

Evidence for a shift in imagination away from environmental disease etiologies and towards microbes and their capacity to invade bodies is found in London, England as early as 1855. By the mid-nineteenth century, the British industrial revolution was well under way, and it provides a window into what would eventually occur in the United States. The datum is a remarkable exchange between Dr John Snow, often called the father of epidemiology, and Sir Benjamin Hall, chairman of a British parliamentary committee charged with drafting a disease prevention plan for London (see University of California, Los Angeles, 2001). Snow was asked to testify on behalf of an industrialist who opposed any legislation that would impose controls on his factory practices.

Snow begins by telling the Committee that he is not aligned in any fashion with this or any other London industrialist. His opinions, he asserts, are derived from science, not politics. The questioning begins.

SIR BENJAMIN: To what points would you desire to draw the attention of the Committee as regards the sanitary question?

DR SNOW: I have paid a great deal of attention to epidemic diseases, more particularly to cholera … and I have arrived at the following conclusion to what are called offensive trades, that many of them really do not assist in the propagation of … diseases, and that in fact they are not injurious to the public health. I consider that if they were injurious to the public health they would be extremely so to the workmen engaged in those trades, and as far as I have been able to learn that is not the case.

Snow was no friend of industry, but he did see a disconnect between industrial practices and health that would, with time, become a normal way of imagining bodies and environments.

The agency of the microbe in explaining disease would shift attention from increasingly chemical-based industrial environments to matters of public and personal sanitation, with a particular emphasis on the individual and his or her own hygienic practices. Cesspools, house sinks, sewage lines, and related public works were often criticized as health hazards, as were undisciplined and ignorant people who failed to take appropriate care of themselves and those in their charge. Health and the avoidance of disease were imagined as bodies disciplined by properly educated selves who sought to regulate the 'smallest fragments' of day-to-day life (Foucault, 1991: 170).

Imagining health as self-regulation rather than the outcome of bodies and their many intersections with industrial environments was truly a win–win for a capital, manufacture-based economy. Not only did a focus on the person and his or her body direct the medical gaze away from increasingly risky industrial environments, it also encouraged a policing of the working class. The habits of this class were surveyed, suggestions were offered, directives were issued, and workplace incentives and punishments were enacted. Mercantile and commercial doctrines became intertwined with medicine in a manner that imagined the industrialist as a benefactor and his factory a wholesome place (Burchell, 1996; Osborne, 1997).

This second cultural imaginary, however, was not destined to remain unchallenged. The hubris of industry yoked to remarkable advances in science would usher in a new era, one marked by the collision of human bodies and industrial environments. This collision would challenge the imaginary of the link between bodies and environments, and force a rethinking about the soma and its biophysical milieu. Recalling the first historical period, bodies were once again joined to environments. But this emerging imagery transposed the body and the environment, locating the biological and physical properties of landscapes, air, water, and soil inside the skin, deep in the interiors of human bodies. If the first figurative and normative image is typified as bodies in environments, the third image is best captured in the phrase: environments *in* bodies. In this third period, environments are thought of and represented as encroaching upon, invading, and indeed, poisoning bodies. But not just any environments are invading bodies; the principal offenders are human-made, synthetic, or what we might call anthropoid environments.

Industrial Environments in Bodies

In 2004, close to 120 years after James wrote *American Resorts with Notes Upon Their Climate*, the U.S. Environmental Protection Agency (EPA) initiated a controversial research project under the unfortunate acronym CHEERS, or the Children's Environmental Exposure Research Study.[3] The description of the project currently posted on its Website is:

1) Participants are not required to use pesticides or to change any of their regular household routines or how they normally use bug sprays (pesticides).
2) Allow two of our researchers to visit you at your home every 3 to 6 months for two years. If pesticides are used, notify researchers to arrange a time at your convenience to conduct study activities before and after the use of pesticides. The visit will take approximately 2 hours per day or per visit.
3) Videotape (the video camcorder will be provided) some of your child's activities and keep an activity diary about your child.
4) Allow your child to wear a small watch size activity sensor during the study period. (Approximately 1 week every 3 – 6 months)
5) Help to collect some samples of food and urine. Our research staff will show you how to do this and provide you with needed supplies.
6) Keep track of your home pesticide and cleaning products use. (U.S. Environmental Protection Agency, 2004)

Please note the two quite different images of environments, bodies, and health fashioned in the words of Bushrod James and the U.S. EPA. James joined climates and weather patterns to bodies and health. And indeed, bodies and climate is one salient way we, today, imagine ourselves in relationship to environments. A room can be 'stuffy'; the outdoor air can be 'heavy' or 'thick'; a certain outdoor 'temperature-humidity number' might trigger asthma symptoms; a particular 'humidex discomfort index' might spark a migraine. James's account, written well over a century ago, resonates with us today. If the humidity is too high, we turn on an air conditioner in search of a better fit between our bodies and the immediate environment.

The CHEERS project, however, conjures another quite different image, one in which places become possible sites for the poisoning of the body. Evoked in the formal cadence of a research project is the idea that invisible chemical matter can enter the body and possibly alter its somatic, psychic, and behavioural habits and routines. Beneath the surface of this study design is evidence of an altered sensibility, new and concrete configurations of environments and bodies, and their unknown consequences for human health.

What is the EPA's primary justification for designing this controversial project? In its own words, 'current information on young children's exposures to chemicals used in consumer products is very limited. [We need] a better understanding of how children are exposed to pesticides and other chemicals found in homes and the factors that affect their exposure.' (U.S. Environmental Protection Agency, 2004). This is a startling admission in light of Rachel Carson's damaging critique of a particularly noxious pesticide – DDT – in 1962. Carson's clarion call to acknowledge the effects of toxins on environments and bodies helped to launch a new era of environmental and public health initiatives. But almost five decades later we are still debating the effects of manufactured environments on human health, with no appreciable end in sight.

Carson's portrait of the vexing migration of DDT, its deleterious effects on a number of species, and its risks to humans created a space to re-imagine a nexus between soma and its biophysical surround. Carson challenged the cultural authority of the microbe and the separation of bodies and environments. Over time, bacteria became secondary to industrial hazards and contaminated municipal waste (Colten, 2005: 109).

Synthetic molecules now vie with nature's microbes as sources of infirmity and disease. But unlike germs, there is no molecular theory of disease. Molecules and bodies await their own Pasteur. In the meantime, there is no agreed-upon protocol for following the molecule in its uncertain and cryptic trek through the body (Casper, 2003: xx). There is no discernible and commonly agreed-upon pathophysiology for most modern toxic exposures, and treatments remain more homeopathic than clinical (Kroll-Smith & Floyd, 1997: 17–23). There are sound reasons medical students are required to take courses in microbiology but can elect to skip courses in environmental toxins. The fact is – as the ill-fated CHEERS study acknowledges – too little is known about the latter to warrant required courses for time-strapped medical students.

When manufactured environments move into bodies they act like quicksilver slipping beyond the reach of most diagnostic medicine. Less certain and harder to see, taking refuge in the body's labyrinthine interior, environments in bodies are occasions for considerable speculation and conflict. Synthetic environments that seep into skin, are inhaled into lungs, or find their way into mouths raise a host of disquieting questions that can be restated as the enigma of misplaced molecules and flesh. Faced with this conundrum, the voice of clinical medicine is audible but often – from the patient's vantage point – confusing, more vexing than clarifying.

If the abstract knowledge of biomedicine becomes concrete and practical at the moment its body of knowledge encounters a body, those bodies allegedly invaded by atoms grouped into chemical clusters effectively foreclose this encounter. What is left, hopefully, is the forbearance of the physician who seeks to legitimate her or his patient's complaints and the stoic resignation of the patient who accepts the good faith – if ultimately unsatisfactory – efforts of her or his doctor. In an odd take on the old idea of cultural lag, the nature of modern bodies is changing more quickly than diagnostic medicine can accommodate. The yawning gap between contemporary bodies, molecules, and clinical medicine is more than a bioscience problem, however. It is also a profoundly personal, social, and political problem.

People who report persistent symptoms that physicians cannot explain often have a personal story or account about the cause of the symptoms (Kroll-Smith & Floyd, 1997; Kroll-Smith & Ladd, 1995). These accounts often narrate a tie or connection between symptoms and local environments. Although many physicians will listen patiently to these accounts, few will treat them seriously. And, over time, as patients persist in connecting their symptoms to environments, many physicians will conclude that the true problems are rooted in either their patients' erroneous beliefs or, perhaps, a psychological disorder. Physician Ronald Gots, for example, describes multiple chemical sensitivity as a label, not a diagnosis, given to people who do not feel well for a variety of reasons and who share the common belief that chemical sensitivities are to blame (Gots, 1993).

This rupture between patients' and doctors' beliefs regarding the nexus between environments and diseases is a comparatively recent development. Throughout most of the nineteenth century, the idea that rotting and decaying matter of all kinds produces both 'noxious vapors' and disease was 'equally intelligible to nearly illiterate subsistence farmers and to trained physicians' (Valencius, 2002: 123). Popular knowledge and medical knowledge recognized the inescapable idea that bodies existed in environments and that not a few of these physical and organic places were potential threats to health. Patient and doctor, for example, both knew that bad air was a source of sickness. The germ theory of disease accompanied by the increasing professionalization of physicians would eventually sunder that relationship, creating a chasm between the experiences and beliefs of patients and the certified wisdom of physicians.

In their thoughtful account of people who suffer from 'medically unexplained physical symptoms,' Zavestoski et al. (2003) identify several strategies that both patients and physicians employ to negotiate the semantic mysteries of somatic anomalies whose etiologies are, apparently, caused by exposures to domestic, industrial, and military toxins. None of these strategies, however, are ideal.

What makes molecular theories of disease open to contradictory interpretations and polarizing opinions is, in part, the absence of coherent etiological explanations of exposures and symptoms and, in part, the peculiar phenomenology of perceiving bodies and low-level chemical exposures. From the vantage point of society, one cannot simply claim to have a disease. Although intensely personal, disease must be confirmed by others authorized to make such pronouncements. It cannot, of course, just be raining from my point of view; the rain, we all know, falls on both the just and the unjust. Contamination by toxins, on the other hand, is more often than not a *from-my-point-of-view* problem. It begins with my recognition that something untoward is happening to my body and at least a faint recognition that it might have something to do with invisible, seemingly undetectable molecules. The problem for the attending physician is whether to confirm the patient's perception of disease caused by a clinical condition defined almost exclusively in subjective terms.

Bodies, Environments, and Cultural Imaginations: A Concluding and a Beginning

This short survey of the varying ways that American culture has imagined bodies and their peculiar relationships with environments begs a few conclusions. It seems, for example, that there is nothing concrete and unalterable about the ways in which a culture will envisage bodies and environments. The fluid character of this imagination and *how* specifically it is formed is a topic of inquiry in its own right. But not far behind the *how* is the *why* question.

The peculiar way in which a culture imagines bodies and environments, it appears, is linked to the varied ways in which we reproduce ourselves through industrial and agricultural practices. The idea of bodies closely connected to climate and topography makes a certain sense in an agricultural economy. Conversely, it is in the interests of an increasingly capital-intensive industrial economy to discourage an examination of the morbidity of the factory floor while promoting the horrors of the germ. Although the germ theory of disease was an unalloyed medical breakthrough, it was a way of looking that did not see the real and potential health problems of industrial practices.

But imagining bodies as separate from manufactured environments would be short-lived. As anthropoid molecules find their way into bodies taking up residence in the bloodstream, tissue, nerve centres and the bones themselves, we are encouraged to picture industrial environments as entering bodies. Imagining industrial environments inside our bodies is, for most people, unsettling, if not terrifying. If we combine the image of invasive environments with the difficulties that physicians experience in identifying the etiologies of environmental diseases and the even greater problem of treating these medical anomalies, we are invited to do some re-imagining of our own.

Diseased or Disabled?

Imagine what might happen were we to borrow from the grammar of disability and picture the environment – as well as bodies – as impaired. What we have in mind is tinkering with the language and practice of disability in a manner that allows us to imagine a more robust and ecological version of the conventional idea of impairment.

Disease is arguably a simpler idea than disability. It is a medical classification, part of the language of physicians who diagnose and treat sick bodies. Differences, of course, are common regarding whether or not a particular cluster of symptoms meets the criteria for disease, but the language of disease is directed specifically at the sick body. Disability, on the other hand, is more complicated. Its language encompasses the body and a far wider array of referents, including – but not limited to – civil rights, social justice, compensation, and social change (Francis & Silvers, 2000; Turner, 1984).

A vocabulary of classification and treatment, disease begins and ends with 'what is.' The body is overweight, is hypertensive, is fevered, is incontinent, and so on. It is a vocabulary rooted in observation and measurement. Disability, as a contemporary rights-based movement, is a vocabulary of acknowledgment and modification (Barnes, Mercer, & Shakespeare, 1999; Linton, 1998). It is a vocabulary rooted in 'what should be.' Entry ways should be modified to allow wheelchair access; public spaces should be smoke- and scent-free zones; public bathrooms should be accessible to the handicapped; monthly wages should be paid to people who are injured or become sick at the job; and so on. The grammar of disability-rights talk is among the important contemporary voices of social parity and justice.

The distinction we are drawing between disease and disability is akin to the distinction that Emile Durkheim (1974: 80) makes between 'judgments of reality' and 'value judgments' and two types of models that Clifford Geertz (1973: 93) develops in his work on religion: 'models of' and 'models for.' Judgments of reality are assertions of facts about the world. 'On average, women live longer than men' is an assertion of fact. Most people will agree that disease is a judgment of reality. It makes sense as fact. Value judgments, on the other hand, are expressions of moral purpose, principled intentions that author a version of the world based on the ideas of good and right. Disability leans strongly towards the idea of principled intention, encouraging action to make the world more livable for others. It assumes, note Francis and Silvers (2000: xiii), that no one should suffer 'an attenuation of the right to be in the world.' In *The Interpretation of Cultures*, Geertz (1973: 93) makes a distinction between symbols, including language, that work as a *model of* reality and those that work as a *model for.* He draws this distinction to illustrate how symbols work, on the one hand, to reveal or make some thing apprehensible, and on the other, to guide the organization of material or non-symbolic things so as to make them conform to the symbol. The first is a model *of*, the second is a model *for*, reality.

Consider, for example, how a model *of* thinking works using the body. The fleshy, boney body is captured, at least in part, through the use of words like healthy and robust, diseased, impaired, anorexic, desirable, and so on. Disease is a word that implies hundreds of related words (a vocabulary) all directed towards rendering the body knowable through images, graphs, charts, tests, measurements, and numbers. These abstractions taken together reveal a body. They open it, uncover it, disclose it. There it is.

Now, consider how a model *for* thinking works with the body. Here the body is not a fleshy, boney object but a symbol or an abstraction that incites new social arrangements or altered physical environments.

A body in training promotes good eating habits and sleep practices. A body with STD (a sexually transmitted disease) becomes a model for changing sexual habits and altering personal relationships.

It is not difficult to see how we are using these two types of modelling in relationship to disease and disability. Disease works as a model *of* the body. It uses what John Dewey called a 'spectator theory of knowledge' (Kulp, 1992) to see the body in its natural state as sick. Disability, on the other hand, uses a model *for* the body. It uses a contextual knowledge to develop enabling technologies, alter routines and environments, and create spaces that house or accommodate impairment. A spectator theory of knowledge is organized around an objective observer assessing and evaluating a part of nature, in this case the human body. Contextual knowledge, by contrast, is the person in the body collaborating with diverse institutional others to call attention to somatic miseries, the need for understanding, and the importance of reordering social and physical landscapes to reduce, if not eliminate, adverse symptoms. If a disease model begins with the discrete, sick body, a disability model begins at a more complicated place: the intersection or ecology of body, places, and knowledge.

From the Sick Role to Ecological Impairment

Environmental health movements are likely to direct criticism to clinical and research medicine for failing to recognize symptoms and their etiologies or for poorly designed studies that fail to find causation. That criticism is all too often well-founded. But perhaps the quest to embrace a legitimate, clinically verifiable sick role should be complemented by the increasing need to examine the intersections of bodies and environments, to acknowledge, in other words, the possibility that these intersections or ecologies might be impaired.

Ecological impairment is a type of disability that acknowledges both the complex exchanges between bodies and environments and the difficulties that these exchanges pose for clinical medicine. It is a language that acknowledges the possibility that (1) environments themselves might be sources of impairment, and (2) at least some bodies exposed to these environments might experience an attenuation of health and loss of function, even though these somatic miseries escape detection by medical nosology.

Ecological impairment imagines a reticulate pattern linking environments, bodies, and disabilities. It begins with the idea that bodies and environments are in a relentless embrace, a dance of sorts that never ends. Moreover, ecological impairment holds out the promise for a reasonable and equitable approach to the increasing numbers of ordinary people who cannot live normal productive lives in mundane, seemingly benign places. As word play, environmental impairment imagines that environments, like bodies, can be injured. But unlike an impaired body that is unlikely to pose a risk to other bodies, an impaired environment, almost by definition, places other bodies in danger.

Imagining ecological impairment should not require too great a leap of faith, however. Both disability rights and Sick Building Syndrome converge as harbingers of this new image. Invoked here is a logic almost identical to that employed in most disability rights discussions. A person in a wheelchair is not disabled when built environments include adequate means of egress and ingress, desk spaces, bathroom facilities, and so on. The idea is to modify the environment to reduce or eliminate loss of function. In the absence of an appropriately modified environment, the person in the wheelchair is impaired. From the vantage point of the individual bound to a chair, however, it is reasonable to see the environment as disabling. Joined together, both the person and the place become ecologically impaired.

Imagining the environment as disabling has its own precursor in the vexing problem of the sick building. Sick Building Syndrome (SBS) emerged in the late 1970s, and by 1984 the World Health Organization reported up to 30 per cent of new and remodelled buildings caused excessive complaints related to indoor air quality (1984). Although the original idea of SBS was to label people who became symptomatic when living or working in specific indoor environments, SBS nevertheless was viewed by many people as a way of identifying the environments themselves as sick. Moreover, solutions to SBS always include redesigning spaces by increasing ventilation rates, removing source point pollutants, and other remedial measures. These actions could be construed as 'healing' the sick building.

The Americans with Disabilities Act, signed into law in 1990, is based on the medical model of disability. Indeed, it is the only piece of civil rights legislation whose justification is based on clinical evaluations. The medicalization of disability grants employers, insurance companies, and state and federal agencies wide discretion in determining a person's relative state of disablement or loss of function. Moreover, it focuses acute attention on the person who becomes an object of medical–legal treatment. Ecological impairment does not ignore the person – indeed, people and their bodies are parts of the ecology – but it complements clinical care with the need to treat the offending or disabling environments. Recognizing the exchange relationships between bodies and environments signals the need to modify or change environments as an integral part of the social and political response to diminished human capacity and loss of well-being.

More a flight of fancy than a genuine cultural imaginary, ecological impairment is nevertheless a starting point for reconfiguring the way that we think about manufactured environments and human health. Ecological impairment rightly begs many questions. For example, by what criteria are environments to be judged impaired and impairing? How does a person enter an environmentally impaired role? What are the rights and responsibilities of the environmentally impaired?

A Summary and Conclusion

The nomenclature and meanings depicting both bodies and environments change over time. As the United States expanded westward working the land for subsistence and capital, bodies were seen as closely tied to nature. Topography and climate, in particular, were imagined to directly affect human well-being. The discovery of the germ and its paramount role in human sickness shifted attention from environments to bodies as the sites for the study of disease etiologies. At the same time, the germ theory of disease was reshaping the way in which we imagined environments and health, the environment itself began to change. Nature found itself in competition with an increasingly industrial economy. At stake was the future of the environment.

The emergence of an industrial environment and a germ theory of disease worked in tandem to reshape how we imagine both bodies and environments. Indeed, commonplace domestic environments and the faulty hygienic habits of ordinary people were far more likely to be imagined as sources of disease than the increasingly molecular environments of an exploding industrial economy. Telltale signs of the effects of industrial environments on human well-being became increasingly apparent and hard to ignore. A new cultural imaginary emerged, one that acknowledged the primacy of industrial environments in human health. Indeed, the synthetic molecule quickly vied with the germ as a source of disease. Industrial environments were increasingly viewed as invading human bodies, creating mysterious and untreatable disorders. Without a molecular theory of disease to complement the germ theory, physicians were left with at best educated guesses about etiologies and possible treatment regimens.

The essentially contested nature of industrial environments and human health invites, if only speculatively, a shift in thinking from a disease to a disability model. Perhaps, like bodies, environments themselves can become impaired. This observation might be followed by a sigh and a simple, 'So what?' Or, if we abandon our common-sense, Enlightenment-inspired, belief in the authority of discrete types and classes, we might be prepared to see bodies and environments as empirically confounded, inseparable.

It is customary to think of bodies and environments as if they are two separate and distinct entities. The pronoun 'my' in front of 'body' signals a possessive interest in human bodies that differs from the typical article 'the' that precedes 'environment.' 'My body' and 'the environment' are linguistic signals that two ontologically discrete things are being discussed. In a world enunciated with discrete categories, all of us simply know where our bodies end and the environment begins (Kroll-Smith & Lancaster, 2002: 205).

But this is not the case. The boundaries between bodies and environments, however, are porous. Indeed, in one sense, the notion of boundaries, as in separating bodies from environments, only makes sense analytically as a way of conceiving or conjuring the two. It is far less useful as an empirical distinction. Impair an environment, in other words, and bodies are also impaired.

The need to re-imagine the relationship of bodies and environments has never been more urgent. 'Nature,' we are now told, is more a human artefact than a pristine world devoid of culture (Giddens, 1991; McKibben, 1990). Nature as a natural phenomenon will survive in our memories and imaginations, but it is no longer the natural nature that nurtured us and ensured our survival as a species. It is a 'socialized nature' (Giddens, 1991); it carries our footprints. We made it, although unintentionally and without a clear understanding of its effects on human well-being. In the absence of an agreed-upon biomedical understanding of synthetic molecular environments and human health, it is, arguably, time that we shift the discussion from medicine to disability.

Ultimately, of course, a civilization has only the impairments it agrees to recognize. To move ecological impairment from imagination to state and federal policy will require a heroic act of political will. Environments have a way of imposing themselves on us, however. As the debate over global warming boils over, we suspect the idea of ecological impairment, or something like it, will, with time, become increasingly difficult to ignore. In the meantime, it is an idea worth imagining.

NOTES

1   Geographers who examine human–environment relations have a long history of studying environment and health connections. Although they do not directly focus on bodies, they do have an awareness of bodies and environments that can lead to the idea of impaired environments. For example, see Cutter (1995), Driedger & Eyles (2003), Hewitt & Hare (1973), Rainham & Smoyer-Tomic (2003). On therapeutic landscapes, see Andrews (2004) and Gesler (1992).
2   Phase 4 weather is defined by Nursall and Philips (1980) as high humidity, high heat, and high particulate matter in the atmosphere.
3   The study is currently on hold, as human subjects panels review the ethical conundrums of paying poor parents a stipend to permit the EPA to conduct research on their children's variable exposures to pesticides in the home.

REFERENCES

Andrews, Gavin J. (2004). (Re)thinking the dynamics between healthcare and place: Therapeutic geographies in treatment and care practices. *Area, 26*(3), 307–318.

Barnes, Colin, Mercer, Geof, & Shakespeare, Tom. (1999). *Exploring disability.* Cambridge: Polity Press.

Burchell, Graham. (1996). Liberal government and techniques of the 'self.' In Andrew Barry, Thomas Osborne, & Nikolas Rose (Eds.), *Foucault and political reason* (pp. 19–36). London: University College London Press.

Casper, Monica. (2003). Chemical matters. In Monica Casper (Ed.), *Synthetic planet* (pp. xv–xx). New York and London: Routledge.

Colten, Craig E. (2005). *An unnatural metropolis.* Baton Rouge: Louisiana State University Press.

Cutter, Susan L. (1995). The forgotten casualties: Women, children, and environmental change. *Global Environmental Change, 5*(3), 181–194.

Deacon, Harriet. (2005). The politics of medical topography: Seeking healthiness at the Cape during the nineteenth century. In Richard Wrigley & George Revill (Eds.), *Pathologies of travel*, Clio Medica, History of Medicine Series #56 (pp. 279–298). Amsterdam and New York: Rodopi.

Driedger, S. Michelle, & Eyles, John. (2003). Different frames, different fears: Communicating about chlorinated drinking water and cancer in the Canadian media. *Social Science and Medicine, 56*(6), 1279–1293.

Durkheim, Emile. (1974). *Sociology and philosophy.* Translated by D.F. Pocock. New York: Free Press. (Originally published in French in 1898.)

Foucault, Michel. (1991). Governmentality. In Graham Burchell, Colin Gordon, & Peter Miller (Eds.), *The Foucault effect* (pp. 87–104). Brighton, England: Harvester Wheatsheaf.

Francis, Leslie P., & Silvers, Anita. (Eds.). (2000). *Americans with disabilities.* New York and London: Routledge.

Geertz, Clifford. (1973). *The interpretation of cultures.* New York: Basic Books.

Gesler, Wil. (1992). Therapeutic landscapes: Medical issues in light of the new cultural geography. *Social Science and Medicine, 34*, 735–746.

Giddens, Anthony. (1991). *Modernity and self-identity.* Stanford: Stanford University Press.

Gots, Ronald E. (1993). *Multiple chemical sensitivities: What is it?* North Bethesda, MD: Risk Communication International.

Hannaway, Carolina. (1993). Environment and miasma. In W.F. Bynum & Roy Porter (Eds.), *Companion encyclopedia of the history of medicine* (pp. 292–308). New York and London: Routledge.

Hewitt, Kenneth, & Hare, F. Kenneth. (1973). *Man and environment: Conceptual frameworks.* Washington: Association of American Geographers.

James, Bushrod. (1889). *American resorts with notes upon their climates.* Philadelphia: F.A. Davis.

Kroll-Smith, Steve, & Ladd, Anthony. (1995). Environmental illness and biomedicine: Anomalies, exemplars, and the politics of the body. *Sociological Spectrum, 15,* 377–396.

Kroll-Smith, Steve, & Floyd, H. Hugh (1997). *Bodies in protest.* New York: New York University Press.

Kroll-Smith, Steve, & Lancaster, Worth. (2002). Bodies, environments, and a new style of reasoning. *Annals of the American Academy of Public Health, 584,* 203-212.

Kulp, Christopher. (1992). *The end of epistemology: John Dewey and his current allies on the spectator theory of knowledge.* Westport, CN: Greenwood.

Ladies' Home Journal. (1999, May). Advertisement for Zyrtec (p. 14).

Linton, Simi. (1998). *Claiming disability.* New York: New York University Press.

McKibben, Bill. (1990). *The end of nature.* New York: Anchor Books.

Mitman, Greg, Murphy, Michelle, & Sellers, Christopher. (2004). A cloud over history. *Osiris, 19,* 1–20.

Nash, Linda. (2003). Finishing nature: Harmonizing bodies and environments in late-19th century California [Electronic version]. *Environmental History, 8,* 1, pars. 53. Retrieved 12 Dec. 2005, from http://www.historycooperative.org/ journals/eh/8.1/nash.html.

Nursall, Allan S., & Phillips, David W. (1980). *The effects of weather on the frequency and severity of migraine headaches in southwestern Ontario. Canadian Climate Centre report 80-7*. Ottawa: Environment Canada. Unpublished manuscript.

Osborne, Thomas. (1997). Of health and statecraft. In Alan Petersen & Robin Bunton (Eds.), *Foucault, health and medicine* (pp. 173-188). New York and London: Routledge.

Rainham, Daniel G.C., & Smoyer-Tomic, Karen E. (2003). The role of air pollution in the relationship between a heat stress index and human mortality in Toronto. *Environmental Research, 93*(1), 9–19.

Steingraber, Saundra. (1997). *Living downstream*. New York: Vintage Press.

Turner, Bryan. (1984). *The body and society*. Oxford: Blackwell.

University of California, Los Angeles. (2001). *Snow's testimony*. UCLA Department of Epidemiology. Retreived 9 Aug. 2004, from www.ph.ucla.edu/epi/ snow/snows_testimony.html.

U.S. Environmental Protection Agency. (2004). *Children's environmental exposure research study* (CHEERS). Retrieved 23 Sept. 2004, from http:// www.epa.gov/cheers.

Valencius, Conevery B. (2002). *The health of the country*. New York: Basic Books.

Valencius, Conevery B. (2004). Gender and the economy of health on the Santa Fe Trail. *Osiris, 19*, 79–92.

Wittgenstein, Ludwig. (1967). *Philosophical investigations*. London: Blackwell.

World Health Organization. (1984). *Report on indoor air quality*. Geneva: Author.

Zavestoski, Stephen, Brown, Phil, McCormick, Sabrina, Mayer, Brian, D'Ottavi, Maryhelen, & Lucove, Jaime. (2004). Patient activism and the struggle for diagnosis: Gulf War illness and other medically unexplained physical symptoms in the US. *Social Science Medicine, 58*, 161–175.

17 Contestation and Medicalization

PETER CONRAD AND CHERYL STULTS

Contestation of illness can have numerous meanings. In social science it is most frequently considered as contested illness, with patients and advocates challenging medical perspectives. But contestation is perceptible in a number of ways with illness, including negotiation between physicians and patients over diagnosis or treatment, patients attempting to bring conditions or etiologies to medical notice, challenges over the meaning of illness, and even as the utilization of alternative medicine. Rarely do we see various representations of contestation collected in a single volume (for an exception, see Kroll-Smith, Brown, & Gunter, 2000).

In this final and reflective chapter of this book we take on several tasks. Our overall goal is to highlight some issues and themes that become more prominent when all the chapters are read together. There are undoubtedly numerous ways that this could be undertaken, but we focus on the overall issue of contestation and medicalization. Thus, we divide our chapter into two major sections. First, we examine how contestation is taken up throughout this volume and conceptualize three major ways that contestation this evident in the various chapters. Second, we focus on one particular contrast, the specific relation between contested illness and medicalization and use the chapters in this volume as a springboard for a broader discussion.

Conceptualizing Contestation

As an alternative to the lens that Pamela Moss and Katherine Teght-soonian provide in Chapter 1 – via authority, bodies, and context – we focus on sorting through the various meanings of contestation that are presented throughout this book. The contributors have all focused on contestation as a specific dimension of power. Reflecting on the collection of chapters as a whole, as well as on each of them individually, we think that contestation may usefully be subdivided into three categories: contesting medicalization, contesting the parameters of illness, and contesting the contours of the illness experience. This conceptualization of contestation is neither exhaustive nor mutually exclusive; rather, it serves to contour the meaning of contestation by drawing out commonalities and differences in the use of contestation by the authors.

Contesting Medicalization

Several chapters in this volume focus, either explicitly or implicitly, on contesting medicalization. *Medicalization* is the process through which non-medical problems are defined and treated as medical problems, usually as illnesses or disorders (Conrad, 1992). Both medicalization and the expansion of medical jurisdiction have become major concerns in many social science disciplines and in interdisciplinary research in recent decades (Conrad, 1992 and 2005; Lock, 2001). More recently, scholarly attention has focused on the various avenues through which these developments have been contested. By *contesting medicalization*, we mean challenging aspects of the creation and application of medical diagnostic categories and treatments.

In Chapter 5, Jan Angus examines the expanding medicalization of coronary heart disease (CHD) as it applies to a new diagnostic category, *coronary candidacy*. This term refers to individuals who have no symptoms of CHD but who do have CHD risk factors that call for lifestyle modification (e.g., smoking cessation, exercise, and dietary alterations) to prevent potential cardiovascular disease in the future. Many laypersons contest their new identities as 'coronary candidates' in response to one or more of three impetuses: (1) this identity is not based on the individual's experience of illness but instead is based on the uncertain possibility of a future cardiac event; (2) accepting coronary candidacy requires difficult behavioural modifications even though the individual feels subjectively healthy, and as a result, many individuals struggle to accept the concept of personal susceptibility to CHD; and (3) even if individuals accept their coronary candidacy, additional contestation may arise in the home from other family members or in the workplace that will prevent or inhibit risk factor modification.

Annie Potts (Chapter 14) reviews the medicalization of women's sexuality in the twenty-first century, specifically the contested illness of Female Sexual Dysfunction (FSD) and the search for a female equivalent of the medication Viagra. Pharmaceutical companies and physician researchers have advanced the concept of FSD as a group of disorders that will benefit from drug therapy. In contrast, the New View Working Group, an anti-medicalization group composed of social scientists, clinicians, and feminist activists, has argued for a more holistic approach to women's sexual issues, incorporating psychological, sociocultural, and relational factors, in addition to biomedical factors. Potts finds that there is similar contestation about the concept of FSD among women themselves: some women support a biomedical, anti-ageing, pro-FSD approach to their sexual issues and advocate pharmacological intervention to remain sexually active, while other women contest the medicalization of sexual changes that commonly occur with advancing age.

In Chapter 11, Sharon Dale Stone contests the medicalization of impairment and disability, what she terms the 'conflation of disability with illness' (p. 201). Stone suggests that biomedicine has focused on impairment and disability as an illness which then implies individual suffering and the consequent need for medical surveillance and intervention. However, Stone argues that this association is problematic because it assumes that all disability and impairment lead to tragedy and suffering. The biomedical perspective fails to consider how the individual self understands impairment and disability. Drawing on interviews with young women who have lived with impairment or disability resulting from hemorrhagic stroke, Stone shows how they do not perceive tragedy and suffering as the primary – or even as a significant – outcome of the event. She found that these women contest being portrayed as 'victims' who have suffered a tragedy, and refer to themselves, instead, as 'survivors' who have used their stroke experience as an opportunity to improve their lives.

Helen Gremillion (Chapter 12) uses the concept of contestation in several ways. As a scholar, Gremillion contests the prevailing medicalized view of anorexia as an almost exclusively white, middle-class disease. She cites evidence for a higher prevalence of eating disorders among Black women and Latinas than has previously been recognized. Gremillion contests the notion that the symptoms of anorexia are the same in individuals from different social groups, that is, the same as in the white, middle-class group, and suggests that there may be alternative, less frequently recognized clinical presentations of anorexia in non-white or marginalized social groups. She also contests the 'racialized and classed power of clinical "expertise"' (220) that facilitates the exclusion of the marginalized from both diagnosis and treatment for anorexia. Gremillion indicates that it is necessary to contest these racialized and classed norms not only to influence clinical practice positively but also to guide new research agendas about anorexia.

In her chapter on Premenstrual Syndrome (PMS) (Chapter 10), Jane M. Ussher contests the medicalization of PMS as a pathological diagnosis, while acknowledging that many women experience significant premenstrual physical and psychological distress. Historical and socio-cultural depictions of women – the 'monstrous feminine' – have led some biomedical practitioners, and even many women themselves, to represent these physiological hormonal changes as an illness in order to make sense of their experience. Social constructions of femininity, which foster a practice of self-silencing by women, force them to suppress their experiences of physical and psychological distress until a 'rupture … occurs premenstrually' that allows 'the expression of both day-to-day frustrations and anger associated with more substantial issues, which are normally repressed' (p. 190). This alleged illness is accompanied by feelings of guilt, anxiety, and the perception of a loss of control. According to Ussher, helping women to understand that these negative feelings are the result of sociocultural factors rather than a bodily illness can reduce premenstrual distress.

Contesting the Parameters of Illness

A second category of contestation involves contesting the parameters of illness, that is, challenging how a problem or set of symptoms comes to be defined as a legitimate illness by the biomedical community, health policy-makers, and the lay public. In some chapters in this book, the authors explore contestation in regard to the parameters of illness – including the possibility of its very existence – that are either controversial or flatly rejected by biomedicine. In other chapters, authors explore controversies and tensions that circulate around the diagnosis of and treatments for widely accepted medical conditions, showing how even these 'obvious' illnesses are also subject to contestation.

Pia H. Bülow (Chapter 7) and Pamela Moss (Chapter 9) examine the contested illness of Myalgic Encephalomyelitis (ME), also known as Chronic Fatigue Syndrome (CFS). Bülow examines the illness narratives of CFS sufferers to explore their experiences of living with a contested illness. The narratives reveal a pattern of repeated contestation and distrust by the health care system and peers. External confirmation of the legitimacy of their symptoms – particularly through the attachment of a diagnostic label, 'Chronic Fatigue Syndrome' – and self-reflection about possible personal responsibility for the genesis of the illness appear to help these patients sustain their personal sense of moral status in the face of contestation. Along a different line of reasoning, Moss argues that biomedicine's approach to diagnosis is inadequate because it does not consider the embodied experience of women who are ill: 'Contestation of a diagnostic category takes place not only within the primary discourse defining the illness, biomedicine in this case, but also within the social practices that clinicians and ill bodies engage in, for example, interpreting symptoms and describing bodily sensations' (173). To improve diagnostic categorization for ME, Moss blurs the conceptual boundary between 'illness' and 'disease' to construct the notion of an 'ill body': defining criteria for ME must include not only the biophysiological disease process or material 'body,' but also the experience of illness by the patient. In this way medicalized authority can be resisted, and contested illness can be reclaimed by ill bodies.

Maren Klawiter (Chapter 15) illustrates the ways in which women's experience of treatment for breast cancer – a legitimate and minimally controversial disease – has been transformed over the past 30 years from one that was closeted, solitary, and brief to one that is public, shared, and prolonged. These changes emerged in the wake of a series of changes in the breast cancer *disease regime*, that is, the set of interrelated practices through which breast cancer has been studied, medically managed, and administered. These changed experiences are reflected in the emergence of support groups composed of women diagnosed with breast cancer. Along with the reframing of such women as permanently marked by some degree of risk of recurrence, support groups have provided a material basis for women's activism to contest important aspects of breast cancer treatment.

Katherine Lippel (Chapter 3) reviews the pursuit of workers' compensation benefits in the province of Quebec, Canada, through an analysis of case law regarding claims made by persons who have controversial – or contested – illnesses. She also draws from a qualitative study of the effects of the compensation process on the mental health of such applicants. Lippel demonstrates that efforts to claim these income support benefits involve contestation regarding the parameters of illness, not only for persons who suffer from controversial illnesses such as Fibro-myalgia, Chronic Fatigue Syndrome, or Multiple Chemical Sensitivity Syndrome, but for all individuals who choose to enter the maze of medi-cal and rehabilitation examinations and legal and juridical deliberations. Lippel reports that, although the experience of the claims and appeal processes generate considerable stress for all claimants, this is particu-larly the case for persons with controversial illnesses.

Like Lippel, Michael J. Prince (Chapter 2) examines the pursuit of income support benefits but focuses his analysis at the federal level by looking at the Canada Pension Plan Disability (CPP-D) program. He finds it to be a field of contestation at multiple levels for all persons with disabilities who apply for income support, regardless of their diagnosis. Since the CPP-D program provides full benefits only for those who qualify as completely 'disabled,' this presents problems because of the contested definition of *disability*. To receive benefits from the CPP-D program, the claimant, physician, and employer have to prove that the claimant's disability is so 'severe in condition and pro-longed in duration' that it prevents these individuals from having *any form* of 'gainful employment' (p. 36). Although this process is difficult enough for those with illness conventionally understood as legitimate, individuals who have a contested illness experience even greater chal-lenges in having their experience validated by their physicians, employers, and the legal system.

Contesting the Contours of the Illness Experience

The authors in the third category take a different approach to the con-cept of contestation. Rather than contesting for (or against) the specific parameters that define an illness, these authors examine con-testation as it applies to selected aspects, or contours, of the illness experience. Even where a particular illness is widely accepted by the biomedical community, the individuals experiencing it must never-theless negotiate significant areas of uncertainty with respect to how they manage their lives and their identities and how their illness is viewed by others.

Mary Ellen Purkis and Catherine van Mossel (Chapter 7) demon-strate that, although cancer is well accepted as an illness, cancer care and the cancer health care system are spaces for significant contestation for individuals with cancer. Analysing narratives provided by current cancer patients, they find that contestation arises in the experiences of

cancer patients throughout their experience following the initial diagnosis of cancer. Cancer patients are confronted repeatedly by a series of
demands for engagement and response related to the new identity that
they must forge in the wake of diagnosis and to the negotiation and
monitoring of their treatment trajectory. Although cancer patients are
continually presented with a number of apparent choices, from among
which they must choose in the face of considerable uncertainty, treatment protocols operate in ways that foreclose significant choice and
make contestation regarding choices more difficult once a diagnosis has
been made.

As with cancer, Hepatitis C is well accepted by biomedicine as a disease, yet as Michael Orsini (Chapter 6) discusses, there are multiple
aspects of contestation visible in the controversies that emerged after
it was discovered that Hepatitis C had been transmitted to a significant number of Canadians through the country's blood supply system. For example, he notes that there are important differences in
terms of treatment outcomes, as well as disagreements among those
who have been infected with the virus regarding how to understand
these outcomes. Orsini suggests that competing interpretations of
treatment outcomes affect whether individuals with Hepatitis C take
up – or refuse – an illness identity, which in turn shapes the possibilities for collective action in response to this issue. Orsini argues that his
research findings indicate the need to revisit our conceptions of contestation – including how persons with a chronic illness act politically
– and of biological citizenship.

In Chapter 13, Joyce Davidson contests diagnostic and clinical practice with respect to Autistic Spectrum Disorders (ASDs). Davidson
contends that because of the much higher prevalence of autism in male
children and the largely male-specific diagnostic criteria, girls and
women with an ASD are frequently misdiagnosed. Drawing on the
written, autobiographical accounts of high-functioning ASD women,
Davidson finds that many have been diagnosed with alternative disorders (e.g., anorexia) or are simply considered to be expressing deviant
or 'neurotic' behaviour. Similar to Moss, she argues for the diagnostic
utility of the experiential 'truths' expressed in such accounts.

In Chapter 4, Katherine Teghtsoonian contests key elements of recent
discourses circulating within the Canadian business and research communities about how best to address and manage depression in the workplace. She examines two documents that propose a number of strategies
for employers to use in identifying and responding to this issue. She

finds that one of the key goals of these strategies is 'to bring the employee's psychological profile and lifestyle choices into alignment with the employer's interest in reducing disability-related costs and ... enhancing the productivity and competitiveness of the organization' (p. 83). Both documents endorse disability case management, which Teghtsoonian suggests serves as a vehicle through which employers are able to 'constrain – under the guise of politically neutral, disinterested expertise – the decisions of family physicians and those of the ill employees for whom they care' (ibid.).

Steve Kroll-Smith and Joshua Kelley (Chapter 16) contest the notion of a static relationship between bodies and the environment. They argue that the interplay between these two entities has varied according to the historical context, creating what they define as three distinct periods: *bodies in environments*, *bodies and industrial environments*, and *industrial environments in bodies*. Each period has been marked by particular conceptualizations of the relationship between disease and health, which in turn has been marked by particular sets of interventions and treatments. In the first period, the belief in the inseparability of bodies in environments facilitated the mobility of individuals, as they came to understand that environments affected their health. The industrial revolution, the second period, separated bodies and environments into distinct entities, thereby linking health to the external factor of 'germs' and minimizing the influence of the surrounding environment. The third, and current phase, reunites the body and the environment. The source of disease, however, is now located in the environment instead of in the body, a situation that permits substances (the environment) to enter the body and affect its processes. As a result, many physicians doubt sufferers' explanations for their ills because they cannot identify the origin or cause of their patients' illnesses.

Medicalization and Contested Illness

Many scholars, especially social scientists, have written widely about the medicalization of society (e.g., Conrad, 1992 and 2007; Lock, 2001; Smith & Easterlow, 2005; Williams & Calnan, 1996). Although some scholars have focused on identifying and describing the rise of medicalization, most have taken a somewhat sceptical or critical view. One might accurately say that most of the scholarly concern is critical of the *over*medicalization in our society (Clarke, Shim, Mamo, Fosket, & Fishman, 2003).

As the chapters in this book attest, there is resistance to and contestation of medicalization. As Potts (Chapter 14) shows, organizations like the New View Working Group contest the medicalization of 'female sexual dysfunction.' Other examples of successful contestation of medicalization include the gay and lesbian movement in demedicalizing homosexuality, and the disability movement in advocating non-medical definitions and treatments of people who have disabilities (see Stone, Chapter 11). Sometimes scholars contest the medicalization of conceptions of problems, such as when Gremillion (Chapter 12) argues that the medicalized diagnosis of anorexia may be too narrow and limiting, and of course, there can be individuals who resist diagnostic categories, such as the Canadian mothers in Claudia Malacrida's (2003) study of Attention Deficit and Hyperactivity Disorder (ADHD). This resistance and contestation has had, however, only a limited effect on the growth of medicalization in our society (Conrad, 2007).

Scholars have written about contested illness for at least two decades. In a study of hypoglycemia, Singer, Fitzgerald, Hadden, von Legat, and Arnold (1987: 151) first identified illnesses that had an 'ambiguous status as disease labels' as *controversial illnesses*. In more recent years these have been commonly called contested illnesses. In comparison with a settled or 'normal' illness, a *contested illness* is a condition that has been at least partially identified and mostly 'dismissed as illegitimate – framed as "difficult," psychosomatic, or even non-existent – by researchers, health practitioners, and policy-makers operating within conventional paradigms of knowledge,' especially biomedicine (Moss & Teghtsoonian, Chapter 1:7). The list of putative contested illnesses is long and itself controversial. Typically included are such disorders as Chronic Fatigue Syndrome, Multiple Chemical Sensitivity Syndrome, Fibromyalgia, hypo-glycemia, Gulf War Syndrome, and Sick Building Syndrome. Sometimes other disorders like Post Traumatic Stress Disorder (PTSD), ADHD, and PMS are considered controversial enough to be contested (see Ussher, Chapter 10). Joseph Dumit has recently called these 'illnesses you have to fight to get' (2006: 577). Dumit suggests that a contested illness has three characteristics:

1 Sufferers describe their experiences of being denied health care and legitimacy through bureaucratic categories of exclusion as dependent on their lack of biological facts;
2 Institutions manage these exclusions rhetorically through exploiting the open-endedness of science to deny efficacy to new facts;

3 Patients respond collectively by insisting on the systematic nature of these exclusions and developing counter-tactics.

Dumit sees the outcomes of these contentions as extensive struggles among sufferers, physicians, and medical institutions. Disease support groups, both organized groups and more informal groups on the Internet (see Barker, 2005), are often central to illness advocacy. The key issue for advocates struggling to gain acceptance of a specific contested illness is to attain some kind of medical legitimacy. Although contested illness ranges widely in its manifestation, Kroll-Smith, Brown, & Gunter (2000) have shown that a large number of illnesses are contested not only with regard to their existence but also with regard to their cause or origin and that such contestation particularly engenders disputes over environmental rather than biogenic causation.

Contested illness provides one of the most interesting contrasts to medicalization. In some ways the issues are similar and overlapping. Both medicalization and contested illness highlight that illness categories (usually, but not always, diagnoses) are socially constructed and not automatically ascertained from scientific and/or medical discoveries. Both medicalization and contested illness draw attention to the fact that advocates for or against the establishment of parameters of particular illness or disease categories are important for their acceptance, legitimation, and utilization. In some cases, contested illness itself can become a medicalized controversy and a subject for scholarly analysis (e.g., Broom & Woodward, 1996). Finally, both contested illness and medicalization can operate on the scale of the collective, that is, the level of the creation and acceptance of medical categories, and on the scale of the individual, the level of the application of illness categories in specific cases.

What is most interesting is how the issues of medicalization and contested illness differ. The biggest difference between them is that *while most studies of medicalization express concerns about overmedicalization, contested illness in general suggests the desire for more medicalization.* Analysts of (and certainly advocates for legitimating) contested illness tend to want to expand medical categories and diagnoses, while critics of medicalization tend to be sceptical of the continual expansion of medical jurisdiction (see Moss, Chapter 9). One could imagine concerns about both contestation and medicalization with problems like PMS (see Ussher, Chapter 10) and adult ADHD (Conrad & Potter, 2000). A scholar concerned with contested illness might, however, see the issues from a different viewpoint than would a scholar whose concerns focus on medicalization (e.g., Moss, 2000).

The roles of physicians and sufferers, whether patients or persons experiencing illness, vary. Advocates of contested illness tend to be sufferers, patients or their supporters, although in some cases physicians, as well. Promoters of medicalized categories are more typically physicians, their professional organizations, and/or the pharmaceutical or biotechnological industry. We do see consumers as promoters of medicalization as well, for example, as promoters of infertility as a medical problem (Conrad & Leiter, 2004). But the role of physicians in contestation and medicalization may be where the contrast is sharpest. For advocates of contested illness, physicians or the medical profession are frequently viewed as an obstacle or hindrance to the acceptance of the contested illness category, diagnosis, or even treatment. With medicalization, physicians are commonly promoters of new medical categories or the expansion of older ones, or at the very least, gatekeepers of diagnosis and dispensers of treatment. Indeed, one could say that physicians are gatekeepers of both contested illness and medicalization: in the one case they keep the gate closed, and in the other, they facilitate traffic through the gate. From a patient's viewpoint, with medicalization patients sometimes resist medical labelling of diagnoses, while with contested illness patients actively seek doctors' diagnoses.

Given the similarity and overlap between some aspects of contested illness in relation to medicalization, we can make a distinction between what might be called *emergent medicalization* and contested illness: they are similar in that they both refer to conditions that are not yet fully accepted as medical disorders by the medical profession (e.g., as official diagnostic categories, as conditions in need of medical treatment). These are medicalized categories that remain in some sense contested, either by advocates or opponents. This might include categories like 'Internet addiction' (Stults, 2006), sexual addiction, or Female Sexual Dysfunction. These categories are largely (although not entirely) promoted by clinicians (e.g., medical claims-makers) rather than sufferers. Claims-makers sometimes have fellow advocates, such as lawyers in the case of sexual addiction and the pharmaceutical industry for FSD. Emergent medicalized categories and contested illness are similar in that they are not fully recognized as medical disorders and are being promoted to become accepted medical categories. The difference is where the energy (and momentum for collective action) for the contestation comes from, and to a degree, what constitutes the context for the contested claims. Physicians can play a part collectively (as in the consensus conference for FSD; see Potts, Chapter 14) or as individual advocates (as with most emergent medicalized disorders). Here we have more of an overlap between medicalization and contestation, although the difference in source of advocacy is still significant.

Although medicalization and contested illness both have to do with the acceptance of diagnosis and the legitimization of illness categories and treatment regimens, advocates for specific contested illnesses essentially want more medicalization, while critics of medicalization tend to favour fewer medical categories and less medical treatment. In sum, contestation and medicalization are linked in a number of different ways. Contestation can serve to limit medicalization, yet much contestation of illness ultimately seeks to increase medicalization. Among the interesting places for continued scholarly research are those sites where the processes of contestation and processes of medicalization rub up against one another.

REFERENCES

Barker, Kristin K. (2005). Electronic support groups and contested chronic illness. Paper presented at Contours of Contestation Conference, University of Victoria, Victoria, BC, 10–12 November, 2005.

Broom, Dorothy H., & Woodward, Rosalyn V. (1996). Medicalisation reconsidered: Toward a collaborative approach to care. *Sociology of Health and Illness, 18,* 357–378.

Clarke, Adele E., Shim, Janet K., Mamo, Laura, Fosket, Jennifer Ruth, & Fishman, Jennifer R. (2003). Biomedicalization: Technoscientific transformations of health, illness, and US biomedicine. *American Sociological Review, 68*(2), 161–194.

Conrad, Peter. (1992). Medicalization and social control. *Annual Review of Sociology, 18,* 209–232.

Conrad, Peter. (2005). The shifting engines of medicalization. *Journal of Health and Social Behavior, 46,* 3-14.

Conrad, Peter. (2007). *The medicalization of society.* Baltimore: Johns Hopkins University Press.

Conrad, Peter, & Leiter, Valerie. (2004). Medicalization, markets and consumers. *Journal of Health and Social Behavior, 45,* 158–176.

Conrad, Peter, & Potter, Deborah. (2000). From hyperactive children to ADHD adults: Observations on the expansion of medical categories. *Social Problems, 47,* 59–82.

Dumit, Joseph. (2006). Illnesses you have to fight to get: Facts as forces in uncertain, emergent illnesses. *Social Science and Medicine, 62,* 577–590.

Kroll-Smith, Steve, Brown, Phil, & Gunter, Valerie. (2000). *Illness in the environment: A reader in contested medicine.* New York: New York University Press.

Lock, Margaret. (2001). Medicalization: Cultural concerns. *International Encyclopedia of the Social and Behavioral Sciences,* 9534–9539.

Malacrida, Claudia. (2003). *Cold comfort: Mothers, professionals and Attention Deficit Disorder.* Toronto: University of Toronto Press.

Moss, Pamela. (2000). Not quite abled and not quite disabled: Experience of being 'in between' ME and the academy. *Disability Studies Quarterly, 20,* 287–293.

Singer, Merrill, Fitzgerald, Maureen H., Hadden, Marilyn Joan, von Legat, Christa E., & Arnold, Carol. (1987). The sufferer's experience of hypoglycemia. In Julius A. Roth & Peter Conrad (Eds.), *Research in the sociology of health care,* vol. 6, *The experience and management of chronic illness* (pp. 147–176). Greenwich, CT: JAI Press.

Smith, Susan J., & Easterlow, Donna. (2005). The strange geography of health inequalities. *Transactions of the Institute of British Geographers, 30,* 173–190.

Stults, Cheryl. (2006, Aug.). *Internet addiction: Emergent medicalization of a behavioral problem.* Paper presented at the meetings of the Society for the Study of Social Problems, Montreal, Quebec.

Williams, Simon J., & Calnan, Michael. (1996). The 'limits' of medicalization? Modern medicine and the lay populace in 'late' modernity. *Social Science and Medicine, 42*(12), 1609–1620.

Index